MEDICAL RADIOLOGY
Diagnostic Imaging

Editors:
A. L. Baert, Leuven
K. Sartor, Heidelberg

Springer
Berlin
Heidelberg
New York
Barcelona
Hong Kong
London
Milan
Paris
Tokyo

R. Hermans (Ed.)

Imaging of the Larynx

With Contributions by

C. Bartolozzi · G.Battaglia · M. Becker · J. A. Castelijns · P. R. Delaere · K. G. Delsupehe
D. Farina · P. Flamen · P. P. Gruca · R. Hermans · V. Joshi · J. Kaanders · P. Maculotti
R. Maroldi · S. K. Mukherji · E. Neri · L. Palvarini · F. A. Pameijer · M. Rijpkema
I. M. Schmalfuss · R. Sigal

Foreword by
A. L. Baert

With 145 Figures in 371 Separate Illustrations, 8 in Color

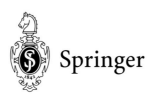

Springer

Robert Hermans, MD, PhD
Professor, Department of Radiology
University Hospitals K. U. Leuven
Herestraat 49
3000 Leuven
Belgium

Medical Radiology · Diagnostic Imaging and Radiation Oncology
Series Editors: A. L. Baert · L. W. Brady · H.-P. Heilmann · F. Molls · K. Sartor

Continuation of
Handbuch der medizinischen Radiologie
Encyclopedia of Medical Radiology

ISBN 3-540-41232-8   Springer-Verlag Berlin Heidelberg New York

Library of Congress Cataloging-in-Publication Data

Imaging of the larynx / R. Hermans (ed.) ; with contributions by M. Becker ... [et al.];
foreword by Albert L. Baert.
   p. ; cm -- (Medical radiology)
   Includes bibliographical references and index.
   ISBN 3540412328 (alk. paper)
   1. Larynx--Radiography. 2. Larynx--Imaging. 3. Larynx--Cancer--Diagnosis. I.
Hermans, R (Robert), 1962- II. Becker, M. (Minerva) III. Series.
   [DNLM: 1. Larynx--radiography. 2. Laryngeal Diseases--pathology. 3. Laryngeal
Diseases--radiography. 4. Laryngeal Neoplasms--diagnosis. 5. Laryngeal
Neoplasms--radiography. WV 500 I31 2002]
RF512 .I434 2002
617.5'3307572--dc21   2001049636

Springer-Verlag Berlin Heidelberg New York
a member of BertelsmannSpringer Science+Business Media GmbH
© Springer-Verlag Berlin Heidelberg 2001

Printed in Germany

Cover-Design and Typesetting: Verlagsservice Teichmann, 69256 Mauer

SPIN: 107 857 17   21/3130 – 5 4 3 2 1 0 – Printed on acid-free paper

To my wife, Isabelle

And our children,
Simon, Lies, Thomas and Tim

Robert Hermans

Foreword

Notwithstanding the important role of direct clinical and endoscopic examination in the modern management of pathological conditions of the larynx, radiological study and, more specifically, cross-sectional imaging by CT and MRI make definite diagnostic contributions by virtue of their potential to display superbly the deeper extent of laryngeal lesions. Indeed, remarkable progress has been achieved during recent years in CT and MRI techniques as applied to the neck region.

This book sets out to provide a sorely needed update of our knowledge of the diagnostic potential of these cross-sectional methods and constitutes a very welcome addition to our series "Medical Radiology", which aims to cover all important clinical imaging fields of modern diagnostic radiology. It will be of great interest to general and head and neck radiologists as well as to ENT surgeons and radiotherapists.

Professor R. Hermans and the other distinguished contributors to this work are internationally renowned experts in the field and they have accumulated vast experience and a wealth of radio-pathological knowledge of the larynx over the years. I would like to congratulate them most sincerely for this outstanding volume, its comprehensive contents and its superb illustrations.

I hope that this book will meet with the same great success as previously published volumes in the series. I would appreciate any constructive criticism that might be offered.

Leuven   ALBERT L. BAERT

Preface

The larynx is an organ of considerable anatomical and functional complexity. Clinical evaluation allows appreciation of the presence of pathology, but it has been known for several decades that cross-sectional radiological techniques allow more comprehensive evaluation of the submucosal extent of pathological processes in the larynx. The introduction of CT and MRI has revolutionised laryngeal radiology. Current radiological modalities provide reliable and fast cross-sectional visualisation of laryngeal structures to a unprecedented level of detail.

During the past decade, numerous studies have clarified the significance of imaging abnormalities in the larynx. Mainly in the management of patients with laryngeal cancer, the most frequent cancer in the head and neck region (apart from skin cancer), this enhanced knowledge has strengthened the impact of imaging in patient care. For example, significant progress was achieved by obtaining more sophisticated radio-pathological correlations, and the added value of imaging to monitor tumour response after therapy has been scientifically established.

This purpose of this book is to provide a comprehensive review of state-of-the-art laryngeal imaging. Several distinguished head-and-neck radiologists have contributed to this book, allowing full coverage of advanced laryngeal imaging. The technological evolution continues, and new possibilities in the evaluation of pathological processes, including laryngeal diseases, are still emerging; at the end of the book, a number of chapters demonstrate these newer developments and their potential impact on patient care.

Progress has not only been made in diagnostic imaging of the larynx; clinical diagnostic techniques, as well as therapeutic strategies, have undergone significant changes over the past years. Care has been taken to portray the role of imaging within these developments.

The ultimate goal of all medical actions is to provide our patients with the best possible therapy for their health problems; it is hoped that this book contributes to this purpose.

Leuven   ROBERT HERMANS

Contents

1 Clinical Evaluation of the Larynx

Kathelijne G. Delsupehe and Pierre R. Delaere

CONTENTS

1.1
Functional Anatomy

The larynx is a complex and delicate structure consisting of a cartilage backbone and fine muscular structures. Together they act to serve the three main functions of the larynx:
- Protection of the airway during deglutition
- Provision of an overpressure of air in the lungs (the so-called "subglottal pressure").
- Production of voice

1.1.1
Laryngeal Framework

The laryngeal framework consists of the thyroid cartilage, suspended by the thyrohyoid membrane to the hyoid bone, the cricoid cartilage and the epiglottis. Posteriorly the arytenoid cartilages complete the framework (Figs. 1.1 and 1.2).

Eight intrinsic laryngeal muscles connect the different cartilages and enable fine coordinated movements required for its functions. All these muscles have an adductor ("closing") function except the posterior cricoarytenoid muscle. The latter is an important muscle since it is the only one which can open the glottis (abductor) (SUNDBERG 1987).

The lining of the vocal folds consists of stratified squamous epithelium. The other parts of the larynx are covered by a ciliated pseudocolumnar epithelium (GRAY 2000; HIRANO 1991).

1.1.2
Supraglottis and Glottis

In order to protect the airway during deglutition, constriction of the glottis can be done at three different levels. These three levels form functional sphincters capable of closing off the trachea completely from the

K.G. DELSUPEHE, MD
Department of Otolaryngology, Head and Neck Surgery, University Hospitals Leuven, Kapucijnenvoer 33, 3000 Leuven, Belgium
P.R. DELAERE, MD, PhD
Professor, Department of Otolaryngology, Head and Neck Surgery, University Hospitals Leuven, Kapucijnenvoer 33, 3000 Leuven, Belgium

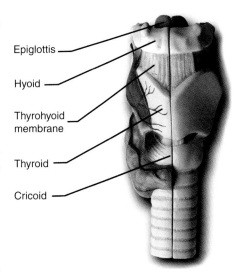

Epiglottis

Hyoid

Thyrohyoid membrane

Thyroid

Cricoid

Fig. 1.1. Laryngeal cartilage structure: frontal view

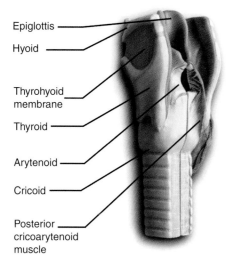

Epiglottis
Hyoid
Thyrohyoid membrane
Thyroid
Arytenoid
Cricoid
Posterior cricoarytenoid muscle

Fig. 1.2. Musculoskeletal composition of the larynx: postero-lateral view

pharynx thereby preventing food and liquid penetrating during swallowing (Logemann 1983).

- *Epiglottis and aryepiglottic folds:* These contain the aryepiglottic muscles, the quadrangular membrane and the cuneiform cartilages. They are attached to the lateral margins of the epiglottis and run laterally, posteriorly and inferiorly to surround the arytenoid cartilages (Fig. 1.3)
- *False vocal folds:* These consist of two shelves of muscle and connective tissue running anteriorly to posteriorly immediately above the level of the true vocal folds (Fig. 1.3)
- *True vocal folds:* These are composed of the vocalis and thyroarytenoid muscles. They are attached to the vocal process of the arytenoids posteriorly, to the inside surface of the thyroid lamina laterally and to the thyroid notch anteriorly (Figs. 1.3 and 1.4) (Hirano 1991).

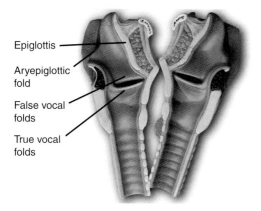

Epiglottis
Aryepiglottic fold
False vocal folds
True vocal folds

Fig. 1.3. Inner view of the larynx (split on the midline)

The same three functional sphincters can generate, together with the diaphragm muscle and abdominal wall muscles, an increased air pressure, the so-called "subglottal pressure". This is required for coughing, and to provide the Valsalva's maneuver and the gag reflex (Jiang et al. 2000; Scherer 1991; Sundberg 1987).

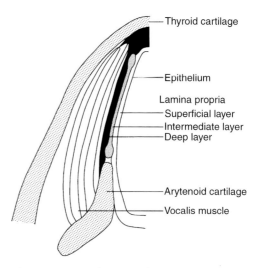

Thyroid cartilage
Epithelium
Lamina propria
Superficial layer
Intermediate layer
Deep layer
Arytenoid cartilage
Vocalis muscle

Fig. 1.4. Horizontal section of the true vocal fold

1.1.3 Voice Dynamics

The most delicate and complex function of the larynx is of course phonation or voice production. This requires fine neuromuscular control and coordination. During phonation pulmonary air power supplied to adducted vocal folds is transduced into acoustic power as the vocal fold vibrates passively (Scherer 1991). This vibration is enabled through an ingenious three-layer structure of the true vocal fold. The "body of the vocal fold" consists of the vocal muscle, the epithelium and the superficial layer of the lamina propria acting as a "cover", and the intermediate and deep layers of the lamina propria (consisting of collagenous and elastic tissue) forming a "transitional zone" (Fig. 1.5). Because of the different stiffness characteristics of these layers, they are somewhat decoupled mechanically from each other during phonation, enabling the mucosa to oscillate with a certain freedom from the ligament and the muscle (Hirano 1991; Hirano and Bless 1993). Finally, glandular structures produce a mucociliary blanket which lubricates the vocal fold, assisting in its vibration, and protects it (GRAY 2000).

The vibration of the vocal fold runs in cycles. A simple overview of a vibratory cycle is depicted in Fig. 1.6.

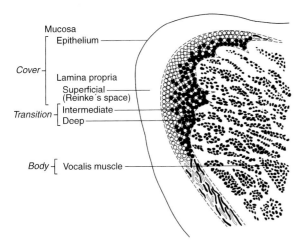

Fig. 1.5. The histopathology of the vocal fold results in three functionally dynamic layers (frontal section)

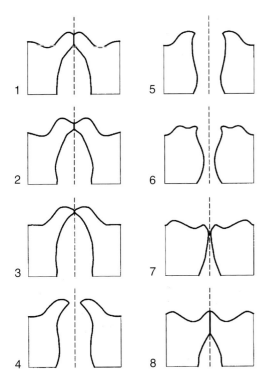

Fig. 1.6. Schematic depiction of a simple vocal vibratory cycle. Frontal section through the glottis and subglottis at different time frames

1.2
Clinical Evaluation of the Patient

1.2.1
History and Risk Factors

There is no substitute for a thorough medical and vocal history when evaluating dysphonia.

Most adults and older children with laryngeal disease present with a voice abnormality and most infants with stridor. However many other symptoms may relate to abnormalities of the larynx (see Table 1.1) (SIMPSON and FLEMING 2000).

A printed questionnaire may be helpful to assist in history taking. Specifically, besides the usual items in the complete medical history, the voice history should reveal the onset and duration of vocal symptoms, known causes or exacerbating influences, nature and severity of symptoms, personality, and vocal commitments and activities. Special attention should be given to several known risk factors for benign and malignant laryngeal conditions as shown in Table 1.2. Finally the patient should be asked what his/her vocal aspirations are, thus establishing the consequent motivation for rehabilitation, in order to tailor therapy to his/her individual needs (BASTIAN 1998).

Table 1.1. Main symptoms relating to the larynx

Hoarseness, vocal fatigue
Breathiness, shortness of breath
Odynophonia
Persistent cough
Globus sensation
Laryngospasm
Painful or difficult swallowing
Aspiration causing coughing or choking
Hemoptysis
Lump in neck

Table 1.2. Important risk factors for laryngeal conditions

Smoking
Alcohol consumption
Gastro(esophageal)laryngopharyngeal reflux
Overuse (increased talkativeness)
Vocal commitments/vocal activities
Environmental irritants (air conditioning, smog, chemical or volatile agents)
Recent upper respiratory tract infection
History of laryngeal trauma including endotracheal intubation

1.2.2
Clinical Examination of the Neck

Inspection and palpation of the head and neck region should be included in the clinical evaluation of the larynx. The palpation is mainly intended to detect lymph nodes. Cervical lymph nodes can be detected in five different areas; each of these areas should be examined carefully. In case of malignancy, the location of the lymph nodes will help to locate a primary tumor (Fig. 1.7). Carcinomas of the supraglottic larynx metastasize bilaterally to the deep cervical lymph nodes of regions II, III and IV. Small primary glottal tumors rarely give lymph node metastasis. Larger glottal tumors can metastasize to regions II, III and IV (see also Chap. 6).

1.2.3
Auditory Perceptual Assessment of the Vocal Capabilities

The vocal capability battery plays a crucial role, along with a sophisticated patient history and laryngeal examination, in making the diagnosis and directing subsequent management. This often neglected part of the evaluation provides multidimensional information concerning the nature and severity of the voice disturbance. Voice clinicians must model

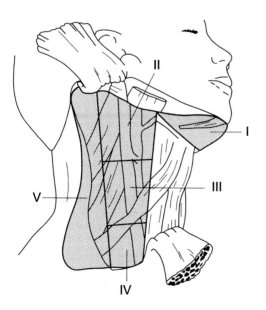

Fig. 1.7. Cervical lymph node areas (*I* submental and submandibular region, *II, III, IV* upper. mid and lower deep cervical lymph nodes around the internal jugular vein, *V* posterior neck region)

and elicit spoken and sung vocal tasks with their own voices and then analyze these sounds for basic vocal capabilities and limitations by auditory perception (BASTIAN 1998).

A widely used and validated model for making perceptual judgments is the GRBAS (grade, roughness, breathiness, asthenicity and strain) scale. The rating is made on current conversational speech or by reading a passage. G stands for the severity of the hoarseness and the overall vocal quality. Two components of hoarseness are identified: breathiness (B) is the auditory impression of turbulent air leakage through an insufficient glottic closure, and roughness (R) or harshness is the impression of irregular glottic pulses of abnormal fluctuation in fundamental frequency. These three parameters have shown sufficient inter- and intra-rater reproducibility for clinical use. In addition to the vocal capability the clinician also notes the level of effort and the overall "vocal personality". These behavioral parameters, scored as asthenicity (A) and strain (S), are less reproducible for current clinical use. Each of the parameters is graded on a four-point scale (0 = normal, 1 = slight deviance, 2 = moderate deviance, 3 = severe deviance) (DEJONCKERE 2000).

1.3
Technical Evaluation

1.3.1
Office Examination of the Larynx

1.3.1.1
Mirror Examination

The mirror examination (Figs. 1.8, 1.9) method is known universally and has been used for many years. The mirror allows three-dimensional viewing and good color resolution. Due to its limited diagnostic value and limitations in patients with pronounced gag reflexes and absence of permanent documentation, it is now replaced by newer techniques (see below). It should no longer be used as the sole method of evaluation in dysphonic patients.

1.3.1.2
Rigid Laryngeal Telescope

Rigid laryngoscopy is performed using a 70° or 90° angled telescope (Fig. 1.10). It offers an extremely clear and magnified view of the larynx and the vocal

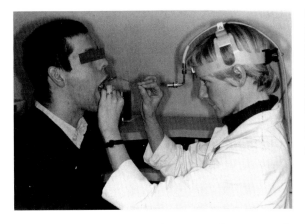

Fig. 1.8. Mirror examination. Indirect mirror laryngoscopy is performed with an external light source reflected by a small dental mirror and directed towards the larynx and pharynx. The mirror is typically positioned at the level of the soft palate while the patient is in the sniffing position and the tongue is drawn forward by the examiner

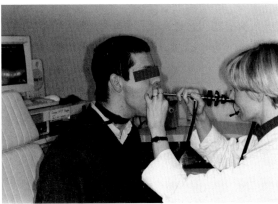

Fig. 1.10. Rigid laryngeal telescope. This technique is also performed in a non-physiological position with the patient in the sniffing position and the examiner assisting with tongue protrusion

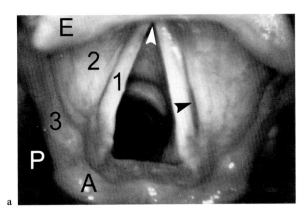

a

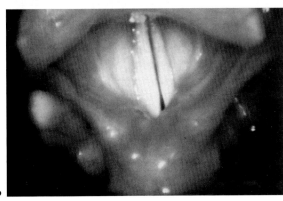

b

Fig. 1.9. Indirect mirror views of the larynx: **a** during respiration (glottis open) and **b** during phonation (glottis closed) (*1* true vocal cord, *2* false vocal cord, *3* aryepiglottic fold, *A* arytenoid cartilage, *E* epiglottis, *P* piriform sinus, *black arrowhead* entrance of laryngeal ventricle, *white arrowhead* anterior commissure)

folds. Some patients require topical oropharyngeal anesthesia. In a small percentage of patients, because of anatomic limitations or a hyperreflexive gag reflex, this technique may be unsuccessful. However, a light source and rigid endoscope are less expensive than a high-quality flexible endoscope.

1.3.1.3
Fiberoptic Nasolaryngoscope

Fiberoptic nasolaryngoscopy (Fig. 1.11) is particularly helpful in patients with exceptionally strong gag reflexes and in pediatric patients. The method is limited by its poorer resolution for subtle to moderate mucosal lesions (unless the tip of the endoscope can be closely approximated to the vocal folds) (BASTIAN et al. 1989) and by the cost (including maintenance and repair) especially for high-quality equipment.

1.3.1.4
Strobe Illumination

Strobe illumination is a specialized method of illuminating the vocal folds quasi-synchronized with vocal fold vibration. The addition of strobe illumination to any of these three examining instruments allows the laryngologist to evaluate mucosal vibratory dynamics in apparent slow motion, for example to understand mucosal scarring. The method requires a stable or nearly stable vocal fold vibratory pattern during phonation and a source to synchronize the stroboscopic light source by a bell microphone applied to the neck. Video documentation can be ob-

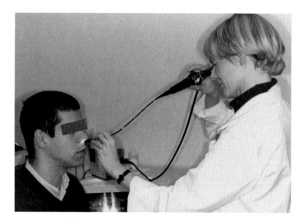

Fig. 1.11. Fiberoptic nasolaryngoscope. Transnasal flexible endoscopy has the distinct advantage of being the only laryngeal examination method that allows the larynx to be visualized in a near-physiological position

tained when using video laryngoscopy yielding a permanent document for teaching the patient and other clinicians (voice therapists and residents) (BASTIAN 1998; BASTIAN et al. 1989; HIRANO and BLESS 1993).

1.3.2
Direct Laryngoscopy

Direct laryngoscopy using a rigid laryngoscope is performed with the patient under general anesthesia. When videostroboscopy is available along with the ability to biopsy suspicious lesions of the larynx and hypopharynx indirectly in the office, direct laryngoscopy will only rarely be needed for diagnostic purposes (BASTIAN and DELSUPEHE 1996; BASTIAN et al. 1989) It is, however, indispensable as part of the management armamentarium plan for voice restoration and is used to obtain tissue in patients in whom indirect procedures have failed.

1.3.3
Objective Measures of Vocal Output

The human voice can be analyzed by devices quantifying the vocal output aerodynamically and acoustically. A detailed description of these techniques is beyond the scope of this chapter. They are reviewed elsewhere (BLESS 1991; DEJONCKERE 2000; ROSEN and MURRAY 2000).

Objective voice analysis is helpful in quantifying and documenting severity and can be used in bio-

feedback applications, but is of little (if any) diagnostic value compared to the above-described careful history and skilful applied auditory perceptual evaluation by the voice clinician (BASTIAN 1998).

1.4
Role of Imaging Studies

The clinical evaluation allows the mucosal layer of the larynx to be appreciated quite well. However, the deep extent of potentially infiltrating lesions can only be judged indirectly. For example, deep spread of a squamous cell carcinoma may cause fixation of a vocal cord. However, the exact submucosal spread and volume of such a lesion can only be determined objectively by sophisticated imaging methods, such as CT or MRI. In malignant lesions, depending on their location, radiological evaluation of the neck is useful, as some adenopathies may not be palpable or are located at sites beyond clinical evaluation (e.g. retropharyngeal or paratracheal adenopathies). Also, information on extranodal tumor spread and the relation to critical structures such as the carotid arteries, is necessary for determining the optimal patient management, and can be deduced from imaging studies.

Imaging is needed in submucosal lesions covered by an intact mucosa. The origin and extent of such lesions is often difficult to determine on the basis of clinical evaluation alone. Imaging may provide important clues to the diagnosis, as representative biopsies may be difficult to obtain in deep-seated lesions.

Also in posttraumatic pathology, imaging is useful for evaluating the laryngeal framework and soft tissues. Laryngeal and tracheal stenoses are objectively documented, helping to establish the indications for and planning of reconstructive surgery.

In most cases, the function of the larynx can be appropriately evaluated in the office. The ongoing evolution of CT and MRI now allows images during phonation and other maneuvers to be obtained. There is growing evidence that in some patients such functional radiological evaluation may provide useful information.

References

Bastian RW (1998) Benign vocal fold mucosal disorders. In: Cummings CW, Frederickson JM, Harker SA, Krause CJ, Richardson MA, Schuller DE (eds) Otolaryngology head and neck surgery. Mosby Year Book, St Louis, pp 2119–2123

Bastian RW, Delsupehe KG (1996) Indirect larynx and pharynx surgery: a replacement for direct laryngoscopy. Laryngoscope 106:1280–1286

Bastian RW, Collins SL, Kaniff T, Matz GJ (1989) Indirect videolaryngoscopy versus direct endoscopy for larynx and pharynx cancer staging: toward elimination of preliminary direct laryngoscopy. Ann Otol Rhinol Laryngol 98:693–698

Bless DM (1991) Assessment of laryngeal function. In: Ford CN, Bless DM (eds) Phonosurgery assessment and surgical management of voice disorders. Raven, New York, pp 95–122

Dejonckere PH (2000) Perceptual and laboratory assessment of dysphonia. Otolaryngol Clin North Am 33:731–750

Gray SD (2000) Cellular physiology of the vocal folds. Otolaryngol Clin North Am 33:679–698

Hirano M (1991) Phonosurgical anatomy of the larynx. In: Ford CN, Bless DM (eds) Phonosurgery assessment and surgical management of voice disorders. Raven, New York, pp 25–42

Hirano M, Bless D (1993) Videostroboscopic examination of the larynx. Whurr, London

Jiang J, Lin E, Hanson DG (2000) Vocal fold physiology. Otolaryngol Clin North Am 33:699–718

Logemann J (1983) Evaluation of swallowing disorders. Pro-ed, Austin, Tex, pp 9–36

Rosen CA, Murry T (2000) Diagnostic laryngeal endoscopy. Otolaryngol Clin North Am 33:751–758

Scherer RC (1991) Physiology of phonation: a review of basic mechanics. In: Ford CN, Bless DM (eds) Phonosurgery assessment and surgical management of voice disorders. Raven, New York, pp 77–94

Simpson CB, Fleming DJ (2000) Medical and vocal history in the evaluation of dysphonia. Otolaryngol Clin North Am 33:719–730

Sundberg J (1987) The science of the singing voice. Northern Illinois University Press, Dekalb, Ill

2 Imaging Techniques, Radiological Anatomy, and Normal Variants

FRANK A. PAMEIJER and ROBERT HERMANS

CONTENTS

2.1 Introduction

The role of modern imaging techniques in imaging the larynx has continued to evolve over the last 10 years as a result of technological advances which have decreased scan acquisition time and otherwise improved our ability to obtain high resolution, thin section (1–3 mm) images. These technical developments permit the radiologist to visualize and assess the laryngeal anatomy free of motion artifacts.

Optimized patient care requires close cooperation between the radiologist and the physician (oto-

F.A. PAMEIJER, MD, PhD
Department of Radiology, The Netherlands Cancer Institute, Antoni van Leeuwenhoek Hospital, Plesmanlaan 121, 1066 CX Amsterdam, The Netherlands
R. HERMANS, MD, PhD
Professor, Department of Radiology, University Hospitals Leuven, Herestraat 49, 3000 Leuven, Belgium

laryngologist) in charge of the patient. While the otolaryngologist uses modern laryngoscopy to evaluate the mucosal surface, it is the radiologist's role to show the depth of penetration of a lesion. Findings of both examinations should be discussed together, preferably in an interdisciplinary setting. To be an effective consultant, the radiologist must know and describe the laryngeal anatomy from an otolaryngologist's perspective (Chap. 1).

In the first part of this chapter the various techniques available for imaging the larynx are described together with comments concerning their currency or obsolescence. In the second part the normal radiological anatomy of the larynx is described from an "ENT perspective", focusing on CT and MRI. In the third section the (minimal) requirements for a diagnostic CT or MRI study of the larynx are outlined. Finally, normal variants that may be encountered in laryngeal imaging are discussed.

2.2 Imaging Techniques

In the past, a variety of conventional methods have been applied to evaluate the larynx, including soft tissue views of the neck, xeroradiography, plain film tomography, laryngography and barium swallow. CT and MRI have replaced most of these studies. CT or MRI has become essential for the correct pretherapeutic staging and proper treatment of laryngeal tumors (ZBAEREN et al. 1996).

Plain radiography was the first technique used to image the larynx. Soft tissue lateral views of the neck are still valuable as a survey study to assess gross airway patency. These films also show the thickness of the retropharyngeal soft-tissue and can be used to evaluate patients suspected of having a retropharyngeal abscess. However, most of these patients will undergo an additional CT or MRI study. Plain radiography can be used as a screening study to search for a foreign body. In daily practice, these films are still done, but modern laryngoscopy is the mainstay of diagnosis and therapy in this situation. Moreover, the variability of calcification of the laryngeal cartilages creates a diagnostic problem and may be the source of "false" foreign bodies. In the past, image contrast of soft-tissue plain films was enhanced using xeroradiography. Recently, digital radiographic techniques have been introduced. Images acquired by these systems can be postprocessed. Advantages include changing of brightness and contrast interactively and magnifying regions of interest. Repeat films become unnecessary and film and film storage cost is reduced. Plain films of the larynx are still indispensable in radiotherapy planning.

Conventional tomographic techniques were used on a large scale into the 1980s. Coronal tomograms were useful for studying the area of the true vocal cords. However, only surface deformity can be visualized by this technique which, in addition, has a relatively high radiation exposure. At present, conventional tomography has become obsolete because the information derived from this examination is now routinely available from "modern" cross-sectional techniques, such as CT and MRI.

Fluoroscopic techniques employ an image intensifier with links to videotape recording or plain film technique (spot filming). With the introduction of digital fluoroscopic units, it became possible to acquire images with very high frame rates (4–8 per second). The examination is recorded on videotape and allows review without additional patient exposure. This technique has been used in various contrast examinations. Laryngography and tracheography were developed to provide a better definition of the mucosal abnormalities of the larynx and to visualize areas not well seen by endoscopy. Just as bronchography for the evaluation of pulmonary disease has been rendered obsolete, so has laryngo- and tracheography by the combination of modern endoscopy and cross-sectional imaging. Nowadays, fluoroscopy in combination with oral contrast administration is most often used for the evaluation of speech and swallowing disorders.

2.2.1
Ultrasonography

Ultrasonography has no primary role in the radiological evaluation of the adult larynx. The ossification of the laryngeal cartilages in the adult prevents ultrasound imaging of the endolaryngeal soft tissues in most patients. When there is an acoustic window, some normal structures such as the thyroid cartilage may be identified. Sometimes the true vocal cords are well seen and vocal cord mobility can be assessed using phonation. However, clinical usefulness is low because the cords are (almost) always accessible to endoscopic evaluation.

Ultrasonography in combination with fine needle aspiration cytology (FNAC) has an important role in nodal staging of the neck in head and neck cancer, including laryngeal carcinoma (VAN DEN BREKEL et al. 1991).

2.2.2
Angiography

A laryngeal paraganglioma may be confirmed if this is suspected on other studies (KONOWITZ et al. 1988), but otherwise the role of diagnostic angiography of the larynx is very limited. Angiography of the larynx (and pharynx) is increasingly used in chemoradiation protocols for patients with advanced head and neck cancer. In this approach, a very high dose of cisplatin is delivered to the primary laryngeal or pharyngeal tumor using a transfemoral selective intra-arterial catheter. Simultaneously, a cisplatinum-neutralizing agent (sodium thiosulfate) is administered intravenously for systemic protection (ROBBINS et al. 1996).

2.2.3
Cross-sectional Imaging

Pretreatment cross-sectional imaging, either CT or MRI, has become essential for the correct pretherapeutic staging and proper treatment of laryngeal tumors (ZBAEREN et al. 1996). Usually, when a patient is referred for cross-sectional imaging of a laryngeal abnormality the histological diagnosis has already been established by endoscopic biopsy. Therefore, cross-sectional imaging should primarily supply additional information regarding the depth of penetration of a lesion, including its relationship to surrounding critical neurovascular structures.

In determining which imaging modality should be the first choice, various arguments can be applied (CURTIN 1989; SOM 1997):
- Both CT and MRI (state-of-the-art) can supply all the information needed by the otolaryngologist for adequate treatment planning.
- Soft tissue contrast of MRI is superior.
- CT is more available, lower in cost and shorter in duration (with spiral CT, the entire larynx can be examined in less than 20 s).

- Coronal (and sagittal) extension of pathology is (potentially) better depicted by MRI.
- Multidetector (spiral) CT generates high quality coronal and sagittal reconstructions.
- Shorter data acquisition time for CT results in less motion degradation caused by swallowing and respiration, or in marginally cooperative patients.
- Most radiologists prefer CT for evaluation of cervical metastatic disease.
- CT performs slightly better than MRI in staging of neck metastases (Curtin et al. 1998).

In this era of concern about cost it seems to be a good principle to do one cross-sectional study that accurately answers the clinical questions for the lowest price. Personally, the authors follow the approach advocated by Mancuso (1994). For laryngeal imaging, they prefer CT as a first choice. In less than 10% of cases, an additional MRI study is needed to resolve specific issues that would have consequences for treatment (Mancuso 1994).

2.2.4
Nuclear Imaging Techniques

Nuclear imaging techniques such as single photon emission computed tomography (SPECT) and positron emission tomography (PET) are recent additions to the range of investigations available to the head and neck surgeon (McGuirt et al. 1998; Mukherji et al. 1996; Valdes Olmos et al. 1997). PET and SPECT offer information on metabolic processes, while cross-sectional techniques, such as ultrasound, CT and MRI (mainly) supply morphological information. Potentially, metabolic techniques can detect subtle mucosal and submucosal abnormalities that do not change gross morphology, and therefore are invisible on CT and MRI studies.

In a pretherapeutic setting, (Thallium) SPECT and CT/MRI show comparable results for detection of occult primary tumors of the head and neck (Van Veen et al. 2001). Following treatment, anatomical changes, edema and scarring caused by surgery and radiotherapy often make it very difficult to assess whether recurrent or residual disease is present using clinical examination and conventional cross-sectional techniques. Various authors have reported promising results of post-treatment PET in this setting (Davis et al. 1998; Hoh et al. 1997; McGuirt et al. 1998). More detailed information on PET imaging in head and neck cancer is provided in Chapter 10.

2.3
Radiological Anatomy
from an "ENT Perspective"

A discussion of laryngeal anatomy includes the mucosa, laryngeal cartilages, muscles, nerves, blood vessels and lymphatics. Instead of this "traditional" type of discussion, in the following section an attempt is made to highlight only those anatomical structures that the radiologist should be familiar with to be an effective consultant for the otolaryngologist.

The larynx is part of the respiratory tract and houses the human voice. The craniocaudal extension is from the base of the tongue to the trachea. The larynx consists of three elements: a cartilaginous skeleton, mucosa, and the paraglottic/paralaryngeal space.

- The larynx is supported externally by a *cartilaginous skeleton* consisting of the hyoid, epiglottic, thyroid, arytenoid and cricoid cartilages (Fig. 2.1).

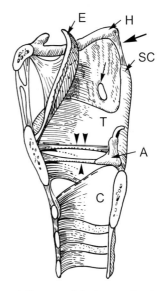

Fig. 2.1. Lateral diagram of the larynx showing the cartilaginous skeleton (mucosa, intrinsic laryngeal muscles, and paraglottic fat removed). The vocal ligament (*single arrowhead*) stretches from the vocal process of the arytenoid (*A*) to the anterior thyroid cartilage. The ventricular ligament (*double arrowhead*) runs from the upper arytenoid to the anterior thyroid cartilage (*T* thyroid lamina, *SC* superior cornu of thyroid). The superior cornua are attached to the hyoid by the thyrohyoid ligament (*unlabeled thick arrow*) which forms the posterior margin of the thyrohyoid membrane (*C* cricoid cartilage, *E* epiglottis, *H* hyoid bone). *Note:* The small structure at the upper tip of the arytenoid is the corniculate cartilage. It has no clinical significance, but is occasionally seen on CT. The small hole (*unlabeled thin arrow*) in the thyrohyoid membrane transmits the internal branch of the superior laryngeal nerve that provides sensation to the laryngeal mucosa

These cartilages are connected by membranes, ligaments and joints.

- Internally the laryngeal *mucosa* (squamous epithelium) is draped over the cartilaginous framework (Fig. 2.2).
- The *paraglottic/paralaryngeal space* lies between the cartilaginous skeleton and the mucosa (Fig. 2.3). This compartment consists of (varying amounts of) fat, lymphatics and intrinsic laryngeal muscles.

The sound-making ability of the larynx is created through various mucosal folds (false and true vocal cords) that contract or relax in response to the joint action of the arytenoid cartilages and several intrinsic laryngeal muscles that are innervated by the recurrent laryngeal nerve (branch from the vagus nerve).

The following discussion includes the normal anatomy of the *hypopharynx*. The hypopharynx is part of the gastrointestinal tract and is situated below the oropharynx and cranial to the cervical esophagus. The hypopharynx and larynx are anatomically and functionally intimately related. This close association is important both from a clinical and from an imaging standpoint. Imaging studies of the hypopharynx must always include the larynx (PAMEIJER et al. 1998).

2.3.1
Nomenclature

The original Latin nomenclature is very helpful in understanding the laryngeal anatomy. The first part of the name identifies the nature of a structure; the second part its origin and insertion. "*Membrana thyrohyoidea*" is a membrane running from the thyroid to the hyoid cartilage (thyrohyoid membrane). "*Plica aryepiglottica*" is a mucosal fold running from the arytenoid cartilage to the epiglottis (aryepiglottic fold). "*Musculus thyroarytenoideus*" is a muscle running from the thyroid to the arytenoid cartilage (thyroarytenoid muscle, i.e., part of the true vocal cords; Fig. 2.4).

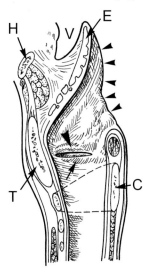

Fig. 2.2. Lateral diagram of the larynx sectioned sagittally in the midline. The slit-like ventricle separates the true vocal cords (*unlabeled arrow*) and the false vocal cords (*large arrowhead*) (*small arrowheads* aryepiglottic fold, *T* thyroid cartilage, *C* cricoid cartilage (lamina), *dashed line* projection of the arch of the cricoid cartilage, *E* epiglottis, *H* hyoid bone, *V* vallecula)

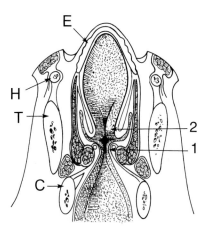

Fig. 2.3. Coronal diagram of the larynx showing the laryngeal subsites. The true vocal cords (*1*) consist mainly of the bellies of the thyroarytenoid muscle. The false vocal cords (*2*) consist mainly of fatty tissue. The true vocal cords and false vocal cords are separated by the slit-like laryngeal ventricle (sinus of Morgagni), extending superolaterally as the sacculus laryngis or appendix (*E* epiglottis, *H* hyoid bone, *T* thyroid cartilage, *C* cricoid cartilage)

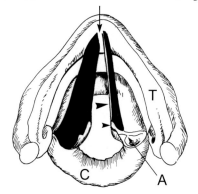

Fig. 2.4. Inner view of the larynx seen from above after removal of most soft tissues (*A* arytenoid cartilage, *C* cricoid lamina, *T* thyroid cartilage). The bulk of the true vocal cords is made up of the thyroarytenoid muscle (*in dark*) running from the inner aspect of the thyroid lamina to the arytenoid cartilage parallel to the vocal ligament (*large arrowhead*). The thyroarytenoid muscle can be separated in two bellies. Only the medial portion (vocalis muscle) is seen on the right. The vocal ligament extends from the vocal process (*small arrowhead*) to the anterior commissure (*unlabeled arrow*)

2.3.2
"ENT Landmarks" Seen on Endoscopy and/or CT and MRI (Fig. 2.5)

2.3.2.1
Cartilaginous Skeleton

2.3.2.1.1
Hyoid Bone

U-shaped bone that acts as a "rafter" from which the larynx is suspended. Muscles acting on the hyoid elevate the larynx, which is an essential part of swallowing.

2.3.2.1.2
Epiglottis

Leaf-shaped cartilage that serves as a lid to the laryngeal "voice-box". The "stem" of the leaf, which attaches in the midline to the inner aspect of the thyroid cartilage, is called the *petiole*. The epiglottis can be divided into a cranial part above the level of the hyoid (suprahyoid portion or free margin) and a caudal part (infrahyoid portion or fixed portion).

2.3.2.1.3
Thyroid Cartilage

Double-winged cartilage, with prominent superior and inferior cornua (*cornu* = horn) projecting from the posterior margin of each side of the thyroid wings (lamina). Cranially, the superior cornua are attached to the hyoid by the thyrohyoid ligament. Caudally, the inferior cornua articulate with the cricoid, forming the cricothyroid joint. The remaining spaces between the thyroid and hyoid and the cricoid and thyroid are filled by membranes, cranially the thyrohyoid membrane, caudally the cricothyroid membrane. The anterior thyroid cartilage has a deep notch in its upper surface (i.e., superior thyroid notch). On axial imaging, this may simulate a local defect (Fig. 2.5c). In general, the angle made by the two thyroid alae is wider in women than men.

2.3.2.1.4
Cricoid Cartilage

Signet ring-shaped cartilage, with the larger "signet" part (lamina) facing posteriorly and the narrower arch anteriorly. The cricoid forms the foundation of the laryngeal skeleton and is the only complete cartilaginous ring in the respiratory tract. The inferior surface of the cricoid cartilage is the border between the larynx and the trachea.

2.3.2.1.5
Arytenoid Cartilages

Pyramid-shaped, paired cartilage. The base of the pyramid articulates with the upper margin of the cricoid lamina. This cricoarytenoid joint demarcates the level of the true vocal cords. The base of the arytenoids has two processes. The *muscular process*, pointing posterolaterally, is the attachment for several intrinsic laryngeal muscles. The *vocal process*, projecting anteromedially, forms the attachment of the vocal ligament.

2.3.2.2
Mucosa

2.3.2.2.1
Aryepiglottic Fold

Mucosal fold running from the arytenoid to the lateral margin of the epiglottis. The aryepiglottic fold "plays on two teams" (Fig. 2.5d). Its anterior surface is endolaryngeal and defines the lateral boundaries of the supraglottic larynx (respiratory tract). At the same time, its posterior surface forms part of the piriform sinus and is part of the hypopharynx (digestive tract). Because of its relationship to both the larynx and the (hypo)pharynx, tumors centered on the free edge of the aryepiglottic fold are referred to with the terms *junctional* or *marginal*.

A modified Valsalva's maneuver (blowing air against closed lips, puffing out the cheeks) produces a substantial dilatation of the hypopharynx (ROBERT et al. 1993). In selected cases, obtaining images during such a maneuver may be useful to delineate the aryepiglottic folds better.

2.3.2.2.2
Vocal and Ventricular Ligaments

Two paired ligaments extending anteriorly from the arytenoids to the inner thyroid lamina. The more inferior *vocal ligament* forms the medial support of the true vocal cords. The more superior *ventricular ligament* forms the medial support of the false vocal cords. The true vocal cord is separated from the false vocal cord by a slit-like lateral out-pouching, the *laryngeal ventricle*. The laryngeal ventricle is the anatomically defined border between the glottic and the supraglottic larynx (Fig. 2.2). Otolaryngologists use the term "sinus of Morgagni" for this slit-like opening. Not visible to the endoscopist, the laryngeal ventricle extends superolaterally under the surface of the false vocal cord as the *sacculus laryngis* or *appendix*. Dilatation of the sacculus laryngis causing a submucosal supraglottic mass is called laryngocele.

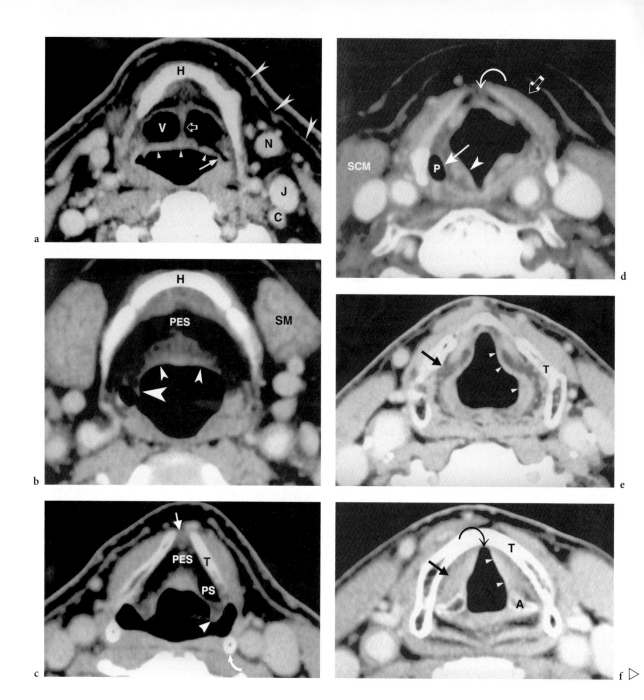

2.3.2.2.3
True Vocal Cord

The true vocal cord is a paired mucosal fold. The bulk of the true vocal cords is made up of the thyroarytenoid muscle running from the inner aspect of the thyroid lamina to the arytenoid cartilage parallel to the vocal ligament. The thyroarytenoid muscle can be separated into two bellies. The medial portion is called the *vocalis muscle* (Fig. 2.4). On CT and MRI, the true vocal cord is recognized by its muscle density (signal intensity). Both true vocal cords meet anteriorly in the midline at the anterior commissure. On normal cross-sectional imaging (quiet breathing), the

mean width of the soft tissues at the anterior commissure is 1.02±0.56 mm (KALLMES and PHILIPS 1997).

The appearance of the cords varies with the phase of respiration. In quiet breathing the cords are slightly abducted and the airway is open (Fig. 2.5f). During phonation (usually the vowel 'e' is used), the vocal cords will appear adducted and during breath-holding the vocal cords are apposed. Acquiring images during phonation may give a better visualization of the laryngeal ventricle and produces some dilatation of the piriform sinuses (Fig. 2.6). However, with the cords together, it is impossible to evaluate the thickness of the anterior commissure.

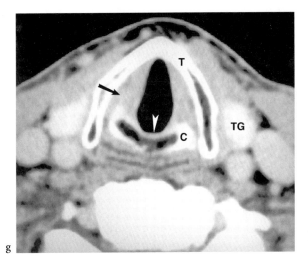

g

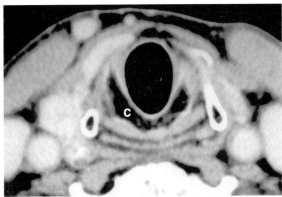

h

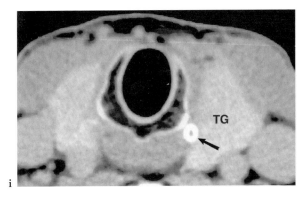

i

Fig. 2.5a–i. Axial CT scan through the larynx from cranial to caudal (different patients) demonstrating normal anatomy (*H* hyoid bone, *T* thyroid cartilage, *A* arytenoid cartilage, *C* cricoid cartilage, *PES* preepiglottic space). **a** CT image at the level of the hyoid bone (*V* vallecula, *C* common carotid artery, *J* internal jugular vein, *N* lymph node, *small arrowheads* free margin of epiglottis, *open arrow* glossoepiglottic fold, *arrow* pharyngoepiglottic fold, *large arrowheads* platysma muscle). **b** CT scan through upper aryepiglottic fold (*large arrowhead* aryepiglottic fold. *small arrowheads* fixed portion of epiglottis, *SM* submandibular gland). **c** Supraglottic larynx (*arrow* superior thyroid notch, *arrowhead* aryepiglottic fold, *curved arrow* superior cornu of thyroid cartilage, *PS* paraglottic space). **d** Supraglottic larynx (*arrowhead*, anterior (endolaryngeal) surface of aryepiglottic fold, *arrow* posterior (endopharyngeal) surface of aryepiglottic fold, *curved arrow* petiole of epiglottis, *open arrow* strap musculature, *SCM*, sternocleidomastoid muscle, *P* piriform sinus). *Note:* The left common carotid artery is in a retrolaryngeal-pharyngeal position (tortuosity). This normal variant causes asymmetry of the piriform sinuses. **e** Supraglottic larynx. Level of the false vocal cords (*arrowheads* false vocal cord, *arrow* paraglottic space predominantly filled with fatty tissue). **f** Glottic larynx. Level of the upper surface of the true vocal cords (*white arrowheads* true vocal cord, *arrow* paraglottic space predominantly filled with thyroarytenoid muscle, *curved arrow* anterior commissure). **g** Glottic larynx. Level of the true vocal cords (*arrow* paraglottic space almost completely filled by thyroarytenoid muscle, *arrowhead* posterior commissure, *TG* thyroid gland, upper pole). **h** Glottic larynx. CT image through the undersurface of the true vocal cords as the airway widens. Cricoid cartilage assumes a more ring-like configuration. **i** Subglottic larynx. Cricoid ring almost completely visible (*arrow* inferior cornu of thyroid cartilage, *TG* thyroid gland)

The term "posterior commissure" describes the mucosa covering the area between the arytenoid cartilages (Fig. 2.5g).

2.3.2.2.4
False Vocal Cord

The false vocal cord is a paired mucosal fold. The false vocal cord runs from the inner aspect of the thyroid lamina to the arytenoid parallel to the ventricular ligament. It is predominantly made up of fat (Fig. 2.5e), and on CT and MRI is recognized by its fat density (signal intensity).

2.3.2.3
Paraglottic/Paralaryngeal Space

2.3.2.3.1
Paraglottic Space

The paraglottic space is a paired fat-containing space between the cartilaginous skeleton and the mucosal surface of the larynx. Sometimes the name "paralaryngeal" space is used, but this name is misleading as it suggests that the space is along and not within the larynx. At the level of the false vocal cord the paraglottic space is predominantly filled with fat. At the true vocal cord level only a narrow band of fatty tissue is present lateral to the thyroarytenoid muscle. The laryngeal ventricle extends laterally into the paired paraglottic spaces. However, a narrow band of paraglottic fat is present between the most lateral extension of the laryngeal ventricle and the inner surface of the thyroid cartilage (Fig. 2.3). Thus, the paraglottic space is continuous from the false cord to the true cord levels. This continuity is a natural "gateway" for (submucosal and therefore endoscopically occult) spread of disease from the glottic to the supraglottic larynx. The paraglottic space extends cranially to the level of the epiglottis. In an anatomical study, it has been shown that the paraglottic spaces are continuous superomedially with the preepiglottic space in most specimens, while in some cases they are completely separated by a conspicuous collagenous fiber septum (REIDENBACH 1996).

2.3.2.3.2
Preepiglottic Space
The preepiglottic space is a C-shaped fat-containing space (Fig. 2.5b, c) between the epiglottis (posteriorly) and the hyoid bone, thyrohyoid membrane and thyroid cartilage (anteriorly). The preepiglottic space is primarily filled with fat and lymphatic vessels. On imaging studies, the preepiglottic space appears continuous on either side with the paraglottic spaces (REIDENBACH 1996).

Comment: The preepiglottic space and the paraglottic spaces cannot be evaluated endoscopically and can harbor extensive submucosal disease. These fatty spaces should be carefully analyzed by the radiologist because clinically occult, submucosal disease at these locations will frequently alter therapeutic decisions in these patients.

2.3.3
Laryngeal Subsites and Boundaries

2.3.3.1
Subsites

The larynx can be subdivided (from cranial to caudal) into three subsites: the *supraglottis*, *glottis*, and *subglottis* (Fig. 2.3). This subdivision is based on the TNM ruling recommendations for staging of laryngeal carcinoma by the AMERICAN JOINT COMMITTEE ON CANCER (1988). The larynx is subdivided by two theoretical horizontal (axial) planes. The more superior plane is at the level of the laryngeal ventricle (sinus of Morgagni) and separates the supraglottic larynx from the glottic larynx. The second

plane is 1 cm caudal to the first plane and separates the glottis from the subglottic larynx. For accurate staging it is mandatory that the radiologist is able to correctly localize abnormalities seen on CT and MRI studies in these laryngeal subsites.

The supraglottis includes the following ENT landmarks:
- Epiglottis
- Aryepiglottic fold
- False vocal cords
- Laryngeal ventricle
- Arytenoid cartilage (upper part)

The glottis includes:
- True vocal cords
- Anterior and posterior commissures
- Arytenoid cartilage (lower part)
- Cricoid cartilage (upper part)
- Cricoarytenoid joint

The subglottis includes:
- Cricoid cartilage (lower part)

2.3.3.2
Boundaries

The upper larynx (i.e., supraglottis) ends at the level of the glossoepiglottic fold and pharyngoepiglottic folds (Fig. 2.5a). Above these folds is the oropharynx (i.e., tongue base and valleculae). The laryngeal ventricle is the clear anatomical boundary between the supraglottic and glottic larynx. In contrast, there is no distinct anatomical boundary between glottis and subglottis. The subglottis is defined as the area from the undersurface of the true vocal cords stretching to the inferior surface of the cricoid cartilage. Caudal to the subglottis begins the trachea. The aryepiglottic fold forms a boundary between the supraglottic larynx (anteriorly), i.e., the respiratory tract, and the hypopharynx (posteriorly), i.e., the digestive tract.

2.3.4
Hypopharyngeal Subsites and Boundaries

The hypopharynx (Latin: *hypo* = lower) is the most caudal portion of the pharynx that extends superiorly from the level of the hyoid bone to the caudal part of the cricoid cartilage, inferiorly. Above the hyoid is the oropharynx. Below the cricoid cartilage, the hypopharynx becomes the cervical esophagus. The main function of the hypopharynx is the transportation of the food bolus from the oropharynx to the cervical esophagus. The hypopharynx can be divided into three subsites: the (paired) *piriform sinuses*, the *posterior hypopharyngeal wall*, and the *postcricoid region*.

2.3.4.1
Piriform Sinus

Two pear-shaped (piriform is derived from the Latin *pirum* = pear) grooves of the hypopharynx created by the impression of the larynx into the anterior aspect of the pharynx. A frontal view of a barium study will often show these as two symmetric stalactite-like structures. Each piriform sinus is made up of a medial, an anterior, and a lateral wall. The medial wall is the free edge of the aryepiglottic fold, separating the piriform sinus from the larynx. The anterior wall of the piriform sinus is in direct contact with the posterior paralaryngeal space. The lateral wall is formed superiorly by the thyrohyoid membrane and inferiorly by the thyroid cartilage. A posterior wall of the piriform sinus is anatomically not defined, since this area is in direct continuity with the posterior pharyngeal wall. The upper limit of the piriform sinus is the pharyngoepiglottic fold. The lowermost boundary of the piriform sinus, called the apex, lies at the level of the true vocal cords. The apex is well visualized in the frontal view of a barium study. In cross-sectional images, the apex is located at the level of the cricoarytenoid joint (i.e., true vocal cord level).

2.3.4.2
Posterior Hypopharyngeal Wall

The posterior wall of the hypopharynx, which is 4 to 5 cm wide and 6 to 7 cm high, starts at the level of the valleculae. Above this, the posterior wall is continuous with the posterior wall of the oropharynx. Caudally, the posterior wall extends to the level of the inferior surface of the cricoid cartilage where it merges with the mucosa covering the cricopharyngeus muscle and then with the cervical esophagus (Fig. 2.6).

2.3.4.3
Postcricoid Area

This area, also called the pharyngo-esophageal junction, extends from the level of the arytenoid cartilages to the inferior border of the cricoid cartilage. It is composed of the mucosa covering the posterior aspect (lamina) of the cricoid cartilage (Fig. 2.5). This area is the interface between the hypopharynx posteriorly and the larynx anteriorly, sometimes referred to as the party wall. Directly caudal to this the esophageal verge or esophageal inlet is found. This is the junction between the postcricoid portion of the hypopharynx and the cervical esophagus. At this junction, the inferior pharyngeal constrictor fibers merge with the circular muscles of the upper cervical esophagus. It can be seen on endoscopy, but also on cross-sectional imaging, recognized by its flat ellipsoid shape in contrast to the cervical esophagus, which has a rounded appearance (SCHMALFUSS et al. 2000).

2.4
Imaging Strategies for CT and MRI of the Larynx

We cannot supply the ideal imaging protocol, since available imaging resources and local experience may vary. However, we will outline the (minimal) requirements for a diagnostic study. Irrespective of the equipment used (incremental slice-to-slice CT, spiral CT or MRI) there are a few technical details regarding positioning of the patient and scan angulation that are essential.

The images are obtained with the patient supine and during quiet respiration. The head is carefully aligned in the cephalocaudal axis in order to make it possible to compare symmetric structures (e.g., the true vocal cords). Malposition may result in an appearance that simulates disease or asymmetry.

The endoscopist will always classify his/her findings according to the clinical subdivisions of the larynx: the supraglottis, glottis and subglottis. To be an effective consultant, the radiologist will have to do the same. Therefore, the axial plane of section *must* be parallel to the true vocal cords. Ideally, this angle is selected from the preliminary lateral scout view by identification of the air in the laryngeal ventricle, which is in the same plane as the true vocal cords. Alternatively, a plane parallel to the C4-5, or C5-6 disk space can be used as an estimate.

2.4.1
CT Technique

Even in this era of spiral CT, it is still possible to use slice-to-slice CT and produce a fully acceptable scan

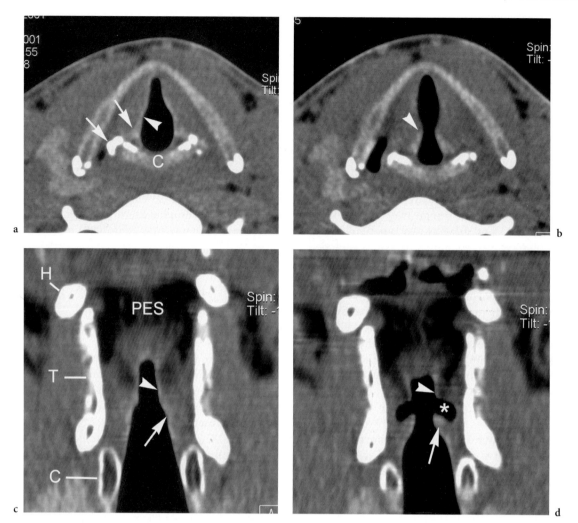

Fig. 2.6. Multislice CT images reformatted along the plane of the true vocal cords (**a, b**), and perpendicular to this plane (**c, d**). The images were obtained during quiet breathing (**a** and **c**) and during phonation of 'e' (**b** and **d**). Images **a/b** and **c/d** were obtained in different patients. **a, b** Only the posterior part of the arytenoid cartilages (*arrows*) is ossified in this young patient (*C* cricoid lamina). During phonation, the vocal cords are adducted, narrowing the glottis. Note the medial rotation of the arytenoid cartilages apparent from the position of the vocal process of the arytenoid cartilage (*arrowhead*). **c, d** The laryngeal cartilages are more heavily calcified in this older patient (*T*, thyroid cartilage; *C*, cricoid arch; *H*, hyoid bone). During quiet respiration, the true (*arrow*) and false vocal cords (*arrowhead*) are apposed. During phonation, the laryngeal ventricle (*asterisk*) is filled with air and separates the two cords (*PES* preepiglottic space)

quality if certain basic requirements are fulfilled. The neck should be slightly hyperextended so that the larynx is drawn higher in the neck to help avoid artifacts produced by the shoulders. If possible, the examination is performed with the administration of intravenous contrast material. This increases the conspicuousness of primary tumors and allows the best possible differentiation of nodes from vessels. The field of view (FOV) must be magnified to optimize spatial resolution. The recommended FOV varies between 16 and 18 cm, depending on the size of the patient.

The CT examination is performed as contiguous 3-mm scans from the skull base to the manubrium, or as a helical study reconstructed as contiguous 3-mm sections. The helical technique uses 3-mm thick scans with a 3–5 mm/s table speed and a pitch of 1:1 to 1:1.6. These parameters may vary slightly according to the CT machine.

Experience with multislice CT of the larynx is still limited. The imaging parameters currently used at the University Hospitals of Leuven are: 4×1 mm collimation, 2 mm slice width, 4 mm feed/rotation. Multislice CT allows high-quality reformations along any plane to be obtained, including along that of the true vocal cords (Fig. 2.6).

The CT images should be filmed in soft-tissue window settings. In addition, images of the larynx (hyoid bone to the inferior border of the cricoid cartilage) should be reconstructed on a smaller FOV (12–14 cm). These should be filmed in two different window settings, one suitable for evaluation of soft tissue, and the other for evaluation of cartilage and bone (SCHMALFUSS and MANCUSO 1998).

As already mentioned, dynamic maneuvers during scanning of the larynx and hypopharynx can enhance visualization of particular anatomic structures. During phonation arytenoid mobility can be judged and a better visualization of the laryngeal ventricle can be obtained; the slight distention of the piriform sinuses also allows better delineation of the aryepiglottic folds. A modified Valsalva's maneuver (blowing air against closed lips, puffing out the cheeks) produces a substantial dilatation of the hypopharynx, which may allow better evaluation of the piriform sinuses, including the postcricoid region (ROBERT et al. 1993). The success rate of these dynamic maneuvers in incremental CT is variable, strongly depending on the cooperation of the patient: consistent repetition of the maneuver for each incremental scan is difficult, spatial misregistration being an important drawback. Furthermore, the incremental acquisition of these additional scans during phonation or modified Valsalva's maneuver is time consuming.

These problems can be largely overcome by spiral CT, as the patient has to do the maneuver only once during one rapid acquisition. It is difficult for most patients to sustain such a dynamic maneuver for a long time – therefore these dynamic spiral acquisitions are, depending on the patient, restricted to a scan time between 15 and 24 s; shorter scan times are feasible with multislice CT technology. The level scanned is determined on the images acquired during quiet respiration; one should compensate for the fact that the larynx descends somewhat during modified Valsalva's maneuver and rises during phonation – the distance over which this occurs, varies but is usually between 0,5 and 1 cm. The patient has to be well informed about what is expected from him or her during the spiral CT study. The dynamic maneuvers need to be practiced with the patient before the examination starts. Often the patients need to be accompanied and encouraged during the actual examination. This small time investment yields good results in the majority of cases (DUBRULLE et al. 1997) (see also Chap. 11).

2.4.2
MRI Technique

MRI of the larynx should not be attempted unless a neck surface coil is available. Careful instruction of the patient by the technologist, or supervising radiologist, is even more crucial than with CT because respiratory and/or swallowing artifacts may seriously degrade the MR study. The patient is instructed to breathe quietly and to practice doing so without moving the neck. Patients should be encouraged to use "abdominal", instead of "thoracic" respiration and not to swallow or at least to swallow as seldom as possible during acquisitions. The neck should not be hyperextended because this makes swallowing more difficult.

The larynx should be studied in both the axial and coronal plane. In cases of midline pathology, a sagittal acquisition may be helpful (Fig. 2.7). It is recommended that the examination be started with a sagittal T1-weighted (T1 W) localizer series to identify the laryngeal ventricle (Fig. 2.8) or the C4-5, or C5-6 disk space. The subsequent axial series can then be angled in a plane parallel to the true vocal cords (Fig 2.9).

MRI images should be no thicker than 5 mm. The recommended section thickness is 4 mm or less with

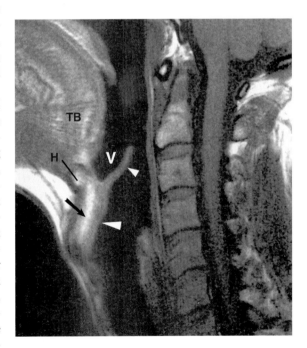

Fig. 2.7. MRI T1-weighted sagittal image in the midline demonstrating the normal anatomy of the supraglottic larynx (*TB* tongue base; *V* vallecula; *H* hyoid bone; *small arrowhead* suprahyoid portion, i.e., free margin, of epiglottis; *large arrowhead* infrahyoid portion, i.e., fixed portion, of epiglottis). The preepiglottic space shows bright fat intensity (*black arrow*)

a 1-mm interslice gap. The optimal FOV for the axial views is 16–18 cm for T1-weighted sequences and 18–20 cm for T2-weighted sequences. This slightly larger FOV with the T2-weighted sequences results in a better signal-to-noise ratio. Pixel size should be kept under 1×1 mm (0.5 mm desirable); acquisition matrix between 256×256 and 512×512.

Due to inherent signal intensity differences between tumor, fat, and muscle, accurate delineation of a primary tumor is often possible using T1-weighted images only. However, administration of intravenous paramagnetic contrast material frequently increases the conspicuousness of primary tumors and is essential for the evaluation of the cervical nodes. We suggest that T1-weighted images be obtained before and after injection of intravenous paramagnetic contrast material. The non-enhanced T1-weighted sequence should be performed in the same plane before contrast material administration so fat or proteinaceous fluid with a high signal intensity will not be confused with enhancement. Fat-saturation techniques, which permit better identification of the tumor margins, may be used for the post-contrast images (ESCOTT et al. 1997; MUKHERJI et al. 1997).

2.5
Normal Variants

2.5.1
Ossification Pattern of the Laryngeal Cartilages

The appearance of the laryngeal cartilages can vary considerably, depending on the degree of ossification and the amount of fatty marrow in the ossified medullar space. In children and adolescents, only the hyoid bone is ossified. In this age group, the CT density of the laryngeal cartilages will be similar to that of soft tissue, making the interpretation more difficult. On average, before the age of 18 years in men and 23 years in women, the laryngeal cartilages are composed entirely of hyaline cartilage. Only the epiglottis and vocal process of the arytenoids are composed of yellow fibrocartilage that usually does not ossify. Ossification of hyaline cartilage starts early in the third decade of life. This is an endochondral type of ossification. A precise pattern of ossification is difficult to define because a high degree of variation exists between individuals (YEAGER et al. 1982). In general, the thyroid cartilage shows great variability in ossification both between individuals and in

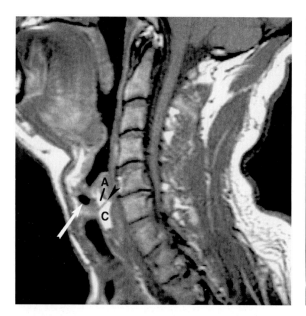

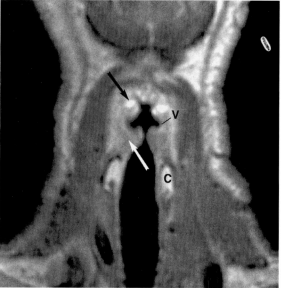

Fig. 2.8. MRI T1-weighted sagittal image, off midline, demonstrating the true and false vocal cords separated by the air-filled (*dark*) laryngeal ventricle (*arrow*). The ossified cricoid (*C*) and arytenoid (*A*) cartilages display bright fat intensity (*arrowhead* cricoarytenoid joint). *Note:* The upper part of the arytenoid cartilage is part of the supraglottis, while the lower part is part of the glottis (Courtesy I.M. Schmalfuss, MD, Gainesville, Florida)

Fig. 2.9. MRI T1-weighted coronal image demonstrating the normal anatomy of the larynx. The thyroarytenoid muscle at the level of the true vocal cords shows muscle intensity (*arrow*). The paraglottic space at the level of the false cords shows bright fat intensity (*black arrow*) (*V* ventricle, *C* cricoid cartilage) (Courtesy I.M. Schmalfuss, MD, Gainesville, Florida)

the same individual. The cricoid and arytenoids show less-pronounced variability in ossification.

In CT images, ossified laryngeal cartilage shows a dense outer and inner cortex and a central hypodense medullary space (Fig. 2.5). In MRI images, the cortex of ossified parts can be seen as a low signal intensity (SI) margin on all pulse sequences, whereas the fat-containing medullary space has an SI similar to that of fat.

2.5.2
Variations in Vascular and Bony Anatomy

A tortuous common or internal carotid artery may present as a (pulsatile) submucosal mass during laryngopharyngoscopy. On (contrast-enhanced) CT, an enhancing vessel is seen in a retrolaryngeal-pharyngeal position. Usually, the CT diagnosis is straightforward (Fig. 2.5d).

When very large, vertebral osteophytes may present as a submucosal bulge of the posterior pharyngeal wall. This finding may lead to imaging evaluation, frequently CT or MRI. Cross-sectional findings are usually straightforward showing the osteophyte(s) in a retropharyngeal position.

References

American Joint Committee on Cancer (1988) Manual for staging of cancer, 3rd edn. Lippincott-Raven, Philadelphia

Curtin HD (1989) Imaging of the larynx: current concepts. Radiology 173:1–11

Curtin HD, Ishwaran H, Mancuso AA, et al (1998) Comparison of CT and MRI imaging of neck metastases. Radiology 207:123–130

Davis JP, Maisey MN, Chevretton EB (1998) Positron emission tomography – a useful imaging technique for otolaryngology, head and neck surgery? J Laryngol Otol 122:125–127

Dubrulle F, Robert Y, Delerue C, et al (1997) Intérêt du scanner spiralé dans la pathologie du larynx et de l'hypo-pharynx. Feuill Radiol 37:118–131

Escott EJ, Rao VM, Guitterrez JE (1997) Comparison of dynamic contrast-enhanced gradient-echo and spin-echo sequences in MR of head and neck neoplasms. AJNR Am J Neuroradiol 18:1411–1419

Hoh CK, Schiepers C, Seltzer MA, et al (1997) PET in oncology: will it replace the other modalities? Semin Nucl Med 27:94–106

Kallmes DF, Phillips CD (1997) The normal anterior commissure of the glottis. AJR Am J Roentgenol 168:1317–1319

Konowitz PM, Lawson W, Som PM, et al (1988) Laryngeal paraganglioma: update on diagnosis and treatment. Laryngoscope 98:40–49

Mancuso AA (1994) Imaging in patients with head and neck cancer. In: Million RR, Cassisi NJ (eds) Management of head and neck cancer: a multidisciplinary approach. Lippincott, Philadelphia, pp 43–59

McGuirt WF, Greven KM, Williams DW, et al (1998) PET scanning in head and neck oncology: a review. Head Neck 20:208–215

Mukherji SK, Drane WE, Mancuso AA, et al (1996) Occult primary tumors of the head and neck: detection with 2-[F-18] fluoro-2-deoxy-D-glucose SPECT. Radiology 199:761–766

Mukherji SK, Pillsbury HR, Castillo M (1997) Imaging squamous cell carcinomas of the upper aerodigestive tract: what clinicians need to know. Radiology 205:629–646

Pameijer FA, Mukherji SK, Balm AJM, et al (1998) Imaging of squamous cell carcinoma of the hypopharynx. Semin Ultrasound CT MR 19:476–491

Reidenbach MM (1996) The paraglottic space and transglottic cancer: anatomical considerations. Clin Anat 9:244–251

Robbins KT, Fontanesi J, Wong FSH, et al (1996) A novel organ preservation protocol for advanced carcinoma of the larynx and pharynx. Arch Otolaryngol Head Neck Surg 122:853–857

Robert YH, Chevalier D, Rocourt NL, et al (1993) Dynamic maneuver acquired with spiral CT in laryngeal disease. Radiology 189:298–299

Schmalfuss IM, Mancuso AA (1998) Protocols for helical CT of the head and neck. In: Silverman PM (ed) Helical (spiral) computed tomography. Lippincott-Raven, Philadelphia, pp 11–57

Schmalfuss IM, Mancuso AA, Tart RP (2000) Postcricoid region and cervical esophagus: normal appearance at CT and MR imaging. Radiology 214:237–246

Som PM (1997) The present controversy over the imaging method of choice for evaluating the soft tissues of the neck. AJNR Am J Neuroradiol 18:1869–1872

Valdes Olmos RA, Balm AJM, Hilgers FJM, et al (1997) Thallium-201 SPECT in the diagnosis of head and neck cancer. J Nucl Med 38:873–879

Van den Brekel MWM, Castelijns JA, Stel HV (1991) Occult metastatic neck disease: detection with US and US-guided fine-needle aspiration cytology. Radiology 180:457–462

Van Veen SAJM, Balm AJM, Valdes Olmos RA, et al (2001) Occult primary tumors of the head and neck. Accuracy of thallium 201 single-photon emission computed tomography and computed tomography and/or magnetic resonance imaging. Arch Otolaryngol Head Neck Surg 127:406–411

Yeager VL, Lawson C, Archer CR (1982) Ossification of the laryngeal cartilages as it relates to computed tomography. Invest Radiol 17:11–19

Zbaeren P, Becker M, Lang H (1996) Pretherapeutic staging of laryngeal carcinoma: clinical findings, computed tomography, and magnetic resonance imaging compared with histopathology. Cancer 77:1263–1273

3 Benign Pathology of the Adult Larynx

ROBERT HERMANS and ILONA M. SCHMALFUSS

CONTENTS

3.1 Introduction

Benign pathology of the larynx requiring radiologic evaluation is uncommon. Laryngocele, traumatic pathology and vocal cord paralysis are the most frequent conditions imaged. In this chapter, the imaging findings of benign pathology of the adult larynx are reviewed.

3.2 Congenital Lesions

Congenital lesions of the larynx are rare. As they often cause severe respiratory distress, they usually are diagnosed early in childhood. These entities are thoroughly discussed in Chapter 4 on pediatric lesions.

Few congenital lesions at the laryngeal level may present later in life. The most frequent one is thyroglossal duct cyst. It arises from remnants of the thyroglossal duct, an embryonal canal between the foramen cecum and the anlage of the thyroid gland. Normally, this duct obliterates early in fetal life. In nearly all subjects, a fibrous remnant of the thyroglossal duct is present. Thyroglossal duct cysts are usually located in or near the midline, and have a close relationship to the hyoid bone. In most cases they are below the level of the hyoid bone, typically embedded within the prelaryngeal muscles (Fig. 3.1). They usually become symptomatic when superinfected. Sometimes they invaginate between the thyroid cartilage and hyoid bone, into the preepiglottic space (Fig. 3.2).

As thyroglossal duct cysts contain microscopic foci of thyroid tissue, very rarely a carcinoma may originate from such a cyst. Theoretically, a thyroglossal duct carcinoma may also be a metastasis from an occult carcinoma of the thyroid gland (KENNEDY et al. 1998). Most of these thyroglossal duct cyst carcinomas are not suspected preoperatively, and are diagnosed at the histologic examination of the resection specimen. Radiologically, the presence of a mural nodule or calcification (or both) in a thyroglossal duct cyst should be considered suspicious for malignancy (BRANSTETTER et al. 2000).

R. HERMANS, MD, PhD
Professor, Department of Radiology, University Hospitals Leuven, Herestraat 49, 3000 Leuven, Belgium
I.M. SCHMALFUSS, MD
Department of Radiology, University of Florida, 1600 SW Archer Road, Gainesville, FL 32610, USA

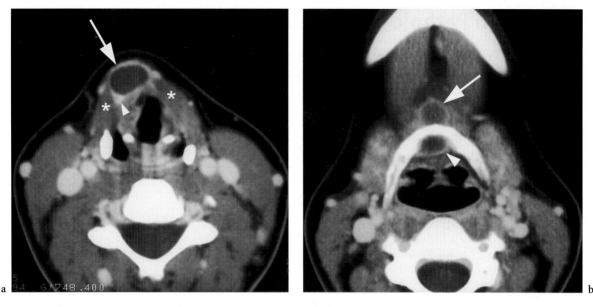

Fig. 3.1a, b. Axial contrast-enhanced CT images in a patient with painful anterior and paramedian swelling of the neck. **a** Cystic lesion (*arrow*) with an enhancing wall, embedded in the prelaryngeal muscles (*stars*). The lesion lies in close proximity to the lobus pyramidalis (*arrowhead*) which could be followed inferiorly to the isthmus of the thyroid gland (not shown). Some small prelaryngeal veins are seen on both sides of the cyst. **b** The cyst (*arrow*) abuts the undersurface of the hyoid bone, its posterior part (*arrowhead*) is prolapsed into the preepiglottic space. Superinfected thyroglossal duct cyst

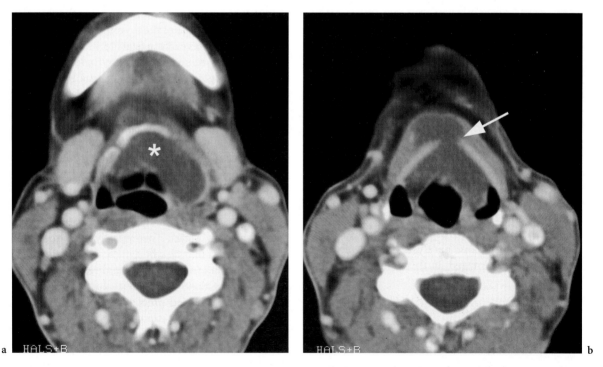

Fig. 3.2a, b. Axial contrast-enhanced CT images in a patient with anterior neck swelling. **a** A thin-walled cystic lesion (*star*) is seen within the preepiglottic space abutting the hyoid bone posteriorly. **b** The cyst extends anteriorly between the hyoid and thyroid cartilage (*arrow*) to become embedded within the prelaryngeal muscles. Thyroglossal duct cyst

3.3
Inflammatory Pathology

3.3.1
Infection

3.3.1.1
Acute Laryngitis

Acute laryngitis is nearly always viral in origin, and a self-limiting condition. Bacterial superinfection may occur. A laryngeal abscess is a rare entity, usually secondary to endotracheal intubation or direct trauma.

Children with epiglottitis or croup are the patients with laryngeal inflammation most commonly seen by the radiologist. The imaging findings in these diseases are discussed in Chapter 4 on pediatric lesions. Epiglottitis may also affect adult patients. Due to the higher airway reserve of adults, the disease usually has a less critical course than in children, although cases of rapid airway obstruction have been described. An epiglottic abscess develops in about 15% of adult patients with epiglottitis. Formation of an epiglottic abscess is much rarer in children. Such an abscess most commonly involves the lingual surface of the epiglottis (WITTE and NEEL 2000) (Fig. 3.3).

3.3.1.2
Tuberculosis

Tuberculosis is one of the diseases that may affect the larynx. Tuberculosis is caused by *Mycobacterium tuberculosis*. Head and neck tuberculosis is most commonly seen in the neck lymph nodes, and represents about 15% of the cases of extrapulmonary tuberculosis and about 1.5% of all new cases of tuberculosis (MOON et al. 1997). Nowadays, neck tuberculosis outside the lymph nodes is rarely seen, but there seems to be an increasing frequency due to the increasing number of immunocompromised patients (HOUGHTON et al. 1997). The most common extranodal localization is the larynx, followed by the temporal bone and the pharynx; other sites such as the sinonasal cavity, thyroid gland and skull base are only rarely affected. Laryngeal tuberculosis may be seen in patients with advanced, but also in those with limited, lung disease. The larynx is infected through bronchogenic spread with direct infestation from the active pulmonary focus, or by hematogenous or lymphatic spread. The supraglottic larynx is affected most commonly.

The presenting symptoms of laryngeal tuberculosis may be dysphonia, dysphagia, swallowing difficulties, sore throat and foreign body sensation. Laryngo-

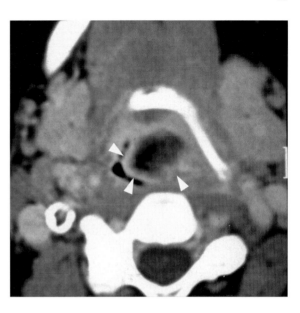

Fig. 3.3. Adult patient with progressive throat pain, dysphagia and dyspnea. Indirect laryngoscopy demonstrated a red, cystic swelling of the epiglottis. Axial contrast-enhanced CT image reveals a hypodense mass along the lingual side of the epiglottis (*arrowheads*). The mass shows peripheral contrast enhancement. Epiglottic abscess

scopic examination shows mucosal swelling and a "dirty" exudate, but may also reveal a fungating tumor-like lesion, mimicking laryngeal carcinoma.

The imaging findings in laryngeal tuberculosis are non-specific, and include bilateral soft tissue thickening, with or without infiltration of the preepiglottic and paraglottic spaces, but usually without a focal mass (Fig. 3.4). However, a focal soft tissue thickening may be seen, especially in more chronic cases. Soft tissue calcifications are uncommon. The laryngeal framework remains intact in most cases, although tuberculosis may cause arthritis of the cricoarytenoid joint. The main differential diagnosis includes laryngeal carcinoma, as well as other types of granulomatous laryngitis (MOON et al. 1996, 1997).

The diagnosis is confirmed by identification of acid-fast bacilli on histopathologic examination of laryngeal biopsies. The treatment is primarily by anti-tuberculous medication (YENCHA et al. 2000). Inadequate treatment may result in laryngeal stenosis and fixation of the vocal cords.

3.3.1.3
Other Causes of Infectious Granulomatous Laryngitis

Rhinoscleroma is an infectious disease of the upper respiratory tract, caused by *Klebsiella rhinoscleroma-*

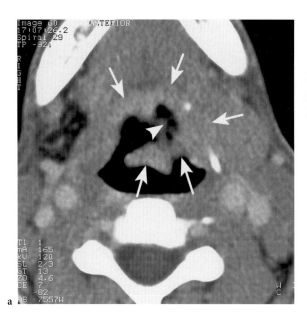
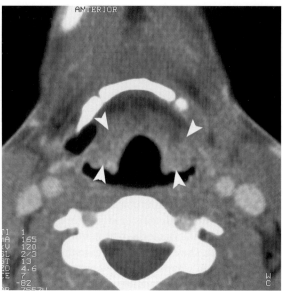

Fig. 3.4a, b. Axial contrast-enhanced CT images. **a** Enhancing soft tissue thickening involving the tongue base and left vallecula (*arrows*) with focal ulceration (*arrowhead*). **b** Symmetric thickening and infiltration of the aryepiglottic folds (*arrowheads*), suggesting an inflammatory etiology. However, based on these imaging findings, carcinoma cannot be definitely excluded. Laryngeal tuberculosis. (Reprinted with permission from HERMANS 2000, p 483)

tis. Apart from the nose, mouth, paranasal sinuses and pharynx, it may also affect the larynx and trachea. Rhinoscleroma evolves through three stages: after an initial stage of mucosal atrophy, a granulomatous stage may appear, eventually followed by fibrosis leading to stenosis. The imaging findings are non-specific, usually showing soft tissue thickening only. The subglottic area is typically involved in laryngeal rhinoscleroma (ABOU-SEIF et al. 1991) (Fig. 3.5).

Syphilis is an infectious disease caused by *Treponema pallidum* and transmitted by direct contact,

usually through sexual intercourse. The chancre, the first symptom of primary syphilis, can develop in the oral region after orogenital contact. During the stage of secondary syphilis, condylomata lata develop. These have been reported to occur in the larynx as well. In congenital syphilis, several head and neck abnormalities may be present, such as saddle nose deformity, frontal bossing, maxillary and dental malformations, but the larynx may also be involved. Syphilis may cause arthritis of the cricoarytenoid joint and laryngeal stenosis.

Leprosy and several mycotic infections have also been reported to involve the larynx. The imaging findings in all these entities are non-specific.

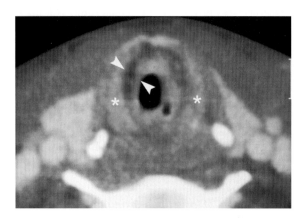

Fig. 3.5. Axial contrast-enhanced CT image. Superficially enhancing circular soft tissue thickening (*between arrowheads*) is seen in the subglottic region, significantly compromising the airway (*stars* cricoid cartilage). Rhinoscleroma

3.3.2
Non-infectious Laryngeal Inflammation

3.3.2.1
Inflammatory Pathology Secondary to Voice Abuse

Voice abuse may lead to persistent hoarseness by formation of nodules on the true vocal cords. Especially in children, this is a frequent cause of chronic hoarseness. These areas of focal inflammation and fibrosis commonly develop bilaterally, at the junction of the anterior one-third and posterior two-thirds of the true vocal cords. Solitary or multiple vocal polyps may develop secondary to voice abuse; such polyps may also be seen secondary to endotracheal intubation, typically at the level of the vocal process of the arytenoid cartilage.

Laryngoscopy reveals a characteristic nodularity of the true vocal cords in the case of vocal nodules. The vocal polyps also have a characteristic appearance. Sophisticated imaging is not necessary. Treatment is by voice rest; polyps can be removed endoscopically.

3.3.2.2
Angioneurotic Edema

In atopic individuals, irritative substances may cause laryngeal edema and hoarseness, sometimes causing obstructive symptoms. In some patients, attacks of laryngeal soft tissue swelling may be life-threatening, and occur as a response to a wide range of provocative substances, the most common of which are food agents, inhalants and drugs (such as aspirin), but cosmetics or insect bites may also cause such an attack. This condition is known as allergic angioneurotic edema. As well as this non-hereditary (allergic) type of angioneurotic edema, a hereditary type is also known.

Hereditary angioneurotic edema is a rare autosomal dominant disease caused by deficiency of the inhibitor of the first component (C1) of the complement cascade. The disease is characterized by recurrent, circumscribed, non-pruritic subepithelial swellings of sudden onset, which usually fade in 2–3 days, but can persist for up to 1 week. Lesions can be solitary or multiple and primarily involve the extremities, larynx, face, and bowel wall. The attacks are frequently induced by trauma, stress or anxiety, and may be aggravated by pregnancy and menstruation (Strome et al. 1985). The diagnosis is suggested by family history, lack of accompanying pruritus or urticaria, the presence of recurrent attacks of gastrointestinal colic, and episodes of laryngeal edema. A reduced concentration of C4 during symptomatic periods is highly suggestive of the diagnosis (Ebo and Stevens 2000).

Imaging of the larynx is usually not performed, as the clinical history and findings are indicative of the diagnosis and immediate treatment is required in the acute situation. Some patients with long-standing disease may show more chronic laryngeal symptoms, such as dysphonia, and submucosal swelling during laryngoscopy. Imaging may be requested in such patients to exclude a non-inflammatory space-occupying process. However, the deep inflammation and edema may mimic an infiltrative malignant lesion, necessitating deep tissue biopsy (Fig. 3.6).

3.3.2.3
Systemic Inflammatory Diseases with Possible Laryngeal Involvement

Rheumatoid arthritis is an inflammatory synovial proliferation with secondary bony erosions. As the cricoarytenoid joint is a synovial joint, rheumatoid arthritis is the most common cause of cricoarytenoid arthritis. Rheumatoid arthritis may also cause dysphonia by the formation of submucosal rheumatoid nodules, and in rare instances such a nodule may become large enough to also cause dysphagia (Sorensen et al. 1998). Other causes of arthritic changes to the cricoarytenoid joint include gout, lupus erythematosus, tuberculosis, syphilis and trauma (Strome et al. 1985).

Wegener's granulomatosis is a systemic disease primarily affecting the upper respiratory tract, lungs and kidneys. It is characterized by necrotizing granuloma, vasculitis and glomerulonephritis. The patients usually present with constitutional symptoms such as fever and weight loss. They may also have nasal discharge and sinusitis. Clinical examination reveals a crusted, granular mucosa, with ulceration and bone destruction. Wegener's granulomatosis may affect the larynx, causing subglottic or glottic stenosis (Fig. 3.7).

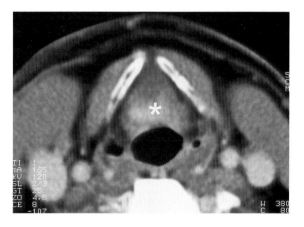

Fig. 3.6. Patient with known angioneurotic edema. Because of dysphonia and submucosal soft tissue swelling at laryngoscopy, a CT study was performed. Axial contrast-enhanced CT image at the supraglottic level shows infiltration of the preepiglottic space by enhancing tissue (*star*). Deep biopsies revealed only chronic inflammatory changes. The lesion remained more or less stable on follow-up CT studies over a 2-year period

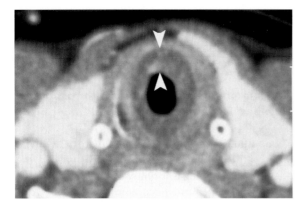

Fig. 3.7. Axial contrast-enhanced CT image of larynx in a patient with known Wegener's granulomatosis. Concentric subglottic soft tissue thickening (*between arrowheads*); note the resemblance to rhinoscleroma, shown in Fig. 3.5. (Reprinted with permission from HERMANS 2000, p 492)

Sarcoidosis is a systemic granulomatous disease of unknown cause. In the head and neck, the orbits and parotid glands are most frequently involved. Laryngeal sarcoidosis is rare. Sarcoidosis can affect the larynx as a manifestation of systemic disease or as isolated laryngeal involvement. It usually affects the supraglottis, and less commonly the subglottis; involvement of the true vocal cords is rare. Recurrent exacerbations and remissions of hoarseness is the main clinical finding in patients with laryngeal sarcoidosis; in some patients it may be associated with vague complaints and constitutional symptoms (MCLAUGHLIN et al. 1999). Sarcoidosis may present as an isolated submucosal mass, possibly mimicking malignancy, requiring deep biopsy for diagnosis. More diffuse thickening and infiltration of the laryngeal soft tissues may also be seen (Fig. 3.8).

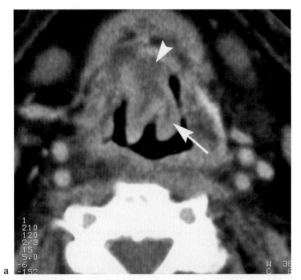

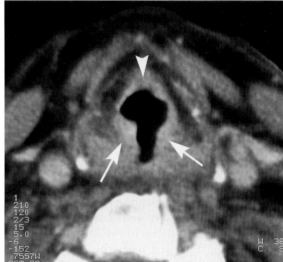

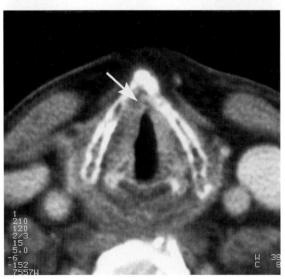

Fig. 3.8a–c. Patient with known sarcoidosis now presents with dyspnea and hoarseness. Laryngoscopically, diffuse laryngeal edema was seen. Axial contrast-enhanced CT images. **a** Thickening and superficial enhancement of the free edge of the epiglottis (*arrow*), with marked infiltration of the preepiglottic fat (*arrowhead*). **b** Slightly thickened infrahyoid epiglottis (*arrowhead*); the aryepiglottic folds (*arrows*) also appear thickened and show superficial enhancement. **c** The true vocal cords also show some increased enhancement; soft tissue thickening of the anterior commissure (*arrow*)

Lupus erythematosus is an inflammatory connective tissue disease with variable features, frequently including fever, weakness, joint pains or arthritis resembling rheumatoid arthritis, and diffuse erythematous skin lesions. Laryngeal involvement is rarely reported. As rheumatoid arthritis, it may cause arthritis of the cricoarytenoid joint or submucosal nodules.

Relapsing polychondritis is a rare inflammatory disease of cartilage of unknown origin, producing a bizarre form of arthritis. It may involve the cartilages of the ear, nose and respiratory tract. Involvement of the airway is present in about half of the patients and causes hoarseness, dyspnea, and possible airway obstruction due to edema and cartilage collapse. The imaging findings seem to be variable. Cartilage destruction as well as cartilage sclerosis, cartilage expansion and calcification have been reported (CASSELMAN et al. 1988). Laryngotracheal edema and fibrosis may also be seen (Fig. 3.9).

3.4
Benign Tumors

Benign tumors are rarely seen in the larynx compared to malignant tumors. They may originate from any of the laryngeal soft tissue components. Typically, benign laryngeal tumors grow beneath the mucosal layer. Radiologically, it may be difficult to distinguish such a submucosal lesion from a primary mucosal lesion with secondary submucosal extension. Therefore, correlation of the imaging findings

with the clinical and endoscopic findings is essential. Rarely, a squamous cell carcinoma originating from the laryngeal ventricle may present as a purely submucosal lesion, as the small mucosal component may be overlooked at endoscopy.

A submucosal laryngeal tumor may correspond to a non-squamous cell neoplasm or some kind of inflammatory lesion. Imaging is essential to determine the extent of the lesion and guide the clinician to the optimal biopsy site. Due to the submucosal localization of these lesions, an endoscopic biopsy may not be successful. In some of these cases, a percutaneous ultrasound- or CT-guided biopsy may be feasible. In some instances, a specific diagnosis can be made based on imaging findings alone.

3.4.1
Hemangioma

Hemangiomas are vascular tumors that may enlarge by rapid cellular proliferation. These ubiquitous lesions are predominantly seen in the skin, subcutaneous tissue, liver, bone, and head and neck region (GREENSPAN et al. 1992). Only a minority are deeply seated. Laryngeal and hypopharyngeal hemangiomas are very uncommon but may be of considerable clinical importance, since they may cause dysphagia, recurrent bleeding, and airway obstruction.

Histologically, they can be subclassified into capillary, cavernous, and "mixed" types. Laryngeal hemangiomas are divided clinically into pediatric and adult types. Pediatric hemangiomas account for about 10%

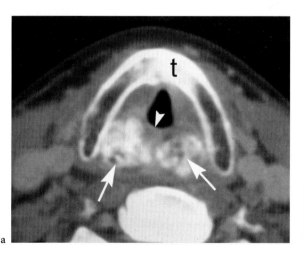
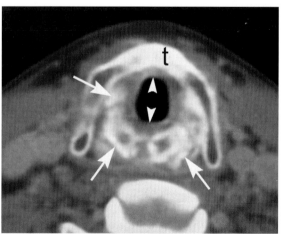

Fig. 3.9a, b. Axial contrast-enhanced CT images in a patient with relapsing polychondritis of the larynx. The thyroid cartilage (*t*) appears broadened; the arytenoid cartilages are expanded and irregularly calcified (**a** *arrows*). In the cricoid cartilage similar areas of sclerosis and irregular calcification are apparent (**b** *arrows*). The airway is also narrowed by concentric soft tissue thickening (*arrowheads*)

of all laryngeal hemangiomas, are more common in girls than in boys and are usually described as subglottic mucosa-covered masses (BECKER et al. 1998) (see also Chap. 4 on pediatric laryngeal pathology). Symptomatic laryngeal hemangioma in adults causes symptoms either by enlargement of a previously a-symptomatic lesion present since infancy, or by formation of a hemangioma de novo in adult life. In contrast to pediatric hemangiomas, the adult type presents as a glottic or more frequently as a supraglottic mass. Men are affected more often than women.

While diagnosis is often possible on a clinical basis, especially with more superficially localized lesions, deep lesions may cause diagnostic problems. Further evaluation, including cross-sectional imaging, is useful for diagnosis and adequate planning of therapy. The appearance on CT is variable; usually a well-demarcated soft tissue mass is seen. Laryngeal hemangiomas usually show strong enhancement after administration of contrast material (BECKER et al. 1998), but less pronounced enhancement or a relatively mottled low-density pattern is also possible if a mixture of several tissue elements is present (Fig. 3.10) (GREENSPAN et al. 1992) (see also Fig. 5.20).

On MRI, a high signal intensity mass is often seen in T2-weighted images, but this finding is not specific for hemangiomas. In T1-weighted images they usually have a low to intermediate signal intensity. They may appear inhomogeneous, both in T1- and T2-weighted images, secondary to areas of fibrosis, fat, thrombosis or calcification within the tumor. After administration of gadolinium, a hemangioma usually shows strong enhancement (GREENSPAN et al. 1992; KAPLAN and WILLIAMS 1987). The differential diagnosis of strongly enhancing laryngeal lesions on CT and MRI includes glomus tumor (paraganglioma) and metastasis of a hypervascular primary tumor, such as renal adenocarcinoma; both entities are very rarely seen in the larynx (BECKER et al. 1998).

Numerous management schemes for laryngeal hemangioma have been described, including superselective embolization, laser therapy, and surgical excision.

3.4.2
Lipoma

Lipomas are a benign neoplasm of adipose tissue, consisting of mature fat cells. Laryngeal lipomas are uncommon lesions; most often they are found in the supraglottis. Symptoms may be hoarseness, feeling of a lump in the throat, or dysphagia. Pedunculated tumors may produce acute respiratory distress secondary to airway obstruction.

Endoscopically, a submucosal mass is seen. CT and MRI allow the lesion to be characterized. On CT, a homogeneous non-enhancing soft tissue mass

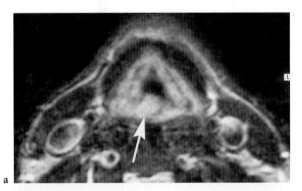
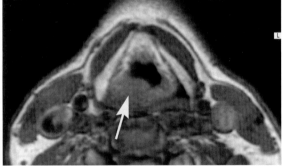
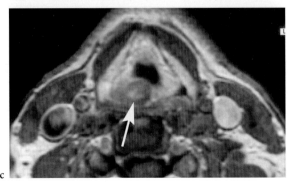

Fig. 3.10a, b. Patient with hemangioma of the right aryepiglottic fold. The lesion (*arrow*) appears relatively hyperintense to muscle on the axial T2-weighted spin echo image (**a**), and isointense on the T1-weighted image (**b**). After injection of gadolinium, moderate to strong enhancement of the lesion is seen (**c**). (Courtesy of M. LEMMERLING, MD, PhD, Gent, Belgium)

with very low density, consistent with fat, is observed (ZBÄREN et al. 1995). On MRI the mass is isointense relative to subcutaneous fat tissue (high signal intensity on T1-weighted images and, depending on the type of sequence used, intermediate to high signal intensity on T2-weighted images). The lesions are usually well encapsulated, but intramuscular and infiltrating laryngeal lipomas have been reported (CHEN and WEINBERG 1984). If a portion of the laryngeal lipoma is isodense or isointense relative to soft tissue, and/or contrast enhancement is seen, the possibility of a liposarcoma should be considered (BECKER et al. 1998).

3.4.3
Neurogenic Tumors

Neurogenic tumors are rarely encountered in the larynx; two cases were found in a series of 1884 laryngeal tumors (BECKER et al. 1998).

Up to 1993, 45 cases of laryngeal neurofibroma have been reported (MARTIN et al. 1995). Patients with neurofibromatosis type I may develop plexiform neurofibromas in the larynx. Plexiform neurofibromas have infiltrating margins, insinuating themselves into adjacent tissue planes, making such lesions difficult to remove completely. On imaging, they appear with indistinct margins, and they may surround and constrict the laryngeal airway. Neurofibromas typically show marked T2 prolongation and variable T1 shortening (MARTIN et al. 1995) on MR studies.

A number of cases of laryngeal schwannoma have been reported. In contrast to plexiform neurofibromas, schwannomas are well-delineated encapsulated tumors. The false vocal cords and the aryepiglottic folds are the most common sites in the larynx to be involved by plexiform neurofibromas and schwannomas since both entities have the tendency to arise from the superior laryngeal nerve and significantly less commonly from the recurrent laryngeal nerve (INGELS et al. 1996; PLANTET et al. 1995).

Laryngeal schwannomas impinge upon the aerodigestive tract, and may cause dysphonia, dysphagia and later also dyspnea. Complete surgical resection is necessary. On CT studies, they may show an unusual appearance, consisting of a denser enhancing inner part (correlating to Antoni A areas containing large vessels) and a lower attenuating outer part (correlating to Antoni B areas, containing fewer cells and a loose myxoid matrix). The MR characteristics may also reflect such tumor inhomogeneity (PLANTET et al. 1995) (Fig. 3.11).

3.4.4
Rhabdomyoma

Rhabdomyomas are benign neoplasms with skeletal muscle differentiation. Rhabdomyomas are considerably less common than rhabdomyosarcomas, representing less than 2% of all striated muscle tumors (VERMEERSCH et al. 2000). They are most commonly seen in the heart. Cardiac rhabdomyomas are regarded as hamartomatous lesions, and are associated with tuberous sclerosis in about 50% of cases.

About 70% of the extracardiac rhabdomyomas occur in the head and neck region. Rhabdomyomas can be classified into an adult type, with a predilection for the oral cavity, pharynx and larynx, and a fetal type predominantly seen in children under the age of 4 years, also mainly affecting the head and neck region. Usually, the lesion is solitary, but multifocal disease occurs in about 20% (HELMBERGER et al. 1996b; VERMEERSCH et al. 2000; ZBÄREN et al. 1995). Laryngeal rhabdomyomas present as submucosal, sometimes polypoid masses, causing hoarseness as the main symptom. On imaging studies, rhabdomyomas appear as well-described, more or less homogeneous soft tissue masses (Fig. 3.12). The treatment of choice is complete surgical excision.

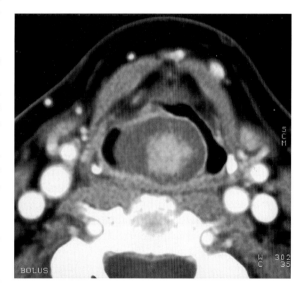

Fig. 3.11. Axial contrast-enhanced CT scan of the supraglottis. Well-delineated exophytic tumor with a low attenuating periphery and enhancing inner part, originating from the right aryepiglottic fold. Schwannoma. (Reprinted from European Journal of Radiology, vol 21, Plantet M-M, Hagay C, De Maulmont C, et al., Laryngeal schwannomas, pp 61–66, copyright 1995, with permission from Elsevier Science)

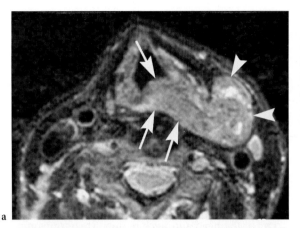

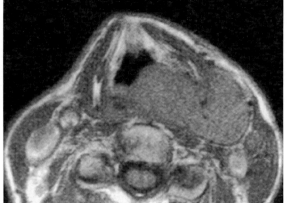

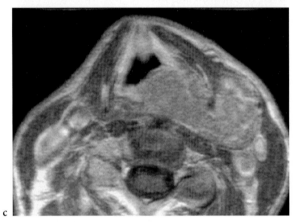

Fig. 3.12a–c. Patient with rabdomyoma originating from the left aryepiglottic fold and pharyngeal wall (*arrows*). A large, sharply demarcated hour-glass shaped lesion is filling up the left piriform sinus and extending through the lateral pharyngeal wall into the soft tissues of the neck (*arrowheads*). The lesion appears relatively hyperintense on the axial T2-weighted spin echo image (**a**), isointense on the T1-weighted image (**b**), and shows overall moderate enhancement after administration of gadolinium (**c**). (Courtesy of M. LEMMERLING, MD, PhD, Gent, Belgium)

3.4.5
Paraganglioma

Paragangliomas or glomus tumors are neoplasms arising from chemoreceptor tissue (glomus formations). Most of the neoplasms of the chemoreceptor system are found in the head and neck. They are classified according to their site of origin as carotid body, glomus jugulare, glomus vagale, or glomus tympanicum tumors. Carotid body tumors are the most frequent. Paragangliomas can occur sporadically or be familial (inherited as an autosomal dominant disease). They can be multicentric, which is more frequently seen in familial cases. Virtually all head and neck paragangliomas are non-secretory (non-chromaffin).

Paragangliomas at locations in the head and neck other than those mentioned above are very rare. They may be encountered in the larynx, associated with the superior (in the anterior aspect of the false vocal cords) and inferior laryngeal paraganglia (in the subglottis) (PETERSEN et al. 1997).

Laryngeal paragangliomas occur more frequently in women, mainly in the fourth to sixth decade, pre-

dominantly in the supraglottis (FERLITO et al. 1994). They often present with hoarseness. Other symptoms include dysphagia or dyspnea, or less commonly hemoptysis and airway obstruction. The presence of throat pain may indicate malignancy (KONOWITZ et al. 1988). Endoscopically, a reddish mass is seen.

These tumors are hypervascular, as can be appreciated on CT and MRI studies. They show significant contrast enhancement, and commonly (but not invariably) intratumoral signal voids on MRI, corresponding to high flow in vessels (Fig. 3.13). Such imaging findings should alert the clinician to the highly vascular nature of these tumors.

Significant bleeding may occur at the time of endoscopic biopsy. Recently, a flow diagram for the diagnosis of vascular laryngeal tumors, exclusive of biopsy, has been proposed. If contrast-enhanced CT or MRI shows enhancement of the lesion, a four-vessel angiogram is proposed. If this study shows a major feeding vessel (usually the superior or inferior thyroid artery), profuse tumor blush and possibly other synchronous lesion(s), the diagnosis of paraganglioma is likely. If the arteriogram does not show such features, one must consider the diagnosis of a neu-

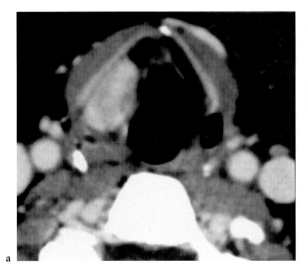
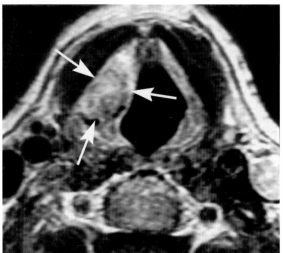

a   b

Fig. 3.13a, b. Patient presenting with hoarseness. **a** Axial contrast-enhanced CT image demonstrates a strongly enhancing mass in the right paraglottic space. **b** Gadolinium-enhanced T1-weighted spin echo image. The soft tissue mass (*arrows*) shows pronounced and inhomogeneous enhancement. Paraganglioma. (Courtesy of R. MAROLDI, MD, Brescia, Italy)

roendocrine carcinoma, an uncommon but more aggressive lesion, requiring radical treatment. Microscopically, neuroendocrine carcinoma may mimic paraganglioma; immunohistochemical and electron microscopic techniques are required for differentiation (SANDERS et al. 2001).

Conservative surgery is the treatment of choice in laryngeal paraganglioma. Preoperative embolization may be considered. Endoscopic resection is not recommended because of the risk of uncontrollable bleeding and of incomplete resection with possible recurrence.

The biologic behavior of laryngeal paragangliomas is benign. Only very rarely may a glomus tumor show a malignant growth pattern with infiltration of surrounding tissues. Such infiltrative behavior is more often seen in carotid body tumors than in those at other locations. Metastatic deposits are even less commonly encountered. In a review of 62 cases of laryngeal paraganglioma, only one possible case of malignant behavior was encountered, a patient who developed a spinal metastasis many years after the initial diagnosis (FERLITO et al. 1994).

3.4.6
Chondroma

Cartilaginous tumors of the larynx account for less than 1% of all laryngeal tumors. Both chondroma and chondrosarcoma are encountered in the larynx, with 70% arising from the cricoid cartilage, with the thyroid cartilage being the next most common site of origin.

Chondromas occur at any age, although they are seen more commonly in adults. They may be asymptomatic, or present with hoarseness, dyspnea or dysphagia. At presentation, a laryngeal chondroma is usually less than 2 to 3 cm in diameter. On pathologic examination, a lobular growth pattern with low cellularity is seen; nuclear atypia and mitoses are not encountered (DEVANEY et al. 1995).

True chondromas of the larynx are probably very rare. It is difficult to firmly establish the diagnosis of benign laryngeal chondroma on a small amount of tissue obtained by biopsy. Low-grade chondrosarcoma may also show a lobular growth pattern. Compared to chondroma, low-grade chondrosarcoma may display only minimally increased cellularity and nuclear atypia, a pattern overlapping with benign chondromas. There is also no appreciable degree of mitotic activity in such lesions (DEVANEY et al. 1995).

On CT studies, cartilaginous tumors of the larynx appear as hypodense, well-circumscribed masses centered within the laryngeal cartilage, with coarse or stippled calcification within the lesion (WANG et al. 1999) (Fig. 3.14). The imaging findings do not allow differentiation of a benign from a malignant chondroid tumor, although in high-grade chondrosarcomas nodal metastasis in the head and neck may rarely be seen. MRI is less specific for diagnosing such a lesion as it does not depict the intratumoral calcifications as well as CT.

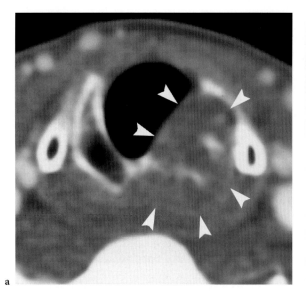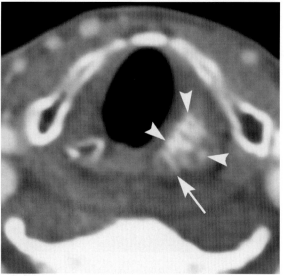

a   b

Fig. 3.14. Axial contrast-enhanced CT images show an expansile, relatively low-density lesion in the left cricoid arch (**a** *arrowheads*); the lesion contains some calcifications. The intratumoral calcifications (**b** *arrowheads*) reveal extension to the level of the true vocal cord and posterior displacement of the arytenoid cartilage (*arrow*). Chondrosarcoma

Surgery is the only curative modality in laryngeal cartilaginous tumors. Low-grade chondrosarcomas may locally recur if incompletely resected, but have only limited risk of metastatic disease. Therefore, in all laryngeal cartilaginous tumors a conservative approach is followed whenever possible, directed towards voice-sparing partial laryngectomy. However, total laryngectomy may be the appropriate treatment in lesions involving larger portions of the cricoid cartilage, interfering with surgical reconstruction of a functional larynx, or when the diagnosis of high-grade chondrosarcoma is established (DEVANEY et al. 1995; WANG et al. 1999).

3.5
Non-tumoral Expansile Lesions

3.5.1
Laryngocele

Laryngoceles are formed by dilatation of the saccule of the laryngeal ventricle. On becoming larger, laryngoceles extend from the level of the laryngeal ventricle superiorly into the paraglottic space.

Laryngoceles may be filled by air or fluid. An air-filled laryngocele occurs when the orifice of the laryngeal ventricle is patent, but functionally obstructed, such as seen in players of a wind-instrument. A fluid-filled laryngocele (also called a saccular cyst) occurs

when the opening of the ventricle is obstructed. Obstruction of the ventricular orifice may be caused by a tumor, inflammation, or scar tissue from previous trauma. In most cases laryngoceles are not caused by an obstructing mass, but an underlying neoplasm has to be excluded, both clinically and radiologically.

On cross-sectional imaging studies, laryngoceles appear as non-enhancing sharply demarcated submucosal laryngeal masses, with air or fluid density/intensity. When limited to the paraglottic space, a laryngocele is called an internal laryngocele (Fig. 3.15), and when extending through the

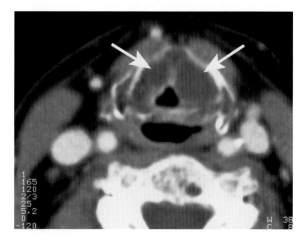

Fig. 3.15. Axial contrast-enhanced CT image through supraglottic larynx. Bilateral fluid-filled internal laryngoceles (*arrows*). (Reprinted with permission from HERMANS 2000, p 403)

thyrohyoid membrane, it is called a mixed laryngocele (consisting of an internal and external part in relation to the laryngeal framework) (Fig. 3.16).

Many small laryngoceles are asymptomatic. An internal laryngocele may cause hoarseness or stridor. An external laryngocele may also present as a mass in the submandibular region. Symptomatic laryngoceles represent about 25% of the entirely submucosally located laryngeal masses (HELMBERGER et al. 1996a). An infected laryngocele, filled with pus, is called a pyolaryngocele. Superinfection may cause respiratory distress and pain. Compared

to a non-infected laryngocele, it additionally shows a thickened and enhancing wall on cross-sectional imaging (Fig. 3.17).

The typical imaging features of a laryngocele allow differentiation from other submucosal laryngeal lesions. Retention cysts, arising from (sub)mucosal glands, may sometimes mimic the appearance of a laryngocele (Fig. 3.18). Very rarely, a deep-seated necrotic tumor may cause diagnostic confusion (Fig. 3.19). In children, a congenital laryngeal cyst may resemble a laryngocele on imaging studies.

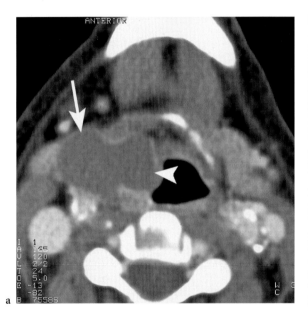

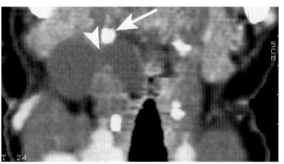

Fig. 3.16. Axial contrast-enhanced CT images through supraglottic larynx (**a**) shows a fluid-filled mixed laryngocele with an intralaryngeal (*arrowhead*) and an extralaryngeal component (*arrow*). A coronal reconstruction (**b**) shows the laryngocele to extend outside the larynx just below the hyoid bone (*arrow*). The waist of the laryngocele (*arrowhead*) is at the thyrohyoid membrane. In this patient the thyroid cartilage is only ossified in its lower aspect. (Reprinted with permission from HERMANS 2000, p 403)

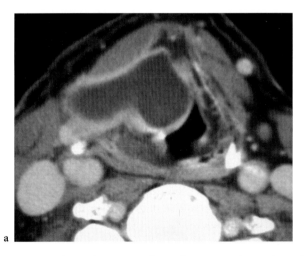

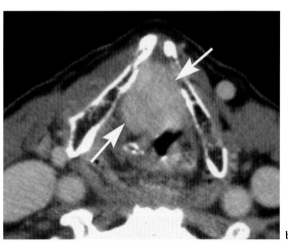

Fig. 3.17a, b. Axial contrast-enhanced CT images in a patient with a history of hoarseness, respiratory distress and dysphagia. **a** Laryngocele with a fairly thick enhancing wall is seen to extend through the thyrohyoid membrane into the neck. **b** Image obtained about 1 cm lower shows an additional contrast enhanced soft tissue mass (*arrows*) obstructing the laryngeal ventricle. Pathologic examination revealed submucosal leiomyosarcoma with secondary pyolaryngocele

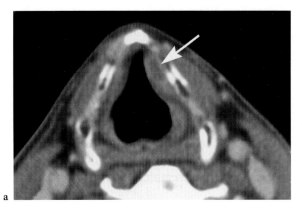 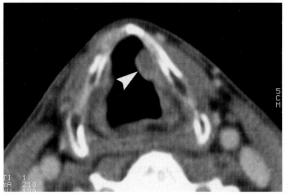

a   b

Fig. 3.18. Axial contrast-enhanced CT-images in a patient with hoarseness and a submucosal swelling in the region of the left false vocal cord and sinus of Morgagni. A small hypodense lesion, showing a faintly enhancing wall, is seen in the left paraglottic space at the level of the false vocal cord (**a**, arrow); it is a bit anterior to the expected location of the laryngeal ventricle. A few millimeters lower, it is seen to bulge in the laryngeal lumen (**b**, arrowhead). During endoscopy, a cystic lesion containing a gelatinous material was removed; pathologic study revealed a retention cyst

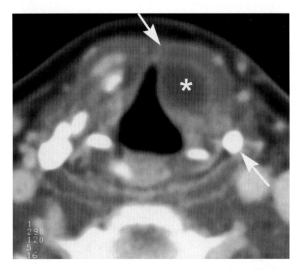

Fig. 3.19. Axial contrast-enhanced CT image demonstrates a submucosal low-density mass (*star*) which initially appears to be centered in the left paraglottic space, but closer inspection reveals that it is actually centered in the partly ossified left lamina of the thyroid cartilage (location indicated by opposing arrows). Necrotic chondrosarcoma

3.5.2
Amyloidosis

Amyloidosis is a disease complex defined by the presence of extracellular deposition of insoluble fibrillary protein material (SCOTT et al. 1986). Amyloidosis is classified according to its clinical and immunocytochemical features. Clinically, amyloidosis is categorized as systemic (80–90%) and localized (10–20%) amyloidosis. Systemic amyloidosis is a serious and usually fatal condition in which accumula-

tion of amyloid fibrils in tissues destroys normal organ structure and function.

The localized form frequently involves the head and neck region (GEAN-MARTON et al. 1991). Another potential site of the localized form is the endocrine system, associated with medullary carcinoma of the thyroid, and the heart and brain in senile amyloidosis (SCOTT et al. 1986). In head and neck amyloidosis, amyloid fibrils are of the AL-type and thus immunocyte-derived. It is suggested that amyloid is formed in loco by excessive precursor light chains produced by plasma cells within foci of the disease (BARNES and ZAFAR 1977). The larynx is affected most frequently (61%), followed by the oropharynx (23%), trachea (9%), orbit (4%) and nasopharynx (3%).

Laryngeal amyloidosis accounts for less than 1% of all benign "tumors" of the larynx. Peak incidence is between 40 and 60 years and men are more often affected than women. The most common sites of involvement are the true vocal cords, followed by the false vocal cords, aryepiglottic folds and subglottic area. Other sites frequently affected together with laryngeal involvement are the trachea, bronchi and tongue in descending frequency.

In laryngeal amyloidosis, the patients usually complain of hoarseness and dyspnea. Although amyloid deposits are submucosal, mucosal ulcerations have been reported due to pressure atrophy of subadjacent amyloid.

An extensive work-up is advised in cases of suspected focal amyloidosis in order to rule out systemic amyloidosis. A fine needle aspiration of abdominal fat or a rectal biopsy are well-established methods for identifying generalized amyloidosis.

On CT, the lesions usually appear as relatively well-defined homogeneous submucosal masses of soft tissue density (DE FOER et al. 1993; MARSOT-DUPUCH et al. 1987). There is no evidence of bone destruction or associated lymphadenopathy. Amyloidosis may also appear as more diffuse intralaryngeal soft tissue infiltration, or a circumferential glottic and/or subglottic soft tissue thickening, possibly associated with a deeper submucosal component (Fig. 3.20). Intralesional calcifications may be seen. A calcified amyloidoma arising from the epiglottis, suggesting the diagnosis of a cartilaginous tumor, has been described (RODRIGUEZ-ROMERO et al. 1996). Enhancement after intravenous administration of contrast is variable. On MRI, contrast enhancement is reported. In T2-weighted images the lesion may appear relatively hypointense (DE FOER et al. 1993), but increased signal intensity has also been observed (ARSLAN et al. 1998) (Fig. 3.21).

Treatment of focal laryngeal amyloidosis consists of surgical resection or endoscopic laser resection (TALBOT 1990).

3.6
Traumatic Pathology

3.6.1
Acute Laryngeal Trauma

Acute laryngeal trauma is rare. By nature, the larynx is relatively protected posteriorly by the cervical spine, superiorly by the mandible and inferiorly by the sternum. In addition, the flexible musculotendinous suspension allows deflection (except backwards) of the larynx, minimizing the impact of an external trauma. On the other hand, laryngeal injury represents a serious threat to critical physiologic functions and may lead to severe long-term complications or even death (ELIACHAR 1996).

The possible etiologies of acute laryngeal injury are very diverse. They may be classified according to the mode of trauma (external or internal, blunt or penetrating, chemical or radiation injuries, burns and smoke inhalation, foreign bodies, and combinations of these), or to the level of injury (supraglottic, glottic, subglottic, hypopharyngeal, or combinations of these).

Most commonly laryngeal trauma is of iatrogenic origin. The larynx is vulnerable to all procedures requiring airway protection, such as endotracheal intubation for elective procedures, emergency intubation, tracheostomy or cricothyroidotomy. Rarely laryngeal injury originates from a complicated endoscopic examination. External laryngeal trauma is less common, and most often seen in motor vehicle accidents. A suicide attempt by hanging is a rare cause (POUQUET et al. 1995). In demographic areas with a high incidence of personal assault, penetrating laryngeal injuries by knife or gunshot wounds may be more often encountered.

Laryngeal injuries present with a variety of symptoms such as respiratory distress, stridor, coughing, hoarseness, pain and tenderness, dysphagia, subcutaneous hematoma and emphysema (ELIACHAR 1996). These signs and symptoms vary depending on the type and severity of the injury, its anatomic loca-

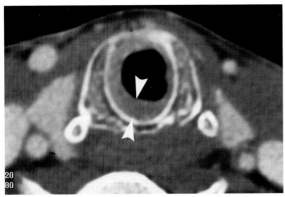 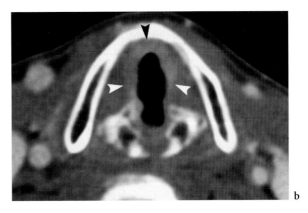

a   b

Fig. 3.20a, b. Axial contrast-enhanced CT images. **a** Circumferential soft tissue thickening (*arrowheads*) in the subglottis. Note the resemblance to rhinoscleroma (Fig. 3.5) and Wegener's granulomatosis (Fig. 3.7). The lesion also extended downwards in the proximal trachea (not shown). **b** There is also soft tissue thickening of both true vocal cords (*white arrowheads*) with involvement of the anterior commissure (*black arrowhead*). There may also be some tissue thickening of the posterior commissure. Amyloidosis

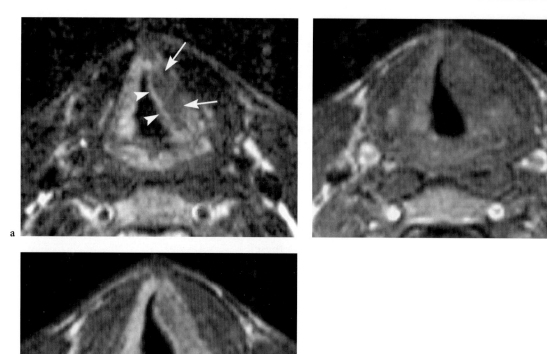

Fig. 3.21. Axial T2-weighted spin echo image at the level of the false vocal cords (**a**) shows a lesion with relatively low signal intensity within the left paraglottic space (*arrows*). The overlying hyperintense rim corresponds to the laryngeal mucosa (*arrowheads*). T1-weighted spin echo image at same level shows that the lesion is slightly hyperintense to muscle (**b**). After injection of gadolinium, moderate lesional enhancement is seen (**c**). Amyloidosis

tion and the time elapsed between the actual injury and presentation of the patient. Careful attention should be given to exclusion of other injuries, such as cervical spine fractures in motor vehicle injuries or damage to adjacent organs, including vessels, in penetrating injuries.

A classification of laryngeal trauma into four groups, ranging from minor voice and airway changes to complete airway disruption, has been proposed (SCHAEFER 1992). Some patients require immediate intervention to establish a controlled airway, such as those with obvious penetrating laryngeal wounds or cartilage fractures. Patients with a stable airway undergo indirect and/or direct laryngoscopy after initial physical examination. Mucosal tears, false passages and tracheal rupture can be identified by laryngoscopy, but extensive soft tissue swelling and injury may limit its diagnostic yield.

CT has proven its value in the evaluation of the traumatized larynx, showing fractures of the laryngeal skeleton and their displacement (Fig. 3.22), as well as outlining hematomas and soft tissue disrup-

tion (Fig. 3.23). CT is indicated in patients with laryngeal tenderness, endolaryngeal edema, or small to medium hematomas. Some authors also recommend obtaining a CT study in patients with only minimal clinical signs and symptoms, planned to be treated conservatively, to definitely rule out laryngeal skeletal injury and other simultaneous neck injuries (ELIACHAR 1996). Surgical laryngeal exploration is dependent on detection of occult cartilage fractures or dislocations, or confirmation of suspected laryngeal skeletal injuries (SCHAEFER 1991). Surgery can be avoided when CT depicts normal laryngeal cartilages or non-displaced fractures in the presence of soft tissue hematoma (SCHILD and DENNENY 1989). Adequate treatment of laryngeal trauma is necessary to avoid stenosis or aspiration, and to restore an acceptable voice quality. There are indications that open reduction and fixation of minimally displaced laryngeal fractures may improve the outcome of glottic function (SCHAEFER 1991). Delay in treatment may lead to suboptimal results.

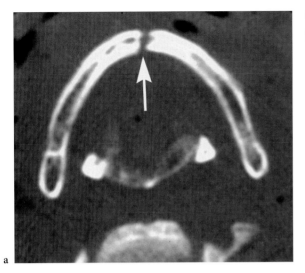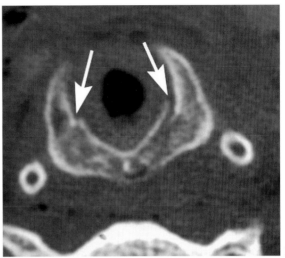

Fig. 3.22a, b. Axial CT images showing a median fracture through the thyroid cartilage (**a** *arrow*) and a bilateral fracture through the posterolateral part of the cricoid arch (**b** *arrows*)

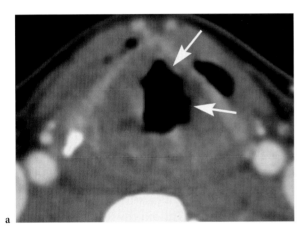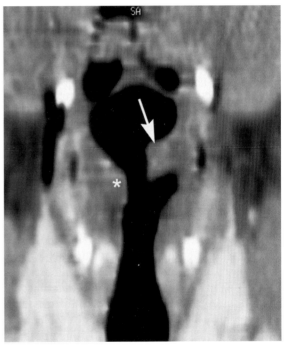

Fig. 3.23a, b. Patient with posttraumatic hoarseness. Clinically, left-sided laryngeal soft tissue laceration was seen. **a** Axial CT image at the supraglottic level, apart from prelaryngeal air emphysema and diffuse intralaryngeal soft tissue swelling, shows laceration of the left true vocal cord (*arrows* compare with opposite side). **b** The coronal reformation shows avulsion and cranial retraction of the left true vocal cord (*arrow*) (*star* right true vocal cord)

3.6.2
Chronic Laryngeal Trauma

Chronic laryngeal stenosis is often the consequence of delayed treatment of the injured larynx or inaccurate evaluation of the extent of the injury. Granulation tissue will progressively become fibrotic and retract, contributing to distortion of the deeper tissue.

Granulation and scar tissue appear on CT studies as a homogeneous soft tissue density, narrowing the airway. Webs may be recognized, usually at the anterior or posterior commissures (Fig. 3.24). At the level of the subglottis, more or less circumferential soft tissue thickening may be visible. Fractures usually remain visible, as they heal by fibrosis. Abnormalities of the cricoarytenoid joint (dislocation or web at the posterior commissure) can be detected as a rea-

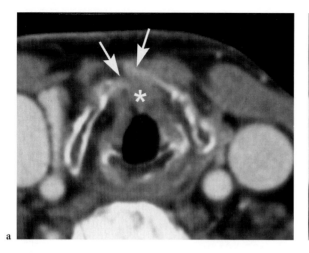
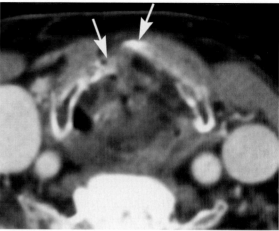

Fig. 3.24a, b. Axial CT images in a tracheostomy-dependent patient who had a laryngeal trauma more than 30 years previously. **a** Distortion of the thyroid cartilage (*arrows*). Scar tissue is seen at the level of the anterior commissure (*star*). **b** Obliteration of the laryngeal lumen at the lower supraglottis level

son for late vocal cord dysfunction (ALEXANDER et al. 1997). Deformation of the cricothyroid joint may point to injury to the recurrent nerve which passes close to the joint capsule. Injury to the cricothyroid joint itself may also result in severe voice dysfunction (SATALOFF et al. 1998).

Postintubation injury is the most frequent cause of chronic subglottic stenosis. Following intubation, tracheal injury (edema, superficial ulcerations) is almost always present initially, but typically heals without sequelae. Stenosis at the cuff-site is caused by scar formation, due to deep ulceration or pressure necrosis. CT is helpful in showing the extent of the stenosis, allowing better planning of surgical resection.

Stenosis sometimes occurs at the tip of the tube, due to granulation tissue formation. After tracheostomy, granulation tissue may project into the lumen at the level of the stoma. The anterior tracheal wall above the tracheostoma may be displaced posteriorly, resulting in suprastomal stenosis preventing successful decannulation. Under these circumstances CT can also be helpful in localizing the problem.

Conventional tomography or MRI may be indicated in chronic laryngeal trauma, if the CT study is significantly degraded by artifacts arising from the shoulders. MR with direct sagittal images has been reported to be useful in the diagnosis of unsuspected epiglottic avulsion at the level of the petiole (DUDA et al. 1996). This diagnosis is more difficult to make on axial CT images, which relies more on secondary signs such as widening of the preepiglottic space; however, sagittal reconstructions based on thin-sliced axial spiral CT images may offer a similar diagnostic accuracy.

3.7
Miscellaneous

3.7.1
Vocal Cord Immobility

Vocal cord immobility is a sign requiring a search for underlying disease. It may be caused by mechanical fixation of the vocal cord, as seen in carcinoma infiltrating the thyroarytenoid muscle, or in fixation of the cricoarytenoid joint by cancer or some other cause. It may also result from neuronal injury, and is then referred to as vocal cord paralysis.

Vocal cord paralysis is caused by palsy of the recurrent laryngeal nerve. This nerve is a branch of the vagal nerve and innervates most intrinsic muscles of the larynx. The offending lesion may be in the course of the recurrent laryngeal nerve itself (distal vagal neuropathy), or more proximal in the suprahyoid course of the vagal nerve (proximal vagal neuropathy).

Distal vagal neuropathy results in isolated endolaryngeal symptoms (hoarseness, and sometimes also aspiration). Imaging should be directed in searching for a lesion in the course of the distal vagal nerve in the carotid space, and along the course of the recurrent laryngeal nerve in the tracheoesophageal groove, extending around the subclavian artery on the right and around the aortic arch within the aortopulmonary window on the left.

At the suprahyoid level, the vagal nerve is quite close to the glossopharyngeal (IX), spinal accessory (XI) and hypoglossal (XII) nerves. Injury to the vagal nerve at this level is commonly accompanied by symptoms related to injury of these cranial nerves.

Imaging should then be directed to the proximal part of the vagal nerve, from its origin in the brain stem to the level of the hyoid bone.

The imaging features of vocal cord paralysis itself are atrophy of the thyroarytenoid muscle (the muscle of the true vocal cord), anteromedial deviation of the arytenoid cartilage, enlargement of the ipsilateral laryngeal ventricle and piriform sinus, and a paramedian position of the vocal cord. Palsy of the recurrent laryngeal nerve may also lead to atrophy of the commonly innervated posterior cricoarytenoid muscle (ROMO and CURTIN 1999) (Fig. 3.25).

Excluding primary laryngeal neoplasms, extralaryngeal malignancies are the most common cause of unilateral vocal cord immobility. About 80% of these tumors are of pulmonary or mediastinal origin and cause vocal cord paralysis by interfering with the function of the recurrent laryngeal nerve (BENNINGER et al. 1998). This explains why left vocal cord paralysis is slightly more common, as the intratho-

racic part of the left recurrent laryngeal nerve is vulnerable to neoplastic invasion by such thoracic malignancies. Less commonly, vocal cord paralysis is caused by esophageal, metastatic or thyroid neoplasms. Invasion of the recurrent laryngeal nerve by adenoid cystic carcinoma originating from the subglottic region or trachea may be encountered.

Rarely, vocal cord paralysis is due to benign disease in or extending to the tracheoesophageal groove. It has been reported to be caused by multinodular goiter (ABBOUD et al. 1999; COLLAZO-CLAVELL et al. 1995), thyroid abscess (BOYD et al. 1997) and parathyroid cyst (SEN et al. 2000).

Iatrogenic causes for vocal cord immobility appear to be increasing (BENNINGER et al. 1998). Procedures such as the anterior approach to cervical spine disease and carotid endarterectomy may be complicated by vocal cord paralysis. Thyroid surgery and esophageal cancer surgery are a relatively common cause of both uni- and bilateral vocal cord paralysis.

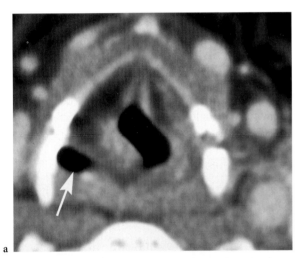

a

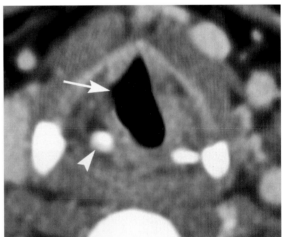

b

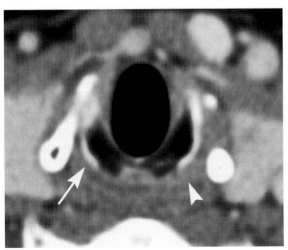

c

Fig. 3.25a–c. Axial contrast-enhanced CT images through the larynx in a patient with right-sided vocal cord paralysis. Relative dilatation of the ipsilateral pyriform sinus (a *arrow*) and ipsilateral laryngeal ventricle (b *arrow*) are seen. The right arytenoid cartilage is slightly anteromedially displaced (b *arrowhead*). c Atrophy of the right posterior cricoarytenoid muscle (*arrow*); compare with normal left posterior cricoarytenoid muscle (*arrowhead*)

Prolonged intubation may cause vocal cord immobility, either by compression injury to the recurrent laryngeal nerve or fixation or disruption of the cricoarytenoid joint.

In a number of patients, no definite explanation for the vocal cord paralysis can be found after thorough examination. These patients with idiopathic vocal cord paralysis typically show spontaneous recovery (BENNINGER et al. 1998).

As treatment of vocal cord paralysis, foreign material may be injected into the paralyzed cord to medialize it. In this way, better glottic closure can be obtained during speech, reducing dysphonia. Some of these materials (such as Teflon) are radiopaque. An alternative treatment is placement of a plastic or Silastic prosthesis beside the paralyzed vocal cord through a window cut in the adjacent thyroid cartilage; such a prosthesis may be visible on CT study (WITTERICK et al. 2000) (Fig. 3.26).

3.7.2
Laryngeal Framework Deformity

The laryngeal cartilages seldom appear perfectly symmetric. On cross-sectional studies, minor asymmetries, particularly in the thyroid cartilage, are often noted. Rarely, such cartilage asymmetry may be quite important and be associated with functional disturbance, such as hoarseness or dysphonia, or even dysphagia. Laryngoscopy shows bulging of the laryngeal soft tissue, mimicking a submucosal tumor. CT (or MRI) excludes the presence of a tumor but reveals bowing of the left thyroid lamina towards the laryngeal lumen, in association with some deformity of the underlying soft tissues (HANSON et al. 1982) (Fig. 3.27). In a number of such cases, some asymmetry in the position of the arytenoid cartilages and cricoid cartilage has also been described (PIEKARSKI et al. 1993).

The pathogenesis of this deformation is unknown. Traumatic etiology has been suggested but is unlikely, as this deformation for some unknown reason always involves the left side of the larynx, and in many cases the patient does not recall a previous trauma to the larynx (PIEKARSKI et al. 1993).

3.7.3
Premalignant Mucosal Lesions

Squamous cell carcinomas can be preceded by a premalignant state, in which the epithelial cells lose their normal appearance and resemble malignant cells; however, infiltration of surrounding tissues is lacking (infiltration or invasion occurs when the basal membrane of the epithelium is disrupted). Clinically, premalignant disease can manifest itself

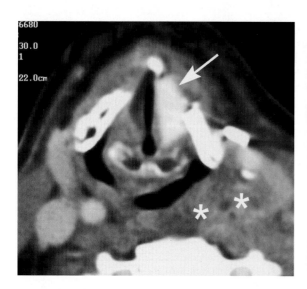

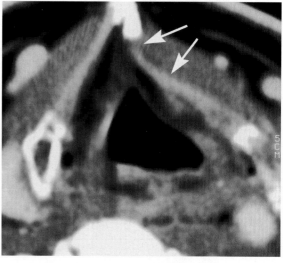

Fig. 3.26. Patient with left-sided vocal cord paralysis caused by anaplastic thyroid cancer. After radiation treatment, a prosthesis (*arrow*) was inserted submucosally, medializing the left vocal cord and correcting dysphonia. Recurrent tumor (*stars*) later developed in the left neck

Fig. 3.27. Axial CT image at the supraglottic level in a patient presenting with hoarseness. The clinical examination suggested a left-sided submucosal lesion. The CT study shows asymmetric appearance of the thyroid cartilage with an inward depression of the left thyroid lamina (*arrows*) but no submucosal lesion

as leukoplakia or erythroplakia, a white to red mucosal lesion.

If performed, the results of cross-sectional imaging studies are usually negative. In some cases slight superficial irregularities and mucosal enhancement may be seen, but differentiation from inflammation or an early invasive cancer is not possible.

References

Abboud B, Tabchy B, Jambart S, et al (1999) Benign disease of the thyroid gland and vocal cord paralysis. J Laryngol Otol 113:473–474

Abou-Seif SG, Baky FA, el-Ebrashy F, et al (1991) Scleroma of the upper respiratory passages: a CT study. J Laryngol Otol 105:198–202

Alexander AE, Lyons GD, Fazekas-May MA, et al (1997) Utility of helical computed tomography in the study of arytenoid dislocation and arytenoid subluxation. Ann Otol Rhinol Laryngol 106:1020–1023

Arslan A, Ceylan N, Cetin A, et al (1998) Laryngeal amyloidosis with laryngocele: MRI and CT. Neuroradiology 40:401–403

Barnes EL, Zafar T (1977) Laryngeal amyloidosis. Ann Otol 86:856–863

Becker M, Moulin G, Kurt A-M, et al (1998) Non-squamous cell neoplasms of the larynx: radiologic-pathologic correlations. Radiographics 18:1189–1209

Benninger MS, Gillen JB, Altman JS (1998) Changing etiology of vocal fold immobility. Laryngoscope 108:1346–1350

Boyd CM, Esclamado RM, Telian SA (1997) Impaired vocal cord mobility in the setting of acute suppurative thyroiditis. Head Neck 19:235–237

Branstetter BF, Weissman JL, Kennedy TL, et al (2000) The CT appearance of thyroglossal duct carcinoma. AJNR Am J Neuroradiol 21:1547–1550

Casselman JW, Lemahieu SF, Peene P, et al (1988) Polychondritis affecting the laryngeal cartilages: CT findings. AJR Am J Roentgenol 150:355–356

Chen KTK, Weinberg RA (1984) Intramuscular lipoma of the larynx. Am J Otolaryngol 5:71–72

Collazo-Clavell ML, Gharib H, Maragos NE (1995) Relationship between vocal cord paralysis and benign thyroid disease. Head Neck 17:24–30

De Foer B, Hermans R, Feenstra L, et al (1993) CT and MRI of laryngeal amyloidosis. Rofo Fortschr Geb Rontgenstr Neuen Bildgeb Verfahr 159:492–494

Devaney KO, Ferlito A, Silver CE (1995) Cartilaginous tumors of the larynx. Ann Otol Rhinol Laryngol 104:251–255

Duda JJ Jr, Lewin JS, Eliachar I (1996) MR evaluation of epiglottic disruption. AJNR Am J Neuroradiol 17:563–566

Ebo DG, Stevens WJ (2000) Hereditary angioneurotic edema: review of the literature. Acta Clin Belg 55:22–29

Eliachar I (1996) Management of acute laryngeal trauma. Acta Otol Rhinol Laryngol Belg 50:151–158

Ferlito A, Barnes L, Wenig BM (1994) Identification, classification, treatment, and prognosis of laryngeal paraganglioma. Ann Otol Rhinol Laryngol 103:525–536

Gean-Marton AD, Kirsch CFE, Vezina LG, et al (1991) Focal amyloidosis of the head and neck: evaluation with CT and MR imaging. Radiology 181:521–525

Greenspan A, McGahan JP, Vogelsang P, et al (1992) Imaging strategies in the evaluation of soft-tissue hemangiomas of the extremities: correlation of the findings of plain radiography, angiography, CT, MRI, and ultrasonography in 12 histologically proven cases. Skeletal Radiol 21:11–18

Hanson DG, Mancuso AA, Hanafee WN (1982) Pseudomass lesions due to occult trauma of the larynx. Laryngoscope 92:1249–1253

Helmberger RC, Croker BP, Mancuso AA (1996a) Leiomyosarcoma of the larynx presenting as a laryngopyocele. AJNR Am J Neuroradiol 17:1112–1114

Helmberger RC, Stringer SP, Mancuso AA (1996b) Rhabdomyosarcoma of the pharyngeal musculature extending into the prestyloid parapharyngeal space. AJNR Am J Neuroradiol 17:1115–1118

Hermans R (2000) Head and neck imaging. In: Pettersson H, Allison D (eds) The encyclopedia of medical imaging, part VI. NICER Institute, Oslo

Houghton DJ, Bennett JD, Rapado F, et al (1997) Laryngeal tuberculosis: an unsuspected danger. Br J Clin Pract 51:61–62

Ingels K, Vermeersch H, Verhoye C, et al (1996) Schwannoma of the larynx: a case report. J Laryngol Otol 110:294–296

Kaplan PA, Williams SM (1987) Mucocutaneous and peripheral soft-tissue hemangiomas: MR imaging. Radiology 163:163–166

Kennedy TL, Whitaker M, Wadih G (1998) Thyroglossal duct carcinoma: a rational approach to management. Laryngoscope 108:1154–1158

Konowitz PM, Lawson W, Som PM, et al (1988) Laryngeal paraganglioma: update on diagnosis and treatment. Laryngoscope 98:40–49

Marsot-Dupuch K, Tubiana JM, Chabolle F, et al (1987) L'amylose laryngée et trachéo-bronchique, cause rare de dyspnée. Ann Radiol 30:347–352

Martin DS, Stith J, Awwad EE, et al (1995) MR in neurofibromatosis of the larynx. AJNR Am J Neuroradiol 16:503–506

McLaughlin RB, Spiegel JR, Selber J, et al (1999) Laryngeal sarcoidosis presenting as an isolated submucosal vocal fold mass. J Voice 13:240–245

Moon WK, Han MH, Chang KH, et al (1996) Laryngeal tuberculosis: CT findings. AJR Am J Roentgenol 166:445–449

Moon WK, Han MH, Chang KH, et al (1997) CT and MR imaging of head and neck tuberculosis. Radiographics 17:391–402

Peterson KL, Fu Y-S, Calcaterra T (1997) Subglottic paraganglioma. Head Neck 19:54–56

Piekarski J-D, Bounatiro Y, Heran F, et al (1993) Les asymétries des cartilages larynges: un problème diagnostique malconnu. Radiol J CEPUR 13:44–47

Plantet M-M, Hagay C, De Maulmont C, et al (1995) Laryngeal schwannomas. Eur J Radiol 21:61–66

Pouquet E, Dibiane A, Jourdain C, et al (1995) Traumatisme fermé du larynx par pendaison. J Radiol 76:107–109

Rodriguez-Romero R, Vargas-Serrano B, Cortina-Moreno B, et al (1996) Calcified amyloidoma of the larynx. AJNR Am J Neuroradiol 17:1491–1493

Romo LV, Curtin HD (1999) Atrophy of the posterior cricoarytenoid muscle as an indicator of recurrent laryngeal nerve palsy. AJNR Am J Neuroradiol 20:467–471

Sanders KW, Abrea F, Rivera E, et al (2001) A diagnostic and therapeutic approach to paragangliomas of the larynx. Arch Otolaryngol Head Neck Surg 127:565–569

Sataloff RT, Rao VM, Hawkshaw M, et al (1998) Cricothyroid joint injury. J Voice 12:112–116

Schaefer SD (1991) Use of CT scanning in the management of the acutely injured larynx. Otolaryngol Clin North Am 24:31–36

Schaefer SD (1992) The acute management of external laryngeal trauma. Arch Otolaryngol Head Neck Surg 118:598–604

Schild JA, Denneny EC (1989) Evaluation and treatment of acute laryngeal fractures. Head Neck 11:491–496

Scott PP, Scott WW, Siegelmann SS (1986) Amyloidosis, an overview. Semin Roentgenol 21:103–112

Sen P, Flower N, Papesch M, et al (2000) A benign parathyroid cyst presenting with hoarse voice. J Laryngol Otol 144:147–148

Sorensen WT, Moller-Andersen K, Behrendt N (1998) Rheumatoid nodules of the larynx. J Laryngol Otol 112:573–574

Strome M, Kelly JH, Fried MP (1985) Manual of otolaryngology. Little Brown, Boston, pp 17–18

Talbot AR (1990) Laryngeal amyloidosis. J Laryngol Otol 104:147–149

Vermeersch H, van Vugt P, Lemmerling M, et al (2000) Bilateral recurrent adult rhabdomyomas of the pharyngeal wall. Eur Arch Otorhinolaryngol 257:24–26

Wang SJ, Borges A, Lufkin RB, et al (1999) Chondroid tumors of the larynx: computed tomography findings. Am J Otolaryngol 20:379–382

Witte MC, Neel HB III (2000) Infectious and inflammatory disorders of the larynx. In: Ferlito A (ed) Diseases of the larynx. Arnold, London, p 259

Witterick IJ, Noyek AM, Kassel EE (2000) Diagnostic imaging of the larynx. In: Ferlito A (ed) Diseases of the larynx. Arnold, London, p 169

Yencha MW, Linfesty R, Blackmon A (2000) Laryngeal tuberculosis. Am J Otolaryngol 21:122–126

Zbären P, Läng H, Becker M (1995) Rare benign neoplasms of the larynx: rhabdomyoma and lipoma. ORL J Otorhinolaryngol Relat Spec 57:351–355

4 Radiology of Pediatric Laryngeal Pathology

Pawel P. Gruca, Varsha Joshi, Suresh K. Mukherji

CONTENTS

4.1 Embryology

Knowledge of the embryology of the larynx and the trachea allows for a better understanding of common congenital anomalies and disease processes involving the pediatric airway.

In the 4th week of gestation, the respiratory system appears as an outpouching from the ventral wall of the foregut (the primitive pharynx). This respiratory diverticulum expands in a caudal direction and becomes separated from the foregut by the development of two longitudinal grooves, eventually merging to form the tracheoesophageal septum during the 7th week of gestation. This septum divides the foregut into a dorsal esophagus and a ventral trachea. The respiratory diverticulum remains in open communication with the primitive pharynx; this opening corresponds with the laryngeal orificium. Incomplete division of the foregut into a respiratory and a digestive portion during the 4th week of gestation gives rise to the formation of tracheoesophageal fistulas. Unequal partitioning of the foregut into the trachea and the esophagus may be the cause of tracheal stenosis, or atresia (Moore 1988).

The laryngeal orifice is surrounded by the mesenchyma of the fourth and sixth branchial arches. Proliferation of this mesenchyma gives rise to the formation of the epiglottic swelling (arising from the fourth branchial arch, and eventually forming the epiglottis) and paired arytenoid swellings (from the sixth branchial arch, and eventually forming the arytenoid cartilages). Also the thyroid (fourth branchial arch) and cricoid cartilage (sixth branchial arch) will arise from the branchial mesenchyma.

The cricoid cartilage develops from two distinct cartilaginous centers: during the 6th week, the anterior ring of the cricoid cartilage fuses, while the posterior ring is fused by the 7th week of gestation. The fusion of the posterior aspect of the cricoid cartilage is aided by the advancing tracheoesophageal septum. A laryngotracheoesophageal cleft results from the arrest in development of the tracheoesophageal septum, which also prevents fusion of the posterior cricoid cartilage.

A the time the laryngeal cartilages are formed, the laryngeal epithelium proliferates rapidly and obliterates the laryngeal lumina. This occlusion is temporary, as resorption of the epithelium leads to recanalization of the larynx during the 10th week of gestation. During this resorption, the laryngeal ventricles are formed, bordered by folds of tissue known as the false and true vocal cords. Laryngeal atresia, subglottic stenosis and laryngeal webs may result from incomplete recanalization.

A ring of mesenchyma derived from the sixth branchial arch gives rise to the intrinsic laryngeal

P.P. Gruca, DO
Department of Radiology, University of North Carolina at Chapel Hill, School of Medicine, Campus Box 7510, Chapel Hill, NC 27599-7510, USA

V. Joshi, MD
Department of Radiology, University of North Carolina at Chapel Hill, School of Medicine, Campus Box 7510, Chapel Hill, NC 27599-7510, USA

S.K. Mukherji, MD
Section Chief, Neuroradiology, Department of Radiology, University of Michigan Health System, 1500 East Medical Center Drive, Ann Arbor, MI 48109-0030, USA

muscles. Therefore, the recurrent laryngeal nerve (the nerve of the sixth branchial arch) supplies these muscles (Stone and Figueroa 2000). The intrinsic muscles are first recognized by the 7th week of gestation. The cricothyroid muscle probably arises from the fourth arch. Thus, the superior laryngeal nerve (the nerve of the fourth branchial arch) supplies the cricothyroid muscle.

4.2
Congenital (Developmental) Lesions

4.2.1
Laryngomalacia (Congenital Flaccid Larynx)

Laryngomalacia (LM) is the most common congenital laryngeal anomaly. LM is also the most common cause of stridor in infants.

Patients with LM present with inspiratory stridor, which usually starts within the first few days to weeks of life. The stridor is of variable intensity and is aggravated with crying, feeding or other periods of excitement. This stridor is worse when the patient is in supine position with the head flexed. The patients are not cyanotic. LM is uncommonly associated with dyspnea or difficulty with swallowing. LM is benign and self-limited. On average it resolves by 12 months of age (between 6 months and 2 years).

There is ongoing debate as to the cause of LM. Several theories regarding its pathophysiology have been proposed. Some authors feel anatomic abnormalities, such as an elongated epiglottis curling upon itself, foreshortened aryepiglottic folds, and bulky arytenoids prolapsing into the airway with inspiration, are the underlying cause (Chung et al. 2000). Other investigators believe that LM is caused by poor neuromuscular control, resulting in inadequate muscular support of the cartilaginous framework of the epiglottis with increased compliance of the supraglottic tissues. Delayed development of the neuromuscular pathways controlling the airway is blamed for poor neuromuscular cartilage support. LM may be associated with other abnormalities of the larynx. In some chromosomal abnormalities such as cri du chat syndrome, LM and laryngeal malformations contribute to the characteristic abnormal cry (Brislin et al. 1995).

Direct endoscopic examination with a flexible laryngoscope provides the definitive diagnosis. The characteristic findings include a narrow elongated epiglottis that may be curved upon itself (omega-shaped epiglottis) with floppy aryepiglottic folds. The arytenoids appear prominent and there is a deep interarytenoid cleft. During inspiration, the supraglottic structures collapse into the lumen of the airway leaving a slit-like opening.

LM is a self-limited condition that typically spontaneously resolves with age. Surgical intervention is reserved for patients who fail to spontaneously improve or have persistent symptoms of sleep apnea, cor pulmonale, feeding difficulties, or failure to thrive.

AP and lateral plain films are the imaging modality of choice for imaging patients suspected of having LM (Fig. 4.1). The anterior bowing and inferior displacement of the aryepiglottic folds during inspiration are the plain film findings. The epiglottis and hyoid bone may be positioned lower due to the imbalance between the suprahyoid and infrahyoid strap muscles (Carpenter and Merten 1991). The intermittent airway obstruction may cause dilatation of the hypopharynx and the valleculae.

Currently, CT and MR play a very limited role in initially imaging patients with LM. CT may be helpful for detecting the presence of associated congenital anomalies, such as subglottic or tracheal stenosis.

4.2.2
Laryngotracheoesophageal Cleft

Laryngotracheoesophageal cleft (LTC) is a rare congenital anomaly resulting in abnormal communication between the larynx and the hypopharynx. LTC has been classified into partial and extensive types. This disorder is associated with a history of maternal polyhydramnios in 30% of the patients. LTC is associated with other congenital abnormalities, with 20% of patients having an associated tracheoesophageal fistula. Affected children usually present in the first weeks to months of life.

LTC is felt to result from lack of development of the tracheoesophageal septum. The absence of the septum inhibits proper formation of the cricoid cartilage and inhibits posterior fusion. This results in the creation of an abnormal communication between the larynx and the hypopharynx. The anomalous communication may be localized to the posterior aspect of the cricoid cartilage or be more extensive and involve the entire common wall between the trachea and the esophagus. The severity of the defect may depend on the gestational age at which the arrest in development occurs.

Patients with LTC present early in life with a variety of symptoms associated with feeding difficulties and

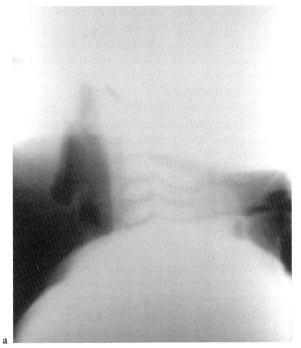

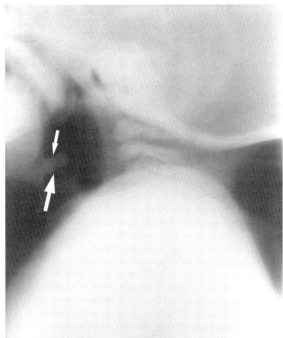

a

b

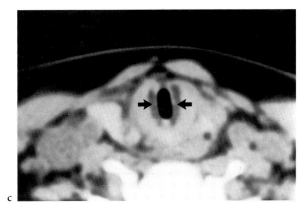

c

Fig. 4.1a–c. Laryngomalacia. **a** Expiratory lateral view of the upper airway shows normal configuration. **b** During inspiration the epiglottis (*smaller arrow*) folds back posteriorly upon itself and the aryepiglottic folds (*larger arrow*) prolapse anteriorly. The hypopharynx is distended (case courtesy of B. Specter, MD, University of North Carolina, Chapel Hill, N.C.). **c** CT reveals loss of the normal configuration of the airway with diminished transverse diameter (*arrows*)

respiratory distress. The severity of the symptoms is usually related to the extent of the cleft. Some patients with very small clefts may be asymptomatic. Affected individuals often present with choking and coughing episodes during feeding which, in severe cases, may be associated with cyanosis. Other symptoms include stridor, recurrent aspiration and voice abnormalities.

Diagnosis is made at direct endoscopy. The management of LTC should be focused on controlling airway function, preventing aspiration and providing indicated surgical repair.

Plain film imaging is the preferred modality for imaging patients suspected of having LTC. The diagnosis of LTC may be confirmed with esophagography, which demonstrates communication between the esophagus and the trachea (Fig. 4.2). The esophogram is best performed with barium, or non-ionic water-

soluble contrast agent with the patient placed in the prone position. Chest films may reveal parenchymal opacities, indicating aspiration pneumonia.

4.2.3
Laryngeal Web and Laryngeal Atresia

Laryngeal web (LW) is a rare lesion that results from an incomplete recanalization of the embryonic larynx during the 7th to 8th week of gestation. LW denotes a spectrum of congenital laryngeal anomalies that result from varying degrees of recanalization of the fetal larynx. At the extreme end of this spectrum is laryngeal atresia. One-third of all patients presenting with LW will have another anomaly of the respiratory tract, most commonly subglottic

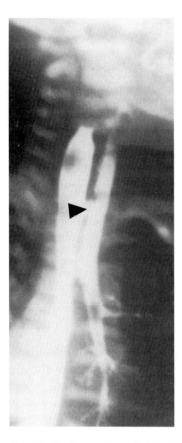

Fig. 4.2. Tracheoesophageal cleft. Oblique radiograph after barium swallow shows barium in the trachea and the bronchus consistent with persistent congenital communication (*black arrowhead*) (case courtesy of L. Fordham, MD, University of North Carolina, Chapel Hill, N.C.)

stenosis. The incidence of an associated abnormality increases with the severity of the LW.

Laryngeal webs are found most commonly at the level of the true vocal cords, the anterior commissure being the most common location. If a LW occurs in the region of the posterior commissure, it may be associated with interarytenoid fixation. Rarely, a LW is seen in the supraglottic larynx. Endoscopically, a LW appears as a soft tissue membrane extending across the laryngeal air column. The thickness of the web is variable and may range from a thin membrane to a thick fibrous band. The larger the web is, the greater the obstruction it creates. The peripheral portion of the web is usually thicker than the free margin, which is typically concave and sharply outlined.

Clinically, a LW presents with signs of airway obstruction detected shortly after birth. Some patients present later with symptoms that may be misdiagnosed as recurrent or atypical croup.

The treatment of LW depends on the thickness of the web. Thin webs may be treated with endoscopic lysis using a carbon dioxide laser or a knife (McGILL 1984). Patients with large webs presenting with severe respiratory distress may require emergent intubation or tracheostomy.

LW may prevent passage of the endoscope thereby preventing adequate examination of the larynx distal to the web. Lateral plain film radiographs may provide valuable information regarding the location and the thickness of the web. Sagittal reformations of spiral CT images may also be beneficial in such cases. Imaging is also useful to detect the presence and extent of associated laryngeal abnormalities such as subglottic stenosis.

Laryngeal atresia (LA) is a rare condition frequently considered to be an extreme form of LW. If not immediately recognized, it is incompatible with life. The majority of patients with LA are stillborn. LA is often associated with various other congenital anomalies. Presence of a tracheoesophageal fistula, if it is large enough to permit ventilation, may aid in survival through the perinatal period. Patients with LA are unable to ventilate their lungs in spite of respiratory movements. Following clamping of the umbilical cord, cyanosis rapidly develops. Attempts to intubate the newborn are unsuccessful. To prevent death, emergent tracheostomy is essential. Once the diagnosis of LA is suspected, laryngoscopy should be performed. The management of LA is dependent on the extent of the atretic region. Occasionally, a small-bore endoscope may be passed through the thin atretic segment. Obviously, more advanced atresia requires tracheostomy.

Conventional radiographic examination in LA, if performed, may reveal no air in the lungs and occasionally may identify the column of air extending to the atretic segment in the larynx or the trachea.

4.2.4
Subglottic Stenosis

Subglottic stenosis (SS) is a narrowing of the air column below the level of the true vocal cords and above the base of the cricoid cartilage. SS may be congenital, or a result of prolonged intubation or laryngeal trauma (MACPHERSON and LEITHISER 1985). Patients with Down's syndrome have increased incidence of congenital subglottic stenosis (CSS).

The normal diameter of the pediatric airway at the subglottic level is 4.5 to 5.5 mm in a full-term and 3.5 mm in a premature infant. CSS in the newborn is defined as a subglottic air column of less than 3.5 mm in diameter in a full-term infant and less than 3 mm in a premature infant.

CSS is felt to result from a defect in the development of the cricoid cartilage or conus elasticus (HOLINGER and OPPENHEIMER 1989). This diagnosis may be difficult to prove, as many patients who require intubation might actually have an underlying CSS that has been aggravated by prolonged intubation.

There are two types of CSS: membranous and cartilaginous. The membranous form typically presents as a circumferential soft tissue thickening within the subglottic region. Histologically, the thickening is felt to be due to increased fibrous connective tissue and hyperplastic mucous glands. This type usually occurs 2–3 mm below the undersurface of the true vocal cords and may extend into the trachea. The cartilaginous form is due to an abnormal cricoid cartilage. The cricoid is thickened and deformed (CARPENTER and MERTEN 1991).

SS usually presents during infancy with signs of airway obstruction. Superimposed infections exacerbate the symptoms involving the upper respiratory tract since mucosal edema further narrows the already compromised airway. The diagnosis is based on endoscopic findings of circumferential narrowing of the subglottic region. Stenosis may be confined to the subglottic region or extend inferiorly into the trachea. It may be difficult, at times, to determine the extent of stenosis by endoscopy alone.

SS is a clinical diagnosis based on a combination of presenting symptoms and clinical findings. AP and lateral plain films of the neck may show airway stenosis in the subglottic region. CT is the imaging modality of choice if the extent of the narrowing cannot be fully appreciated by endoscopy alone. Radiographically SS reveals a circumferential soft tissue thickening involving the subglottic region (Fig. 4.3). Because the cricoid cartilage is not calcified in young children, it is difficult to evaluate by CT. The abnormal soft tissue thickening may extend into and involve the trachea, resulting in narrowing of the tracheal air column. The full extent of the involved area should be determined.

4.2.5
Vocal Cord Paralysis

Vocal cord paralysis (VCP) is the second most common congenital laryngeal anomaly. VCP may be unilateral or bilateral with unilateral paralysis being more common. Left-sided paralysis occurs more frequently. Most cases are diagnosed soon after birth. Unilateral paralysis may remain undiagnosed in some infants as there is usually no respiratory compromise in such cases, and they may have spontaneous recovery. Many cases of VCP are associated with an underlying lesion, where imaging is helpful. Hereditary causes of bilateral VCP are extremely rare.

Unilateral and bilateral VCP differ in etiology. In unilateral VCP, a peripheral lesion is suspected. Therefore, the entire course of the recurrent laryngeal nerve needs to be traced by imaging. Anomalies of the cardiac and great vessels (e.g. ventricular septal defect, tetralogy of Fallot, patent ductus arteriosus) are common causes of congenital unilateral VCP. Unilateral VCP may also result from previous repair of tracheoesophageal fistula or congenital heart defect. In bilateral VCP, an anomaly of the central nervous system is

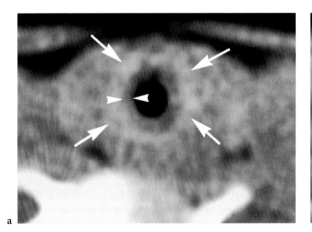
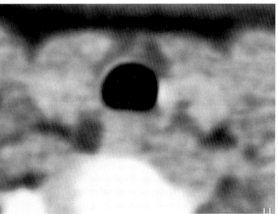

a   b

Fig. 4.3a, b. Subglottic stenosis. **a** CT at the level of the cricoid cartilage (*arrows*) shows narrowing of the subglottic airway by concentric soft tissue thickening (*between arrowheads*). **b** Compare with larger diameter of the cervical trachea in the same patient (case courtesy of R. Hermans, MD, PhD, University Hospitals Leuven, Belgium)

suspected. Frequent abnormalities include myelom-eningocele, hydrocephalus, Chiari malformations, Dandy–Walker anomaly, bulbar palsy, birth trauma, intracranial hemorrhage, encephalocele, cerebral anomalies, or dysgenesis of the nucleus ambiguous. Idiopathic bilateral palsy is unusual.

Patients with unilateral VCP typically present in the newborn period with a weak cry, intermittent cyanosis, aspiration of pharyngeal secretions, and choking during feedings. Stridor and other symptoms of respiratory distress are usually not features of a unilateral VCP. Patients with bilateral VCP classically present with acute respiratory distress and a high-pitched inspiratory stridor that is aggravated by agitation. These patients often have a normal cry. Significant dysphagia caused by pharyngeal lack of coordination (likely due to multiple cranial nerve palsies) is a hallmark of bilateral vocal cord paralysis. Their recurrent pneumonias are due to aspirations from inability to elicit a protective cough reflex.

The diagnosis of VCP is made on endoscopic examination. Fluoroscopy may occasionally be helpful in evaluation of vocal cord motion. Detection of an offending lesion remains the primary goal of imaging these patients. Lesions causing VCP may occur anywhere from the brainstem (nucleus ambiguous) to the upper mediastinum. The course of the vagus and the recurrent laryngeal nerves needs to be traced in all cases of unexplained VCP. The vagus nerve descends in the carotid sheath into the mediastinum. The recurrent laryngeal nerve curve beneath the subclavian artery on the right, and the ligamentum arteriosum on the left. Thus, patients presenting with unilateral left VCP must be imaged to the level below the aortopulmonary window.

No airway support is usually required in patients with unilateral VCP. Although controversial, either direct injection of polytetrafluoroethylene (Teflon) or an external medialization procedure may be of benefit for patients who aspirate (see also Chap. 3). However, this is rarely performed in children, as occasionally unilateral VCP may spontaneously resolve; therefore, efforts should be made to delay all procedures until the age of 4–5 years. Patients with bilateral VCP usually require intubation and possibly tracheostomy.

4.2.6
Laryngeal Cysts

The term laryngeal cyst encompasses several types of air-containing or fluid-filled sacs in the region of the larynx. Included in this classification are both laryngoceles and saccular cysts. Laryngoceles and saccular cysts can be considered to be similar lesions, both representing an abnormal dilatation of the laryngeal ventricle or saccule. The term saccular cyst is also used more generally for any submucosal fluid-filled lesion, isolated from the laryngeal lumen.

Laryngeal cysts may cause stridor in infants and children. They may be seen at all ages. Laryngoceles may be congenital or acquired; in children, these masses are felt to be congenital in origin. Laryngoceles (air- or fluid-filled) may be classified as internal, external or mixed. An internal laryngocele denotes a mass confined to the endolaryngeal structures of the larynx. An external laryngocele extends laterally through the thyrohyoid membrane into the soft tissues of the neck. This extension usually occurs through the natural weakness in the membrane, that is the ostium for the superior laryngeal artery (LEWIS et al. 1990). A mixed laryngocele is comprised of both internal and external components. Laryngoceles may be unilateral or bilateral. These lesions may become infected during periods of upper respiratory tract infection. A pyolaryngocele is an infected laryngocele that contains pus (see also Chap. 3).

Saccular cysts may be congenital or acquired. The congenital form, which is observed in children, results from a simple atresia of the saccular orifice. The exact embryogenesis of the congenital saccular cyst is controversial. Acquired saccular cysts are due to complete occlusion of the saccular orifice secondary to inflammation, tumor or trauma. According to some authors, saccular cysts may arise from retention of mucus in the collecting ducts of submucosal glands located around the ventricle (WARD et al. 1995).

The presenting signs of a laryngeal cyst are dependent on the size and extent of the lesion. Infants and young children may present with signs of respiratory distress. Since the airway is larger in older patients, they may exhibit intermittent hoarseness or aphonia or a muffled cry. Cysts and laryngoceles may be associated with other anomalies including LM and vocal cord paralysis.

Saccular cysts and laryngoceles appear as soft rounded submucosal soft tissue masses on endoscopy. These lesions are covered by mucosa and have a characteristic bluish hue. Large lesions may extend into and obstruct the laryngeal lumen.

On plain films, laryngeal cysts present as soft tissue masses within the glottic and supraglottic region. The presence of air within the lesion suggests that the mass communicates with the airway. On CT and MR, these lesions present as smoothly marginated soft tissue structures, either air- or fluid-filled (Figs. 4.4, 4.5).

The internal attenuation and signal characteristics of a saccular cyst may vary depending on the protein content of the fluid within the lesion. Highly proteinaceous fluid will result in increased attenuation on CT and increased signal on T1-weighted images (MUKHERJI and CASTILLO 2000).

Needle aspiration is the treatment of choice for saccular cysts in children. In cases of recurrent cysts, unroofing may be necessary. Laryngoceles are considered surgical lesions. The exact approach is based on the size of the lesion and whether it has an extralaryngeal component. To exclude the presence of an underlying neoplasm, the region of the orifice of the laryngoceles and saccular cysts should be carefully examined, both endoscopically and radiologically.

4.2.7
Subglottic Hemangioma

Hemangiomas of young children may occur anywhere in the larynx but have a clear predilection for the subglottic region. The lesion is a slow growing and benign tumor, typically presenting during the first year of life, but most commonly before 6 months of age. Subglottic hemangioma (SH) is twice as common in females as it is in males. Cutaneous hemangiomas have been reported with SH in 50% of patients (PRANSKY and SEID 1990).

SH typically presents clinically with signs of airway obstruction with inspiratory or biphasic stridor.

Common presenting symptoms include stridor, dyspnea, cyanotic episodes, hoarseness, cough, and difficult feeding. The symptoms are often exacerbated by excitement, crying or respiratory tract infection. Occasionally, symptoms may progress to acute respiratory distress as continued growth may cause significant airway obstruction.

The diagnosis of SH is made by endoscopy. The typical appearance is that of a red or blue submucosal mass located within the subglottic region, usually arising from just below the posterior commissure. The endoscopic appearance is typical and obviates the need for a biopsy, which is dangerous to perform.

Although spontaneous involution can be expected to occur, a wait-and-see policy is not recommended due to the associated morbidity and mortality. Several therapeutic approaches have been tried, but currently carbon dioxide laser excision is the accepted mode of treatment (HEALY et al. 1984). Steroids or other drugs may be beneficial, although the specific indications are not clearly defined.

SH may be detected on AP and lateral plain films of the neck and present as a soft tissue mass extending into and narrowing the tracheal air column (Fig. 4.6). CT and MR may be useful to define the extent of the mass. Caution must be used in infants with airway compromise as CT and MR may require the child to be sedated. On cross-sectional imaging these lesions present as enhancing, polypoid soft tissues masses, extending into the airway (Fig. 4.7).

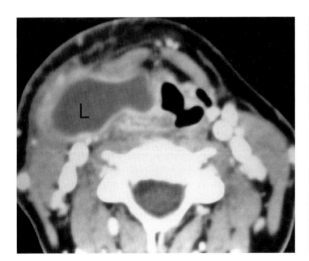

Fig. 4.4. Mixed laryngocele. CT shows a right fluid-filled laryngocele (*L*) simulating a soft tissue mass. There are intralaryngeal and extralaryngeal components. The laryngeal lumen is displaced to the left side by a fluid-containing sac

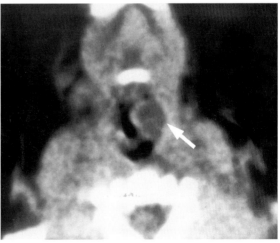

Fig. 4.5. Saccular laryngeal cyst. CT shows a cyst (*arrow*) in the left supraglottic larynx, probably arising at the level of the vallecula (case courtesy of W. Nemzek, MD, University of California, Davis, Calif.)

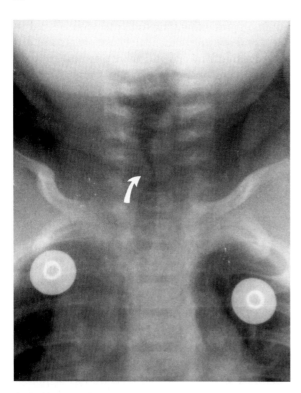

Fig. 4.6. Subglottic hemangioma. Frontal radiograph shows a soft tissue density mass (*arrow*) arising from the right subglottic region and compressing the air column (case courtesy of L. Fordham, MD, University of North Carolina, Chapel Hill, N.C.)

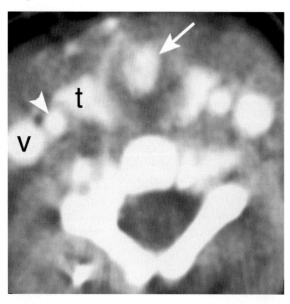

Fig. 4.7. Subglottic hemangioma. Axial contrast-enhanced CT image at the level of the subglottis in a 3-month old child with obstructive breathing, necessitating tracheostomy. A hemangioma (*arrow*) obliterates the subglottic airway (*t* right lobe of thyroid gland, *arrowhead* common carotid artery, *v* internal jugular vein) (reprinted with permission from HERMANS 2000)

4.3
Infections of the Larynx

4.3.1
Epiglottitis (Supraglottitis)

Epiglottitis is an acute infection that involves the supraglottic region, predominantly the epiglottis.

The most common organism causing epiglottitis is *Haemophilus influenzae* type B (HIB), although other microorganisms such as *Streptococcus*, *Candida* and viruses have also been implicated. The incidence of this disease has dramatically decreased with the introduction of HIB vaccination (HICKERSON et al. 1996).

This disease most commonly occurs between the age of 2 and 4 years. The newborn is protected by passive immunity, acquired from the mother, to the capsular antigen. This passive immunity resolves usually by 3 months of age. The child's own immune system does not produce a significant amount of similar antibody until 3 to 5 years of age. This window of diminished antibody levels is responsible for the high incidence of HIB in this age group.

Epiglottitis presents clinically with high fever, and signs of respiratory obstruction. Affected children are often sitting upright (to allow the swollen epiglottis to pull away from the laryngeal inlet) and drooling. These individuals have greater inspiratory than expiratory stridor. The onset of symptoms is often acute and may occur over a 2- to 6-h period (MANCUSO 1996).

Initial clinical examination should be kept to a minimum. Because the patient is susceptible to acute laryngospasm and airway obstruction during forced inspiration, it is critical not to excite the child during initial evaluation (especially with the tongue depressor). In a stable child, able to swallow the secretions, a lateral plain film of the neck can be performed in the emergency room. In many cases, a flexible nasopharyngoscopy can also be performed. On physical examination, the epiglottis is swollen and cherry red. The swelling of the aryepiglottic folds causes narrowing of the supraglottic airway. Thick and tenacious secretions may be present, and a mucous plug in an already compromised airway may cause sudden respiratory arrest (JOHN and SWISCHUK 1992).

If the edema is mild, and the child is being treated in a tertiary center with a well-trained in-house pediatric intensivist, conservative treatment with intravenous antibiotics and steroids can be instigated

(RIMEL 2000). In more serious cases, the affected children will also require nasotracheal or orotracheal intubation under anesthesia; tracheostomy is not currently recommended for achieving airway control.

The findings on plain radiography show a diffusely thickened epiglottis, which is often two to three times the normal size (Fig. 4.8). The aryepiglottic folds and false vocal cords are also thickened. There may be dilatation of the oropharynx if the supraglottic larynx is narrowed because of diffuse edema (GYEPES and NUSSBAUM 1985; ROTHROCK et al. 1990). There is no role for CT and MR in imaging such patients; in fact, these studies may be dangerous to perform since placing the patient in the supine position will further reduce the caliber of an already narrowed airway.

The infection may progress to the formation of an epiglottic abscess, but this is rarely seen in children; abscess formation occurs more commonly in adult epiglottitis. CT with contrast may be used to diagnose such an abscess after the patient has been stabilized (see also Chap. 3).

The clinical differential diagnosis of childhood epiglottitis may include retropharyngeal abscess, tracheitis and foreign body. Patients suffering from such diseases can usually be differentiated based on history and clinical signs (RIMEL 2000).

4.3.2
Croup (Laryngotracheobronchitis)

Croup is a one of the more common diseases of the pediatric larynx. It often occurs between the ages of 1 and 3 years. Croup is a viral infection, most often caused by parainfluenza 1 and 3 and influenza A and B, as well as respiratory syncytial virus (RIMEL 2000).

The patient presents with a low-grade fever, respiratory symptoms such as rhinorrhea, a characteristic barking cough and in severe cases also with inspiratory stridor. Stridor at rest with retractions indicates significant subglottic stenosis and a potentially life-threatening situation.

The infection causes diffuse edema of the mucosa of the subglottic region and trachea. Two characteristics of the subglottic region make this area vulnerable to croup. First, the subglottic region is the narrowest portion of the respiratory tract in children under 3 years of age. Second, the subglottis is the only portion of the upper respiratory tract surrounded by a complete cartilaginous ring. Thus, the lumen of the subglottis is easily compromised by edema caused by this infection (JONES and PILLSBURY 1993).

The diagnosis is usually made clinically. The role of imaging is to confirm the suspected diagnosis of croup and to exclude other causes of stridor, includ-

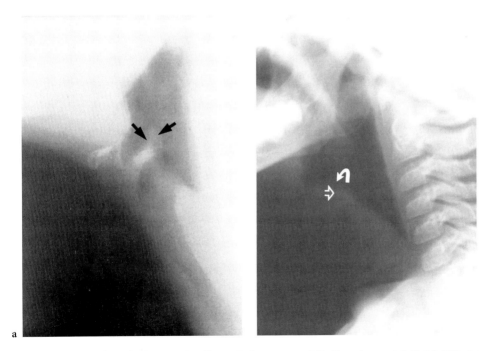

a   b

Fig. 4.8. a Normal epiglottis. Lateral radiograph shows normal findings (*arrows*). **b** Epiglottitis. Lateral radiograph shows a thickened ("thumb-like") epiglottis (*curved arrow*) and edema of the aryepiglottic folds (*open arrow*) (case courtesy of L. Fordham, MD, University of North Carolina, Chapel Hill, N.C.)

ing a foreign body. The preferred imaging method is plain radiography of the neck in AP and lateral projections. Plain films show a loss of the normal subglottic angles resulting in a "steeple-" or a "wine bottle"-shaped appearance of the proximal trachea and the subglottic region on AP projection (Fig. 4.9). On the lateral view there may be loss of distinctness of the normal soft tissue structures in the glottic region due to edema (RENCKEN et al. 1998).

Humidification is felt by some authors to be the primary treatment for most cases of croup, but there is lack of scientific evidence to support this. Some authors have proven the benefit of racemic epinephrine in croup. Recently, steroids have shown to provide therapeutic benefit. Short-term endotracheal intubation is reserved for severe cases. Indications for direct airway control include increasing carbon dioxide levels and a deteriorating neurologic status.

4.3.3
Juvenile Laryngeal Papillomatosis

Multiple papillomas in the pediatric respiratory tract are commonly referred to as juvenile laryngeal papillomatosis (JLP). JLP is the most common tumor of the pediatric airway. This process is usually detected before 3 years of age, but may become symptomatic during the first year of life. The exact age of presentation is based on the location and size of the tumor, and the aggressiveness of the lesion.

The etiologic agent for JLP is the human papillomavirus (HPV). HPV is a DNA virus which promotes epithelial proliferation. HPV-6 and HPV-11 are the common subtypes in JLP. JLP is associated with condyloma acuminata (maternal genital warts). This association is supported by the fact that HPV-6 and HPV-11 are felt to be responsible for 90% of genital warts. The DNA sequences of HPV isolated from JLP and condyloma acuminata are indistinguishable. Additionally, JLP is rarely seen in patients delivered by cesarean section suggesting a protective role of such delivery to the newborn.

Patients with JLP most commonly present with signs of airway obstruction. The most common symptoms are hoarseness, stridor, recurrent "croup", or change in voice quality. Although histologically benign, the danger of JLP is progressive obstruction of the airway. An acute onset of respiratory distress is unusual because JLP results in gradual airway narrowing.

JLP most commonly involves the true vocal cords, although supraglottic or subglottic extent is also reg-

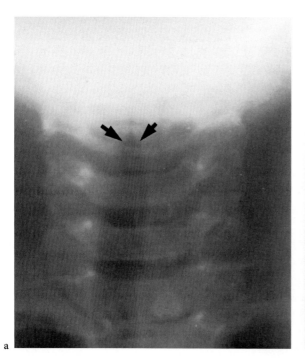
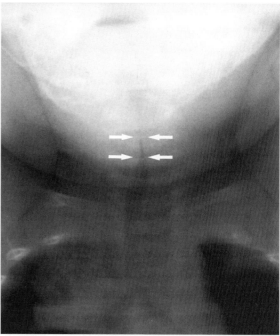

a   b

Fig. 4.9. a Normal subglottis. Frontal radiograph shows a "shoulder-like" appearance of a normal subglottic region (*arrows*) (case courtesy of D. Merten, MD, University of North Carolina, Chapel Hill, N.C.). **b** Croup. Frontal radiograph shows a smoothly tapered subglottic region (*arrows*), also known as a "steeple" or a "wine bottle" sign, secondary to the mucosal edema (case courtesy of L. Fordham, MD, University of North Carolina, Chapel Hill, N.C.)

ularly seen. The tracheobronchial tree is often involved, with tracheal involvement reported at about 26%. The cause of such involvement is attributed to seeding of the viral particles during airway manipulation. Several authors believe tracheostomy increases the likelihood of distal spread and regard this pro-

cedure as contraindicated in affected patients. Distal spread may result in the formation of multiple lung nodules, which have been shown to cavitate (KRAMER et al. 1985).

The diagnosis of JLP is based on endoscopic findings and biopsy. On endoscopic examination, JLP ap-

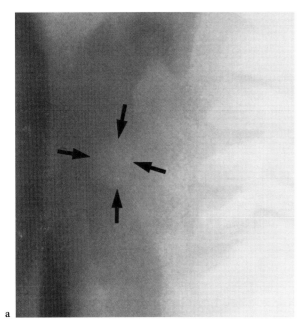

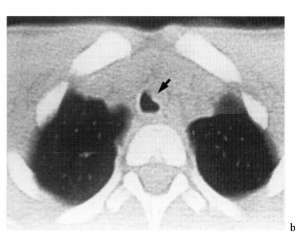

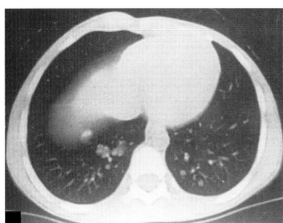

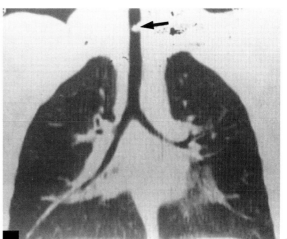

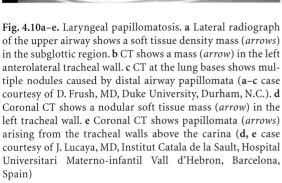

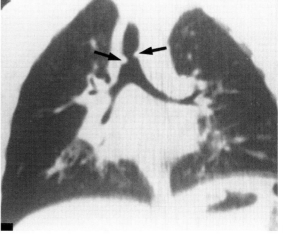

Fig. 4.10a–e. Laryngeal papillomatosis. **a** Lateral radiograph of the upper airway shows a soft tissue density mass (*arrows*) in the subglottic region. **b** CT shows a mass (*arrow*) in the left anterolateral tracheal wall. **c** CT at the lung bases shows multiple nodules caused by distal airway papillomata (**a–c** case courtesy of D. Frush, MD, Duke University, Durham, N.C.). **d** Coronal CT shows a nodular soft tissue mass (*arrow*) in the left tracheal wall. **e** Coronal CT shows papillomata (*arrows*) arising from the tracheal walls above the carina (**d, e** case courtesy of J. Lucaya, MD, Institut Catala de la Sault, Hospital Universitari Materno-infantil Vall d'Hebron, Barcelona, Spain)

pears as pink or red irregular, pedunculated, exophytic masses. These masses may be nodular and vary in size. Histologically, they consist of a highly vascular core of connective tissue covered by stratified squamous epithelium with abnormal keratinization.

JLP has an unpredictable clinical course and shows the tendency to spontaneously regress over time. Malignant transformation occurring in chronic disease has been described, but is the exception rather than the rule (BAUMAN and SMITH 1996).

The treatment of JLP has included medical therapy (interferon, steroids, antiviral agents and various other drugs), but most studies are preliminary and do not have a control arm which would allow judgment of the possible spontaneous remission of the disease. Many authors currently favor the use of the carbon dioxide laser for resection of obstructing laryngeal lesions.

JLP may cause nodular soft tissue masses involving the tracheal air column visible on plain films (Fig. 4.10a). Both CT and MR may be used for evaluating laryngeal disease involving the larynx, showing multiple endophytic nodular soft tissue masses, narrowing the airway and enhancing with contrast (Fig. 4.10b–e). The pulmonary findings consist of multiple bilateral parenchymal nodules. These pulmonary nodules may gradually enlarge resulting in areas of consolidation or distal atelectasis. Solid lesions may eventually cavitate; these cavities are typically thin-walled and may contain air-fluid levels, and are prone to recurrent infections (KRAMER et al. 1985).

References

Bauman NM, Smith RJ (1996) Recurrent respiratory papillomatosis. Pediatr Clin North Am 43:1385–1401
Brislin RP, Stayer SA, Schwartz RE (1995) Anaesthetic considerations for the patient with cri du chat syndrome. Paediatr Anaesth 5:139–141
Carpenter LM, Merten DF (1991) Radiographic manifestations of congenital anomalies affecting the airway. Radiol Clin North Am 29:219–340
Chung CJ, Fordham LA, Mukherji SJ (2000) The pediatric airway: a review of differential diagnosis by anatomy and pathology. Neuroimaging Clin North Am 10:161–180
Gyepes MT, Nussbaum E (1985) Radiographic-endoscopic correlations in the examination of airway disease in children. Pediatr Radiol 15:291–296
Healy GB, McGill T, Friedman EM (1984) Carbon dioxide laser in subglottic hemangioma. An update. Ann Otol Rhinol Laryngol 93:370–373
Hermans R (2000) Head and neck imaging. In: Pettersson H, Allison D (eds) The encyclopedia of medical imaging, part VI. NICER Institute, Oslo, p 387
Hickerson SL, Kirby RS, Wheeler JG, Schutze GE (1996) Epiglottitis: a 9-year case review. South Med J 89:487–490
Holinger LD, Oppenheimer RW (1989) Congenital subglottic stenosis: the elliptical cricoid cartilage. Ann Otol Rhinol Laryngol 98:702–706
John SD, Swischuk LE (1992) Stridor and upper airway obstruction in infants and children. Radiographics 12:625–644
Jones KR, Pillsbury HC (1993) Infections and manifestations of the systemic disease of the larynx. In: Cummings CW, Fredrickson JM, Harker LA, et al (eds) Otolaryngology and head and neck surgery, vol 3. Mosby-Year Book, St Louis, pp 1854–1857
Kramer SS, Wehnut WD, Stocker JT, Kashima H (1985) Pulmonary manifestations of juvenile laryngotracheal papillomatosis. AJR Am J Roentgenol 144:687–694
Lewis CS, Castillo M, Patrick E (1990) Symptomatic external laryngocele in a newborn: findings on plain radiographs and CT scans. AJNR Am J Neuroradiol 11:1002
MacPherson R, Leithiser R (1985) Upper airway obstruction in children: an update. Radiographics 5:339–355
Mancuso RF (1996) Stridor in neonates. Pediatr Clin North Am 43:1339–1356
McGill T (1984) Congenital diseases of the larynx. Otolaryngol Clin North Am 17:57–62
Moore KL (1988) The respiratory system. In: Moore KL (ed) The developing human: clinically oriented embryology, 4th edn. Saunders, Philadelphia, pp 207–213
Mukherji SK, Castillo M (2000) The larynx. In: Orrison WW (ed) Neuroimaging. Saunders, Philadelphia, pp 1411–1459
Pransky SM, Seid AB (1990) Tumors of the larynx, trachea and bronchi. In: Bluestone CD, Stool SE, Scheetz MD (eds) Pediatric otolaryngology. Saunders, Philadelphia, pp 1215–1218
Rencken I, Patton WL, Brash RC (1998) Airway obstruction in pediatric patients: from croup to BOOP. Radiol Clin North Am 36:175–187
Rimel FL (2000) Acquired diseases of the pediatric larynx. In: Ferlito A (ed) Diseases of the larynx. Arnold, London, pp 219–221
Rothrock SG, Pignatello GA, Howard RM (1990) Radiologic diagnosis of epiglottitis: objective criteria for all ages. Ann Emerg Med 19:978–982
Stone JA, Figueroa RE (2000) Embryology and anatomy of the neck. Neuroimaging Clin North Am 10:55–73
Ward RF, Jones J, Arnold JA (1995) Surgical management of congenital saccular cysts of the larynx. Ann Otol Rhinol Laryngol 104:707–710

5   Malignant Lesions of the Larynx and Hypopharynx

MINERVA BECKER

CONTENTS

5.1
Introduction

Imaging is required to evaluate the submucosal extent of malignant laryngeal lesions. Hypopharyngeal malignancies are also included in this chapter, as due to the close anatomical relationship of both structures, malignancies originating in the hypopharynx commonly involve the larynx.

5.2
Squamous Cell Carcinoma

Over 90–95% of laryngeal and hypopharyngeal tumors are squamous cell carcinomas (BATSAKIS 1979; BECKER 1998a, 1998b, 2000; BECKER and HASSO 1996; BECKER and KURT 1999; BECKER et al. 1998a, 1998b; KLEINSASSER 1988a, 1988b). Squamous cell carcinoma of the larynx is primarily related to cigarette smoking. The predisposing role of alcohol in the etiology of laryngeal cancer is less important than it is in cancer of other locations in the head and neck region (KLEINSASSER 1988a 1988c; LEHMAN et al. 1991;

M. BECKER, MD
Priv. Doz., Department of Radiology, Division of Diagnostic and Interventional Radiology, Geneva University Hospital, 24, Rue Micheli-du-Crest, 1211 Geneva 14, Switzerland

TUYNS et al. 1988). The incidence of laryngeal cancer in heavily industrialized cities is two to three times higher than in rural populations with a male to female ratio of 9–10:1 (LEVI et al. 1998). Squamous cell carcinoma of the hypopharynx is less frequent than laryngeal cancer. Predisposing factors are tobacco and alcohol abuse; the male to female ratio is similar to that found in laryngeal cancer.

The most common leading clinical symptoms are hoarseness in laryngeal carcinoma and dysphagia, often associated with palpable cervical lymph nodes, in hypopharyngeal carcinoma. Because squamous cell carcinoma almost always originates at the mucosal surface it is usually first detected endoscopically and then confirmed with endoscopic biopsy. Neither CT nor MR imaging can be used to detect and delineate superficially situated squamous cell carcinoma. The attenuation values of squamous cell carcinoma on CT scans and its signal characteristics on unenhanced and contrast-enhanced MR images are very similar to those of normal mucosa. On the other hand, endoscopy cannot be used to detect tumor infiltration into the submucosal structures, whereas the different characteristics on CT and MR imaging of neoplastic tissue and the adjacent fatty, muscular, and cartilaginous tissues often allow deep tumor infiltration in the horizontal (anterior-posterior) or longitudinal (cranial-caudal) direction to be delineated. Because the prognosis and treatment of squamous cell carcinoma depends on the depth of submucosal infiltration and on the anatomic structures that are involved, cross-sectional imaging with either CT or MR may thus be considered complementary to endoscopy and plays an indispensable role in the pretherapeutic work-up of laryngeal and hypopharyngeal cancer.

Interpretation of CT and MR imaging studies of patients with laryngeal and hypopharyngeal cancer requires an understanding of the typical pathways of tumor spread from the different primary sites and subsites, and knowledge of the criteria for neoplastic invasion of the adjacent structures, particularly the cartilaginous framework of the larynx. In addition, it appears appropriate for the radiologist to be familiar with the implications of imaging findings with regard to the T-classification and options for treatment.

5.2.1
Tumor Sites and Patterns of Tumor Spread

5.2.1.1
Larynx

5.2.1.1.1
Supraglottic Carcinoma
According to their subsite of origin, supraglottic tumors display typical patterns of spread (BECKER

1998a; KIRCHNER and CARTER 1987; MANCUSO 1991; MANCUSO and HANAFEE 1985). Tumors arising from the infrahyoid epiglottis primarily invade the preepiglottic space either along the border of the epiglottic cartilage, or through its preexisting natural perforations or by frank cartilage destruction (Fig. 5.1). Tumors that originate in the region of the petiole often invade the low preepiglottic space (Fig. 5.2), and, via the anterior commissure, extend to the glottis and then the subglottis, thus becoming "transglottic" tumors (see below). Although invasion of the preepiglottic space cannot be detected endoscopically it plays an important role in tumor staging, treatment and prognosis (BECKER 1998b; BECKER and KURT

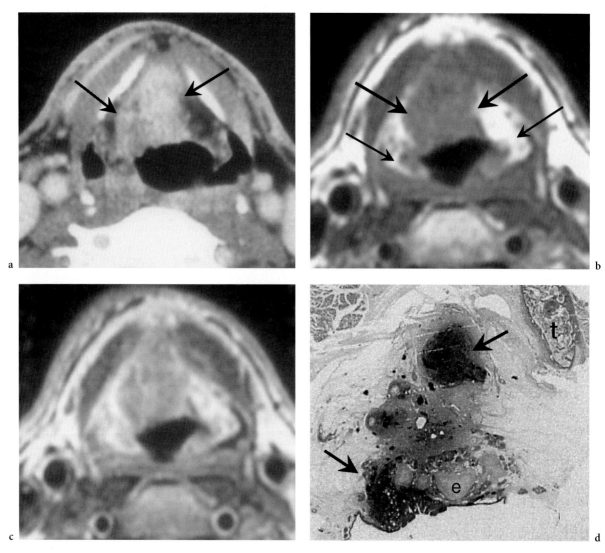

Fig. 5.1a–d. Neoplastic invasion of the preepiglottic space due to anterior supraglottic cancer. **a** Axial contrast-enhanced CT image at the supraglottic level shows an enhancing tumor mass as it invades the preepiglottic space (*arrows*). **b** Axial unenhanced T1-weighted SE image obtained in the same patient at the same level shows a tumor mass with an intermediate signal intensity as it extends into the preepiglottic space (*thick arrows*). Note the high signal intensity of the non-invaded paraglottic space due to the high content of fatty tissue (*thin arrows*). **c** Axial Gd-enhanced T1-weighted SE image at the same level shows enhancement of the tumor mass invading the preepiglottic space. **d** Whole-organ axial histologic slice from supraglottic horizontal laryngectomy specimen confirms tumor invasion of the preepiglottic space (*arrows*; *e* Epiglottis, *t* thyroid cartilage). Hematoxylin-eosin stain

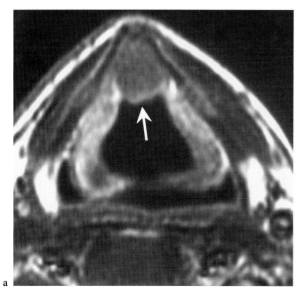

Fig. 5.2a, b. Transglottic spread in an anterior supraglottic cancer underestimated at endoscopy. Patient presenting with a small tumor arising from the mucosa overlying the petiole at endoscopy. Axial (**a**) and sagittal (**b**) contrast-enhanced T1-weighted SE images clearly show that the tumor spreads from the supraglottic mucosa into the inferior preepiglottic space (*arrow*) and downwards into the anterior commissure (*open arrow*) and the anterior subglottic region (*arrowhead*)

1999; Hermanek et al. 1993, 1998; Loener et al. 1997; Mancuso et al. 1999). If the preepiglottic space is invaded, the tumor will be staged T3 according to the UICC and AJCC guidelines. In the presence of extensive neoplastic infiltration of the preepiglottic space by supraglottic laryngeal carcinoma, surgical management may involve a more extensive horizontal supraglottic laryngectomy and sometimes supracricoid laryngectomy with cricohyoidopexy (Maroldi et al. 1997).

Finally, the degree of preepiglottic space involvement by tumor may also affect the outcome of definitive radiation therapy in supraglottic squamous cell carcinoma (Hermans et al. 1999a). Both CT and MRI are well suited to demonstrating replacement of the normal fatty tissue by tumor tissue within the preepiglottic space (Fig. 5.1). Although sagittal images are best suited to delineating the extent of craniocaudal tumor spread within the preepiglottic space, standard axial images are sufficient to establish the diagnosis. Based on data from the literature, as well as on our own results with CT and MRI, the reported sensitivity of CT and MRI in detecting invasion of the preepiglottic space is 92–100%, and the corresponding specificities 93% and 84–90%, respectively (Becker 1998a, 1998b, 2000; Becker and

Hasso 1996; Becker and Kurt 1999; Zbären et al. 1997a, 1997b).

Supraglottic tumors originating from the false cord, laryngeal ventricle, or aryepiglottic fold may grow superficially for some time (Mancuso 1991; Mancuso and Hanafee 1979, 1983, 1985; Mancuso et al. 1977, 1978). By the time they are diagnosed, however, 50% of the tumors will show substantial infiltration of the paraglottic space (Fig. 5.3). Because these tumors tend to spread submucosally along the paraglottic space to the glottic and subglottic region or to other remote areas, cross-sectional images are of particular importance. The primary sign of tumor spread to the paraglottic space on both CT and MRI is replacement of fat by tumor tissue and loss of visualization of the superior extension of the lateral cricoarytenoid muscle in comparison with the opposite side (Fig. 5.3). Our own results with CT and MRI for the detection of neoplastic invasion of the paraglottic space indicate that the sensitivities of CT and MRI are 92–95% and 94–97%, respectively. The specificity of both CT and MRI is, however, limited due to the fact that peritumoral inflammatory changes may lead to overestimation of tumor spread with both methods. The reported specificity for both imaging techniques varies between 43% and 76% (Becker

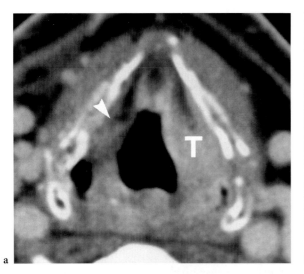

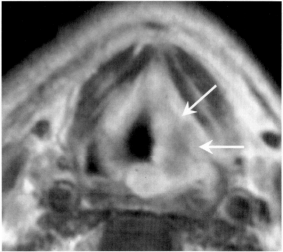

a   b

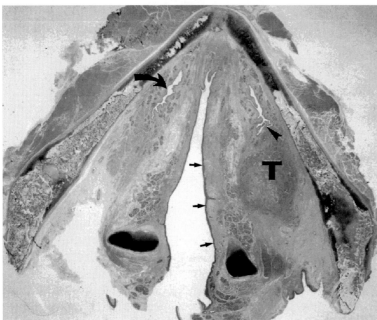

c

Fig. 5.3a–c. Neoplastic invasion of the left paraglottic space due to ventricular cancer. Endoscopically only a very small mucosal lesion was present within the left laryngeal ventricle. **a** Axial contrast-enhanced CT image at the supraglottic level shows an enhancing tumor mass (*T*) obliterating the left paraglottic fat. Note for comparison the normal aspect of the right paraglottic space (*arrowhead*). **b** Axial contrast-enhanced T1-weighted SE image obtained in the same patient at the same level shows an enhancing tumor mass (*arrows*) invading the left paraglottic fat. **c** Whole-organ axial slice from specimen confirms extensive paraglottic space invasion by a predominantly submucosal tumor mass (*T*). The tumor mass originates from the left laryngeal ventricle (*arrowhead*). *Curved arrow* points to the right laryngeal ventricle. Note the normal aspect of the laryngeal mucosa overlying the tumor mass (*small arrows*). Hematoxylin-eosin stain

1998a, 1998b, 2000; Becker and Hasso 1996; Becker and Kurt 1999; Zbären et al. 1996, 1997a).

Tumors arising in the arytenoid or interarytenoid region usually display an aggressive behavior and infiltrate the postcricoid portion of the hypopharynx (Fig. 5.4). Because they tend to spread submucosally, cross-sectional images are the only means of demonstrating the full extent of tumor spread prior to treatment.

The primary lymphatic spread of supraglottic carcinomas is directed toward the superior jugular lymph nodes. Lymph node metastases are common and often bilateral.

5.2.1.1.2
Glottic Carcinoma

Glottic carcinoma typically arises from the anterior half of the vocal cord and primarily spreads ventrally into the anterior commissure (Fig. 5.5). Evaluation of the anterior commissure can be easily done endoscopically and does not warrant cross-sectional imaging. The anterior commissure consists of the anterior attachment of the true vocal cords. Histologically, the anterior attachment of the true vocal cords is composed of dense, avascular fibroelastic tissue which acts as a relative barrier to early glottic cancer (Kirchner and Fischer 1975). Once the tumor has

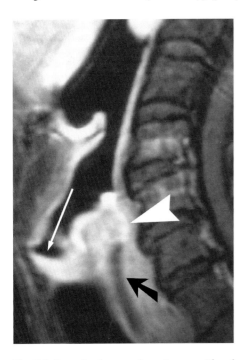

Fig. 5.4. Posterior laryngeal carcinoma with submucosal involvement of the retrocricoid region. Sagittal, contrast-enhanced fat-saturated T1-weighted SE image shows a tumor mass arising from the mucosa overlying the arytenoid with submucosal involvement of the retroarytenoid region (*arrowhead*). The *white arrow* points to the entrance to the ventricle. The *black arrow* points to the posterior portion of the cricoid cartilage. Reproduced with permission from BECKER 1998a

reached the anterior commissure it may easily spread into the supraglottis or subglottis (Fig. 5.5). This type of tumor spread is best evaluated with cross-sectional imaging. On axial CT and MR images neoplastic invasion occurring at the subglottic level below the anterior commissure appears as an irregular thickening of the cricothyroid membrane (BECKER 1998a, 1998b). The prelaryngeal soft tissues may then become invaded via the natural defects formed by the neurovascular bundles within this membrane, or at the line of its attachment to the undersurface of the thyroid cartilage (MANCUSO 1991; MANCUSO et al. 1980; YEAGER and ARCHER 1982). In the presence of significant anterior subglottic spread, invasion of the thyroid cartilage at the anterior commissure is likely.

Posterior extension of early glottic cancer into the anterior process of the arytenoid is relatively uncommon, and initial involvement of the posterior commissure is rare. Nevertheless, advanced glottic carcinomas may spread along the free edge of the vocal cords into the posterior commissure. The posterior commissure comprises the mucosa overlying the medial face of the arytenoids. Because the posterior commissure can be easily evaluated endoscopically, cross-sectional imaging is not warranted to evaluate this structure alone. Nonetheless, the radiologist should be aware of a potential pitfall at the time of CT examination. Because the mucosa of the

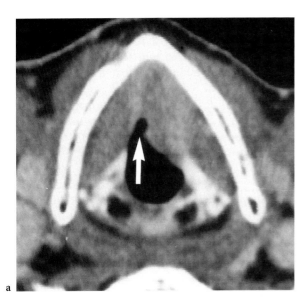

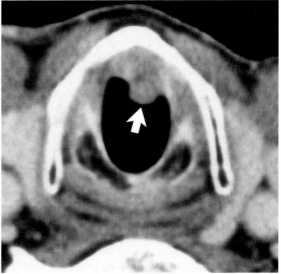

Fig. 5.5a, b. Glottic cancer with invasion of the anterior commissure and subglottis. **a** Axial contrast-enhanced CT scan at the glottic level shows a left-sided mass invading the anterior commissure (*arrow*) and the right vocal cord. The tumor mass also abuts the thyroid cartilage. **b** CT scan obtained at a lower level shows tumor extension into the anterior subglottic region (*arrow*). Reproduced with permission from BECKER 1998a

posterior commissure bunches up during adduction of the vocal cords, it may simulate pathologic thickening due to tumor. CT of the larynx therefore should always be performed during quiet respiration (open glottis). From the posterior commissure tumor may then spread into the arytenoid and cricoid cartilage or into the cricoarytenoid joint. Invasion of the cricoarytenoid joint is difficult to detect with both CT and MRI. Primary posterior glottic tumors may also invade the cricoarytenoid joint as well as the submucosa of the apex of the piriform sinus, thereby gaining access to its lymphatic drainage (MANCUSO 1991; MANCUSO and HANAFEE 1983, 1985; MANCUSO et al. 1978)

When a glottic tumor spreads laterally, it eventually invades the thyroarytenoid muscle thus leading to vocal cord fixation. If the vocal cord is fixed, the tumor will be staged T3 according to the UICC and AJCC guidelines. Subglottic spread is relatively common and may either occur superficial or deep to the elastic cone (KIRCHNER and CARTER 1987; KLEINSASSER 1988c; ZBÄREN et al. 1996, 1997a). Deep subglottic spread is very difficult to detect endoscopically, and underestimation of the tumor may occur unless CT or MR imaging is performed. The degree of subglottic spread and the relationship between tumor and the cricoid are best displayed on axial images (Fig. 5.5). Coronal images are of limited help in assessment of subglottic spread, because they are difficult to interpret except in the midcoronal plane.

Lymphatic metastases from glottic carcinoma are uncommon as long as the tumor is confined to the endolarynx. However, once it has traversed the cricothyroid membrane the frequency of lymph node metastases increases significantly (CURTIN 1996; MILLION et al. 1994).

5.2.1.1.3
Transglottic Carcinoma

The term "transglottic carcinoma" generally refers to tumors that involve both the glottis and supraglottis at the time of diagnosis (MANCUSO 1991; MILLION et al. 1994). Opinions differ, however, as to whether this automatically implies that the tumor has crossed the laryngeal ventricle since transglottic growth can occur either anteriorly or posteriorly to the laryngeal ventricle (Fig. 5.2). Some authors restrict the term "transglottic" to tumors that originate from the laryngeal ventricle and grow primarily submucosally into the paraglottic space. In any case, transglottic involvement implies advanced disease and an unfavorable prognosis (KIRCHNER and CARTER 1987). The submucosal growth pattern is readily recog-

nized on CT and MR images although endoscopically it becomes visible only if it causes the mucosa to bulge but remains entirely occult otherwise. Transglottic carcinoma involving the anterior commissure can display a very aggressive behavior, resulting in infiltration of intact layers of perichondrium and replacement of the thyroid cartilage with neoplastic tissue (KIRCHNER 1984; KIRCHNER and CARTER 1987; MAFEE et al. 1983, 1984; MANCUSO 1991). Such tumors are usually underestimated at endoscopy and CT or MR images are necessary to demonstrate their true extent prior to treatment. Transglottic carcinoma is very often accompanied by lymph node metastases.

5.2.1.1.4
Subglottic Carcinoma

Involvement of the subglottis by laryngeal cancer usually represents inferior spread of a glottic or supraglottic tumor rather than a primary tumor originating in the subglottis. True subglottic tumors are relatively uncommon and are regarded by many investigators as a distinct form of laryngeal carcinoma. According to the literature, 1–8% of all laryngeal tumors are included under this term (KLEINSASSER 1988a). Diagnosis of primary subglottic cancer may be delayed as patients present relatively late in the disease process with symptoms, such as stridor, hoarseness, dysphagia or palpable low cervical lymph nodes. In addition, in our experience, these tumors often present as submucosal masses endoscopically, and initial endoscopic biopsy may be negative.

In our experience, a characteristic circular extension of the tumor taking up almost the entire subglottic lumen may be recognized at cross-sectional imaging (Fig. 5.6). Primary subglottic tumors may also spread superiorly and posteriorly into the posterior commissure or cervical esophagus. Invasion of the extralaryngeal structures is seen in about one-half of all subglottic carcinomas at the time of initial diagnosis.

Lymph node metastases are much more common than in glottic carcinoma. The primary drainage is directed toward the paratracheal and pretracheal nodes. These nodes drain to the lower jugular or upper mediastinal nodes.

5.2.1.2
Hypopharynx

5.2.1.2.1
Carcinoma of the Piriform Sinus

Carcinoma of the piriform sinus is readily detected with endoscopy. Early superficial spreading tumors

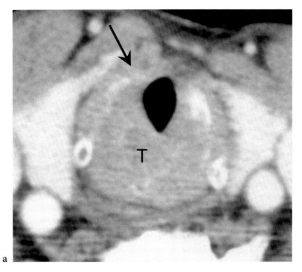
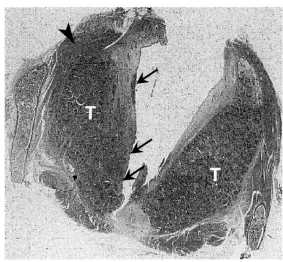

a   b

Fig. 5.6a, b. Primary subglottic cancer. Patient presenting with dyspnea. Endoscopy revealed a relatively small mucosal lesion situated below the posterior commissure and in the right subglottis. The rest of the mucosa appeared tumor-free, but diffuse subglottic narrowing was observed endoscopically. **a** Contrast-enhanced CT at the subglottic level shows circumferential subglottic tumor (*T*) with destruction of the cricoid ring and invasion of paralaryngeal strap muscles (*arrow*). The rest of the larynx was tumor-free. **b** Corresponding histologic slice from specimen confirms circumferential subglottic tumor (*T*) with massive destruction of the cricoid cartilage. Note the relatively small mucosal component (*arrows*) as opposed to the extensive submucosal component (*arrowhead* invasion of the paralaryngeal strap muscles). Hematoxylin-eosin stain. Reproduced with permission from BECKER 1998b

that are limited to the mucosa may be invisible at cross-sectional imaging although more advanced lesions are readily diagnosed on axial CT or MR images. Because the piriform sinus is usually collapsed during quiet respiration the exact tumor location may be difficult to determine. During a CT study, the piriform sinus can be unfolded during image acquisition by means of a modified Valsalva's maneuver. Tumors originating from the lateral wall of the piriform sinus infiltrate toward the common carotid artery. If the tumor encompasses more than 270° of the circumference of the vessel on axial images it becomes unlikely that it can be removed without resecting the artery (YOUSEM et al. 1995). Tumors involving primarily the medial wall or the angle of the piriform sinus may infiltrate the larynx by growing anteriorly into the paraglottic space (BECKER 1998a, 2000; BECKER and HASSO 1996; MANCUSO 1991; MILLION et al. 1994; WEISSMAN and HOLLIDAY 1996) (Fig. 5.7). This tumor growth may be clinically occult. More advanced piriform sinus tumors typically grow caudally into the apex. Once they have reached the apex, they may spread either into the larynx invading the arytenoid, cricoarytenoid joint and subglottis, or they may spread into the postcricoid region of the hypopharynx. Further caudal spread results in invasion of the tracheoesophageal groove and esophageal verge (Fig. 5.8). Invasion of the esophageal

verge may be submucosal and, therefore, undetectable at endoscopy. However, on both axial CT and MR images invasion of the esophageal verge is easy to diagnose. Piriform sinus carcinoma frequently invades the laryngeal framework.

5.2.1.2.2
Carcinoma of the Postcricoid Region

Carcinoma of the retrocricoarytenoid region, also called "postcricoid carcinoma", is a particular tumor type which is uncommon in general but is observed in certain groups at risk, e.g., patients with the Plummer–Vinson (or Paterson–Brown–Kelly) syndrome (BECKER 1998a; KLEINSASSER 1988a, 1988b; MILLION et al. 1994). These tumors spread submucosally, either circumferentially or toward the cervical esophagus. Because tumor growth is mainly submucosal, the true extent only becomes apparent with axial or sagittal CT or MR images (Fig. 5.9). Invasion of the cricoid cartilage is common, and in some cases the tumor may grow beyond the posterior cricoarytenoid muscle into the thyroid gland and cervical trachea.

5.2.1.2.3
Carcinoma of the Posterior Pharyngeal Wall

Carcinoma of the posterior pharyngeal wall commonly presents as a flat, thick tumor spreading at the

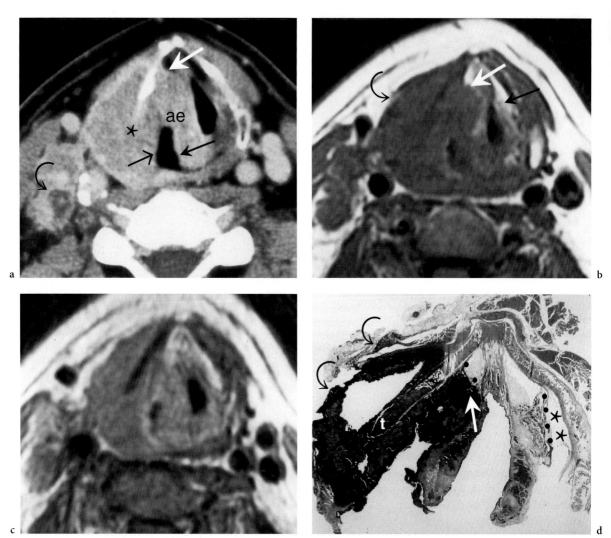

Fig. 5.7a–d. Invasion of the paraglottic space by piriform sinus cancer. **a** Axial contrast-enhanced CT image at the supraglottic level shows a hypopharyngeal tumor mass involving the medial wall (*arrow*) and the lateral wall (*open arrow*) of the piriform sinus and the entire right aryepiglottic fold (*ae*). Invasion of the paraglottic space (*thick arrow*), destruction of the posterior thyroid lamina (*asterisk*) and invasion of the prelaryngeal muscles. A large lymph node metastasis with central nodal necrosis (*curved arrow*) is seen on the right. **b** Axial unenhanced T1-weighted SE image obtained in the same patient at the same level shows a tumor mass with an intermediate signal intensity as it extends into the right paraglottic space (*thick arrow*) and into the soft tissues of the neck (*curved arrow*). Note the high signal intensity of the non-invaded left paraglottic space due to the high content of fatty tissue (*thin arrow*). **c** Axial Gd-enhanced T1-weighted SE image at the same level shows enhancement of the tumor mass invading the right paraglottic space, the thyroid cartilage and the soft tissues of the neck. **d** Whole-organ axial histologic slice from specimen confirms tumor invasion of the right paraglottic space (*thick arrow*) and of the soft tissues of the neck (*curved arrows*) (*t* thyroid cartilage, *asterisks* normal left paraglottic space, *dots* right and left thyroglottic ligaments separating the paraglottic from the preepiglottic space). Note massive anterior displacement of the right thyroglottic ligament by the tumor mass. Hematoxylin-eosin stain. Reproduced with permission from Becker et al. 1995a

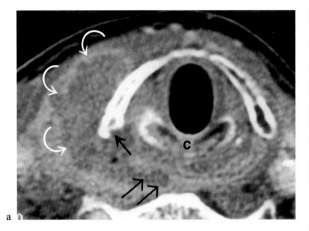
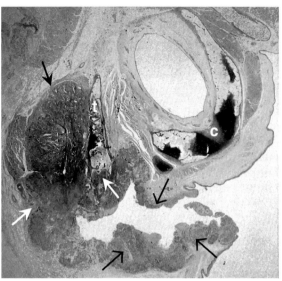

Fig. 5.8a, b. Invasion of the esophageal verge in a piriform sinus cancer. **a** Axial contrast-enhanced CT image at the subglottic level shows a piriform sinus tumor invading the posterior thyroid lamina (*arrow*), the soft tissues of the neck (*curved arrows*) and the esophageal verge submucosally (*open arrows*) (*c* cricoid cartilage). **b** Whole-organ axial histologic slice from specimen confirms submucosal tumor invasion of the esophageal verge (*open arrows*) and invasion of the thyroid cartilage and of the soft tissues of the neck (*arrows*) (*t* thyroid cartilage, *c* cricoid cartilage). Hematoxylin-eosin stain. Reproduced with permission from BECKER and KURT 1999

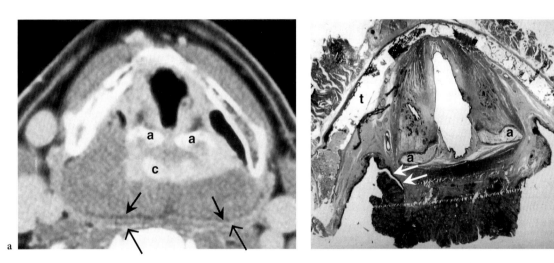

Fig. 5.9a, b. Postcricoid carcinoma of the hypopharynx. **a** Axial contrast-enhanced CT scan at the glottic level demonstrates a large tumor arising from the postcricoid region and extending into the right piriform sinus. The lumen of the hypopharynx is collapsed (*arrows*). Note strong enhancement of the normal mucosa over the posterior pharyngeal wall (*open arrows*) (*c* cricoid cartilage, *a* arytenoid cartilage). **b** Whole-organ axial histologic slice from specimen confirms postcricoid tumor (*T*) with invasion of the medial wall of the piriform sinus (*arrows*) (*t* thyroid cartilage, *a* arytenoid cartilage). Hematoxylin-eosin stain. Reproduced with permission from BECKER 1998a

mucosal surface and often involves both the oropharynx and hypopharynx (BECKER 1998a; MANCUSO 1991; MANCUSO and HANAFEE 1983, 1985; MANCUSO et al. 1978). These tumors are readily diagnosed at endoscopy but cross-sectional imaging is needed to evaluate the degree of submucosal spread. On axial CT or MR images, these tumors appear as asymmetric thickening of the posterior wall (Fig. 5.10). Most posterior pharyngeal wall tumors have a tendency to stop at about the level of the arytenoid cartilages. However, cranial spread to the pharyngoepiglottic fold, glossotonsillar sulcus and posterior oropharyngeal wall is common. Spread to the postcricoid region and invasion of laryngeal cartilages are both uncommon. Although invasion of the retropharyngeal space may be common initially, involvement of the prevertebral muscles is unusual at initial presentation (Fig. 5.10).

5.2.2
Neoplastic Cartilage Invasion

5.2.2.1
Significance of Cartilage Invasion

Neoplastic invasion of cartilage or bone is generally believed to diminish the response to radiation therapy, and to increase the risk of tumor recurrence and radiation-induced necrosis (BECKER et al. 1997a; CASTELIJNS et al. 1996a; 1996b; CURTIN 1989, 1995).

Several recent studies have shown that a variety of CT- and MR-based parameters, such as tumor volume, neoplastic cartilage invasion, tumor invasion of the preepiglottic space, paraglottic space and subglottis appear to be powerful predictors of local outcome in laryngeal and hypopharyngeal cancer treated with radiation therapy (CASTELIJNS et al. 1996b; HERMANS et al. 1999a, 1999b; MANCUSO et al. 1999; PAMEIJER et al. 1997, 1998, 1999). (The prognostic significance of CT- and MR-related parameters is extensively discussed in Chap. 7.) The prognostic implication of invasion of cartilage by laryngeal and hypopharyngeal tumors is reflected in the TNM classification, leading automatically to a T4 classification (see below). For these reasons, the diagnosis of cartilage invasion deserves particular attention.

5.2.2.2
Histologic Mechanisms of Cartilage Invasion

Cartilage invasion occurs preferentially where the attachments of collagen bundles (Sharpney's fibers) interrupt the perichondrium, thus acting as direct pathways for tumor spread into the cartilaginous tissue. These areas typically include the anterior commissure, the junction of the anterior quarter and posterior three-quarters of the lower thyroid lamina, the posterior border of the thyroid lamina, the cricoarytenoid joint and the area of attachment of the cricothyroid membrane (CARTER and TANNER 1979;

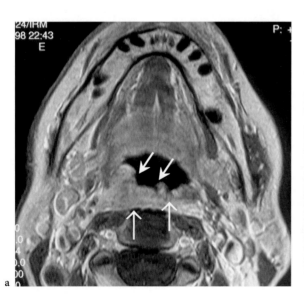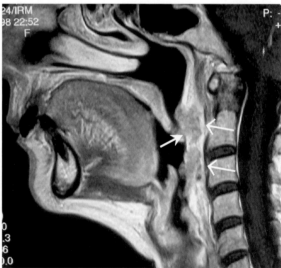

Fig. 5.10a, b. Posterior wall carcinoma. Axial, contrast-enhanced T1-weighted SE image (**a**) and sagittal, contrast-enhanced T1-weighted SE image (**b**) show a moderately enhancing tumor (*arrows*) involving the posterior wall of the oropharynx and hypopharynx. Note infiltration of the pharyngeal constrictor muscles and invasion of the retropharyngeal space (*open arrows*). The prevertebral muscles are not involved

HARRISON 1984; KIRCHNER 1984; YEAGER and AR-
CHER 1982).

A commonly held notion is that ossified cartilage is
much more prone to invasion by cancer than nonossified cartilage. This has been attributed to the activity of
a tumor angiogenetic factor (TAF), whereas nonossified cartilage is thought to be resistant to tumor infiltration due to its capacity to release proteins which in-
hibit TAF and also collagenases (BECKER et al. 1995a;
BENNETT et al. 1980; CARTER and TANNER 1979; GALLO
et al. 1992; GREGOR and HAMMOND 1987; GREGOR et al.
1981; HARRISON 1984). Recent work has indicated,
however, that invasion of nonossified hyaline cartilage
may be more common than previously thought by
showing that in 11% of invaded cartilages, invasion is
limited to nonossified portions, leaving ossified portions intact (BECKER et al. 1997b).

The suggested mechanism of laryngeal cartilage
invasion by neoplastic tissue involves an osteoblastic
phase in which hyaline cartilage is transformed into
bone which is followed by an osteoclastic phase in
which the newly formed bone is eroded. Osteoclasts
are stimulated by prostaglandins and interleukin-1
released by tumor cells. This process is not bound to
the direct presence of tumor cells within cartilage but
occurs also as a reaction within cartilage in the vicinity of tumor. Increased osteoblastic activity and new
bone formation are, therefore, seen even before tumor
penetrates the perichondrium. In summary, the process of neoplastic invasion of laryngeal cartilage involves three distinct phases, namely (1) inflammatory
changes within cartilage adjacent to tumor inducing
new bone formation prior to actual tumor invasion,
(2) osteolysis, and (3) frank invasion by tumor cells.

5.2.2.3
Detection of Neoplastic Cartilage Invasion with CT

The CT features of the laryngeal cartilages in adults
are explained by the different attenuation values of
their three tissue components: cortical bone, marrow
cavity with high fatty content, and nonossified hyaline cartilage. The ossification pattern of laryngeal
cartilage and particularly the thyroid cartilage is
quite variable (CASTELIJNS et al. 1996a; YEAGER and
ARCHER 1982). Although tumor tissue by itself has
very similar attenuation values to those of nonossified cartilage, the presence of tumor may also be the
cause of new bone formation and osteolysis in the
adjacent cartilage. Therefore, patterns of ossification
caused by neoplastic growth must be clearly distinguished from anatomical variants.

The accuracy of CT for the detection of laryngeal
cartilage invasion varies considerably among different reports in the literature (Table 5.1). These dis-
crepancies may in part be explained in terms of variable technical parameters. For example, older studies
were based on scan times of 4–9 s/slice and 4–6 mm
section thickness (CASTELIJNS et al. 1988; SULFARO et
al. 1989) and thus were more prone to motion and volume averaging artifacts than current standard protocols. Of more influence, however, are the diagnostic
criteria used by the different investigators to assess
invasion of each cartilage (Table 5.1). Until recently,
the presence of tumor on both sides of a laryngeal cartilage was the only generally accepted diagnostic sign
for tumor invasion on CT (CASTELIJNS et al. 1988;
CURTIN 1989, 1995, 1996). Because this sign is positive

Table 5.1. Neoplastic invasion of the laryngeal cartilage: CT versus histology. Note: All surgical specimens were evaluated by whole-organ histologic slices. Reproduced with permission from BECKER 1998a

Reference	No. of patients	Sensitivity (%)	Specificity (%)	Negative predictive value (%)
CASTELIJNS et al. (1988)	16	46	91	69
SULFARO et al. (1989)	71	47	88	–
BECKER et al. (1995a)	53	66	94	86
ZBÄREN et al. (1996)	40	67	87	82
BECKER et al. (1997b)	111[a]	61[a]	92[a]	85[a]
	111[b]	91[b]	68[b]	95[b]
	111[c]	82[c]	79[c]	85[c]

[a] Results obtained using a combination of the CT criteria extralaryngeal tumor spread and erosion or lysis applied to all cartilages

[b] Results obtained using a combination of the CT criteria extralaryngeal tumor spread, sclerosis and erosion or lysis applied to all cartilages

[c] Results obtained using a combination of the CT criteria extralaryngeal tumor spread and erosion or lysis applied to all cartilages, and sclerosis applied to the cricoid and arytenoid, but not the thyroid cartilage

only in an advanced stage, CT was long considered to be insensitive to cartilage invasion.

In order to increase the sensitivity of CT, several other diagnostic signs have been proposed, including changes of the cartilage itself, namely sclerosis, obliteration of the medullary cavity, serpiginous contour, bowing, cartilaginous blow-out and the presence of tumor adjacent to nonossified cartilage (BECKER et al. 1995a, 1997b; KAVANAGH et al. 1985; MAFEE et al. 1983, 1984; MUÑOZ et al. 1993; SILVERMAN 1985). In a recent prospective study including 111 patients we have evaluated the usefulness of each of these criteria using cross-sectional histopathologic findings of the resected specimens as

the gold standard (BECKER et al. 1997b). The results of our study indicate that four different diagnostic signs and their combinations can be recommended to detect neoplastic invasion of laryngeal cartilage on CT, namely extralaryngeal tumor spread, sclerosis, erosion and lysis. Each of these CT signs corresponds to distinct histologic findings and has either a high sensitivity or a high specificity (BECKER et al. 1997b, 1998c).

Sclerosis (Fig. 5.11) is a sensitive sign for the detection of neoplastic cartilage invasion and enables diagnosis of early perichondrial invasion or microscopic intracartilaginous tumor spread. The specificity of this sign varies considerably from one cartilage to an-

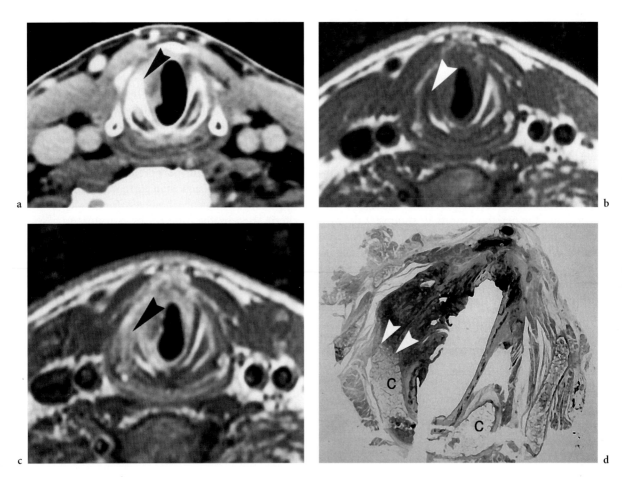

Fig. 5.11a–d. Neoplastic invasion of the cricoid cartilage detected by both CT and MRI. Glottosubglottic carcinoma of the larynx in a 46-year-old male patient. **a** Axial contrast-enhanced CT scan at the subglottic level. A mass with homogeneous contrast enhancement is infiltrating the right subglottic region. The cricoid cartilage shows asymmetric sclerosis (*arrowhead*) indicating cartilage invasion. Note preservation of the inner margin of the cricoid cartilage. **b** Axial T1-weighted SE image. A mass with intermediate signal intensity infiltrates the right subglottic region. The right cricoid cartilage shows a decreased signal intensity (*arrowhead*). **c** Contrast-enhanced axial T1-weighted SE image shows extensive contrast enhancement of the right subglottic tumor mass, as well as of the adjacent cricoid cartilage. The extensive enhancement of the right cricoid cartilage (*arrowhead*) suggests tumor invasion. **d** Axial slice from specimen at the same level shows a large subglottic tumor mass invading the right cricoid cartilage (*arrowheads*) (*C* cricoid cartilage). Hematoxylin-eosin stain. Reproduced with permission from BECKER et al. 1995a

other, being lowest in the thyroid cartilage (40%) and higher in the cricoid and arytenoid cartilages (76% and 79%, respectively) (BECKER et al. 1997b). Therefore, if a tumor mass is seen adjacent to a sclerotic cartilage, this does not automatically imply that tumor cells are found within the remodeled marrow cavity (Fig. 5.12). Conversely, failing at surgery to remove a cartilage that exhibits sclerosis on CT carries a 50–60% risk of leaving tumor behind. As the process of cartilage invasion progresses, minor and major osteolysis is seen within the areas of new bone formation. Minor areas of osteolysis correspond to the CT criteria of *erosion*, while major areas of osteolysis correspond to the CT criteria of *lysis* (Figs. 5.13, 5.14). Histologically, erosion and lysis correspond to de-

struction of bone due to osteoclastic activity, and a direct contact between receding bone and tumor cells is seen within these lytic areas. As a consequence, erosion and lysis can be considered specific criteria for the detection of neoplastic invasion in all cartilages (Figs. 5.13, 5.14). The overall specificity of erosion and lysis is 93%. However, both of these criteria are not very sensitive as they are bound to the presence of more advanced invasion of laryngeal cartilage (BECKER et al. 1997b) (Table 5.1). *Extralaryngeal spread* occurs due to tumor invasion through a cartilage into the extralaryngeal soft tissues (Figs. 5.7, 5.8). This CT criterion is highly specific (overall specificity 95%), but because it is only seen very late in the disease process its sensitivity is as low as 44%.

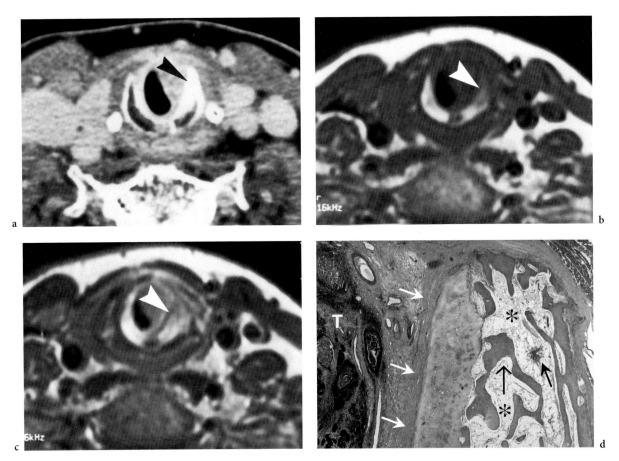

Fig. 5.12a–d. CT and MRI false-positive for neoplastic cartilage invasion due to inflammatory changes in the non-invaded cricoid cartilage. Glottosubglottic carcinoma of the larynx in a 71-year-old female patient. **a** Axial contrast-enhanced CT scan at the subglottic level. A mass with homogeneous contrast enhancement is infiltrating the left subglottic region. The left cricoid cartilage shows extensive sclerosis in the vicinity of the tumor (*arrowhead*) suggestive of cartilage invasion. **b** T1-weighted axial SE image. A mass with low signal intensity infiltrates the left subglottic region. The adjacent left cricoid cartilage shows a decreased signal intensity (*arrowhead*). **c** Contrast-enhanced T1-weighted SE image. Contrast enhancement is seen in the left cricoid cartilage (*arrowhead*) as well as in the subglottic tumor mass. **d** Axial slice from specimen shows a large left-sided subglottic tumor mass (*T*) but no evidence of cartilage invasion. The cricoid cartilage shows extensive inflammatory changes with lymph follicles (*black arrow*), fibrosis (*asterisks*) and bone resorption (*open arrow*), but with an intact perichondrium (*white arrows*). Hematoxylin-eosin stain (original magnification +6.25). Reproduced with permission from BECKER et al. 1995a

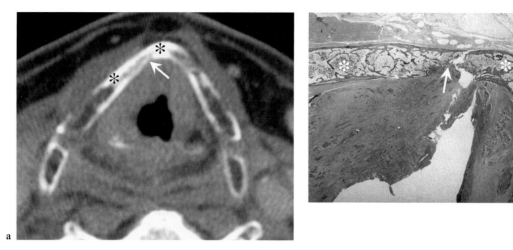

Fig. 5.13a, b. Erosion of the thyroid cartilage in a transglottic cancer. **a** Contrast-enhanced CT scan obtained at the false cord level shows a tumor mass that abuts the thyroid cartilage. The right thyroid lamina demonstrates a small erosion (*arrow*) and extensive sclerosis (*asterisks*). **b** Corresponding axial slice from surgical specimen confirms minor invasion of the thyroid cartilage (*arrow*) corresponding to the small erosion seen on CT. Note increased density of bone trabeculae (*asterisks*) surrounding the area of actual invasion and corresponding to sclerosis seen in **a**. Hematoxylin-eosin stain. Reproduced with permission from BECKER 1998a

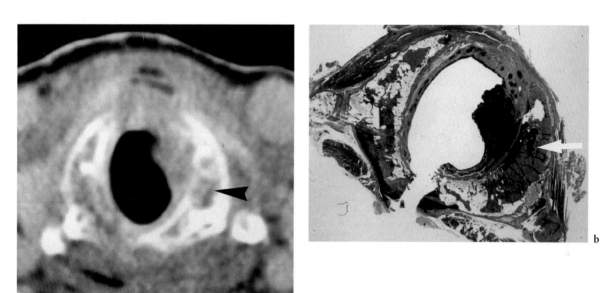

Fig. 5.14a, b. Lysis and sclerosis of the cricoid cartilage in a glottic-subglottic cancer. **a** Contrast-enhanced CT scan obtained at the subglottic level shows a tumor mass that abuts the cricoid cartilage. The left cricoid lamina demonstrates an area of lysis (*arrowhead*) surrounded by extensive sclerosis. **b** Corresponding axial slice from surgical specimen at the same level confirms major intracartilaginous tumor spread (*arrow*) corresponding to lysis seen on CT. Hematoxylin-eosin stain. Reproduced with permission from BECKER 1998a

Using the combination of extralaryngeal tumor, sclerosis, and erosion/lysis applied to all cartilages an overall sensitivity as high as 91% may be obtained (Table 5.1). Because the negative predictive value of this combination is 95%, CT may be considered as an excellent test to exclude cartilage invasion prior to treatment. On the other hand, the associated overall specificity of only 68% appears quite low because it is very difficult and impractical to confirm cartilage invasion by means of biopsy. The use of extralaryngeal tumor and erosion/lysis applied to all cartilages yields a specificity of 92%, but the associated sensitivity is only 61% (Table 5.1).

5.2.2.4
Detection of Neoplastic Cartilage Invasion with MRI

The diagnosis of neoplastic cartilage invasion on MRI is mainly based on an altered signal behavior of hyaline cartilage and fatty marrow on the different pulse sequences. On T2-weighted images hyaline cartilage invaded by tumor displays a higher signal intensity than normal cartilage. On unenhanced T1-weighted images invaded hyaline cartilage and invaded fatty marrow display a low to intermediate signal intensity similar to that of tumor tissue whereas areas of enhancement adjacent to the tumor are seen after injection of gadolinium chelates (BECKER 1998a, 1998b, 2000; BECKER and HASSO 1996; BECKER et al. 1995a; CASTELIJNS et al. 1987, 1988; CURTIN 1996) (Fig. 5.11). If these signs are absent, cartilage infiltration can be ruled out with a high level of confidence (Fig. 5.15), as indicated by a very high negative predictive value (Table 5.2).

Unfortunately, the MR findings suggesting neoplastic cartilage invasion are not as specific as expected initially but may be false-positive in a considerable number of instances as indicated by a positive predictive value of only 68–71% (BECKER 1998a,

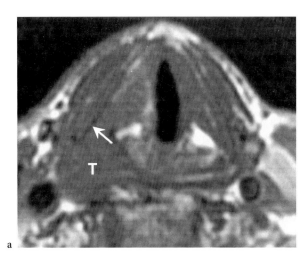
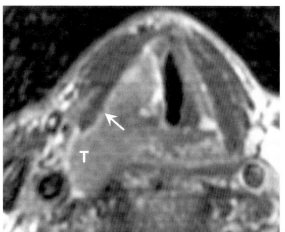
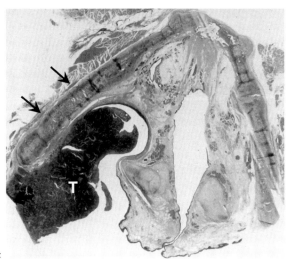

Fig. 5.15a–c. MRI findings true negative for neoplastic invasion of the thyroid cartilage. **a** T1-weighted SE image obtained at the supraglottic level shows a right-sided piriform sinus tumor with intermediate to low signal intensity (*T*). The adjacent right thyroid lamina shows an intermediate to low signal intensity as well (*arrow*). **b** T1-weighted SE image obtained after intravenous administration of contrast material shows enhancement of the tumor mass (*T*), but no enhancement of the adjacent thyroid lamina (*arrow*). This suggests that the thyroid cartilage is composed of nonossified hyaline cartilage and that no intracartilaginous tumor spread is present. **c** Corresponding axial slice from surgical specimen at the same level confirms that the right thyroid lamina is composed of nonossified hyaline cartilage (*arrows*). No cartilage invasion was found at histology. The tumor (*T*) arises from the lateral wall of the right piriform sinus. Hematoxylin-eosin stain. Reproduced with permission from BECKER 1998a

Table 5.2. Neoplastic invasion of the laryngeal cartilage: MRI versus histology. Note: All surgical specimens were evaluated by whole-organ histologic slices. Modified with permission from BECKER 1998a

Reference	No. of patients	Sensitivity (%)	Specificity (%)	Negative predictive value (%)
CASTELIJNS et al. (1988)	16	89	88	92
BECKER et al. (1995a)	53	89	84	94
ZBÄREN et al. (1996)	40	94	74	96
BECKER (unpublished data, 2001)	121	92	74	97

1998b; BECKER et al. 1995a). This is because reactive inflammation, edema and fibrosis in the vicinity of the tumor may display diagnostic features similar to those of cartilage infiltrated by tumor (Fig. 5.12). Inflammatory changes within the fatty marrow associated with the above-mentioned process of bone remodeling that occurs in the vicinity of tumor prior to actual invasion of cartilage may appear as an increased signal on T2-weighted images and contrast material-enhanced T1-weighted images and thus be indistinguishable from neoplastic tissue. Since peritumoral inflammatory changes are most commonly observed in the thyroid cartilage, the specificity of MR imaging in detecting neoplastic invasion of the thyroid cartilage is only 56% as opposed to 87% and 95% in the cricoid and arytenoid cartilage (BECKER et al. 1995a). The positive diagnosis of neoplastic invasion of the thyroid cartilage should, therefore, be made with caution on MR imaging.

On the other hand, extensive tumor invasion involving both inner and outer aspects of the cartilage (i.e., corresponding to the CT criteria of extralaryngeal tumor) can be diagnosed with a high accuracy with MR imaging. The results of MR imaging reported in the literature are summarized in Table 5.2. Because all authors have used the same criteria to assess cartilage invasion by means of MRI, the reported overall results do not vary considerably except for minor differences that may be explained by the influences of sample size and patient characteristics.

5.2.2.5
The Choice: CT or MRI?

Due to their high sensitivity and high negative predictive value both MRI and CT may be used for pretherapeutic evaluation of cartilage invasion if the diagnostic criteria are selected and combined appropriately (BECKER 1998a; BECKER et al. 1995a; 1997b). False-positive results, however, are inevitable with both imaging modalities. Despite the entirely different physical mechanisms by which tissue is interrogated with CT and MRI the tendency toward "over-

reading" tumor involvement is strikingly parallel with regard to each individual cartilage. This may be explained by the fact that the underlying pathologic process leading to overestimation of neoplastic cartilage invasion is the same, namely reactive inflammation.

5.2.3
Tumor Classification According to the TNM System

The purpose of tumor staging according to the TNM system is to help assess the prognosis and facilitate clinical research. The staging criteria for laryngeal and hypopharyngeal carcinoma proposed by the International Union Against Cancer (UICC) and the American Joint Commission on Cancer (AJCC) are now identical (HERMANEK et al. 1993, 1998) (Tables 5.3 and 5.4). The degree of invasion of the primary tumor is most accurately reflected in the postsurgical (pT) classification which is based on histopathologic analysis of the resected specimen. The clinical or pretherapeutic (T) classification of the primary tumor is used in patients who do not undergo surgery. It is based on all information available prior to treatment, including findings on physical examination, endoscopy, biopsy and cross-sectional imaging.

The guidelines of both the UICC and the AJCC recommend the use of imaging, and several studies as well as the experience at our institution have shown that the use of cross-sectional imaging greatly improves the accuracy of pretherapeutic T-classification of laryngeal and hypopharyngeal tumors (Table 5.5). However, no recommendations are made by the UICC or AJCC regarding the preference for one technique or another. In a prospective study we have compared the T and the pT classifications in 111 patients who underwent clinical examination with endoscopy as well as both CT and MR imaging prior to surgery. Using the pT classification as the gold standard, the staging accuracy of clinical examination with endoscopy was only 58%, but it was in-

Table 5.3. Classification of primary tumor (T) for carcinoma of the larynx according to UICC and AJCC

Tx	Primary tumor cannot be assessed
T0	No evidence of primary tumor
Tis	Carcinoma in situ

Supraglottis

T1	Tumor limited to one subsite of supraglottis with normal vocal cord mobility
T2	Tumor invades more than one subsite of supraglottis or glottis, with normal vocal cord mobility
T3	Tumor limited to larynx with vocal cord fixation and/or invasion of postcricoid area, medial wall of piriform sinus or preepiglottic space
T4	Tumor invades through thyroid cartilage or extends to other tissues beyond the larynx, e.g., to oropharynx, soft tissues of neck

Glottis

T1	Tumor limited to vocal cord(s), may involve anterior or posterior commissure with normal mobility
T1a	Tumor limited to one vocal cord
T1b	Tumor involves both vocal cords
T2	Tumor extends to supraglottis or subglottis or with impaired vocal cord mobility
T3	Tumor limited to the larynx with vocal cord fixation
T4	Tumor invades through thyroid cartilage or extends to other tissues beyond the larynx, e.g., to oropharynx, soft tissues of the neck

Subglottis

T1	Tumor limited to the subglottis
T2	Tumor extends to vocal cord(s) with normal or impaired mobility
T3	Tumor limited to the larynx with vocal cord fixation
T4	Tumor invades through cricoid or thyroid cartilage or extends to other tissues beyond the larynx, e.g., to oropharynx, soft tissues of the neck

Table 5.4. Classification of primary tumor (T) for carcinoma of the hypopharynx according to UICC and AJCC

Tx	Primary tumor cannot be assessed
T0	No evidence of primary tumor
Tis	Carcinoma in situ
T1	Tumor limited to one subsite of the hypopharynx and less than 2 cm in size
T2	Tumor invades more than one subsite of hypopharynx or an adjacent site and measures more than 2 cm but less than 4 cm in size, without fixation of hemilarynx
T3	Tumor measures more than 4 cm, with fixation of hemilarynx
T4	Tumor invades adjacent structures, e.g., cartilage, soft tissues of neck, thyroid gland, neck vessels, esophagus

Table 5.5. Overall pretherapeutic staging accuracy for laryngeal and hypopharyngeal cancer, as reported by several study groups. Note: The staging accuracy was evaluated considering the pathologic stage (pT) as gold standard (*CE* clinical evaluation including direct laryngoscopy and biopsy, *CE-CT* combined information from clinical evaluation including direct laryngoscopy and biopsy and CT, *CE-MRI* combined information from clinical evaluation including direct laryngoscopy and biopsy and MRI). Reproduced with permission from Becker 1998a

Reference	No. of patients	Tumor origin	CE (%)	CE-CT (%)	CE-MRI (%)
Sulfaro et al. (1989)	71	Larynx and hypopharynx	59	88	–
Vogl et al. (1991)	28	Larynx and hypopharynx	64	–	86
Dullerud et al. (1992)	51	Larynx	78	84	–
Zbären et al. (1996)	40	Larynx	57	80	87
Thabet et al. (1996)	98	Larynx and hypopharynx	52	84	–
Becker M (1997) (unpublished data, see text)	111	Larynx and hypopharynx	58	80	85

creased significantly when combined with either CT (accuracy 80%) or MR imaging (accuracy 85%) (M. BECKER, 1997, unpublished data). These results underline the usefulness of CT and MR imaging for pretherapeutic staging.

5.2.4
Atypical Forms of Squamous Cell Carcinoma

The term "atypical forms of squamous cell carcinoma" is used for certain distinct histopathologic variants of laryngeal and hypopharyngeal carcinoma with a different biologic behavior, namely, undifferentiated carcinoma of nasopharyngeal type, verrucous carcinoma, spindle cell carcinoma, basaloid cell carcinoma, adenoid squamous cell carcinoma and giant cell carcinoma. According to the literature, 2–7% of all laryngeal and hypopharyngeal tumors are atypical forms of squamous cell carcinoma. These tumors may differ from the common type of squamous cell carcinoma in several aspects regarding diagnosis, prognosis and therapeutic approach (BANKS et al. 1992; BATSAKIS 1979; BECKER et al. 1995b, 1998a, 1998b; FERLITO 1993; FERLITO and RECHER 1980; GLANZ and KLEINSASSER 1987; HYAMS et al. 1988; KLEINSASSER 1988c).

Undifferentiated carcinoma of nasopharyngeal type is an unusual variant of squamous cell carcinoma with a distinct lymphoid component (BECKER et al. 1998b; FERLITO 1993). Synonyms for this tumor include lymphoepithelial carcinoma and lymphoepithelioma Schmincke–Regaud. Infection with the Epstein–Barr virus (EBV) appears to play an important etiologic role. Patients with this type of tumor typically present with supraglottic or piriform sinus masses covered by an intact mucosa at endoscopic examination (Table 5.6). Since the tumor is rather deep-seated, biopsies must be obtained from beneath the mucosa or the lesion will be missed. Therefore, multiple biopsies may be necessary until the correct histologic diagnosis can be made.

Undifferentiated carcinoma of nasopharyngeal type often metastasizes to the cervical lymph nodes and sometimes to the lungs or other organs, and cervical lymph node metastases may be the first presenting symptom. Radiotherapy alone or in combination with chemotherapy appears to be effective in eradicating localized disease (FERLITO 1993; SHANMUGARATNAM et al. 1979; TOKER and PETERSON 1978). At CT and MRI the tumors are very large, display homogeneous enhancement, and do not show cartilage invasion, but very often show lymph node metastases. The characteristic radiologic features of this tumor type are summarized in Table 5.6 and are shown in Fig. 5.16.

Verrucous carcinoma or Ackerman tumor has a reported incidence of 1–4% of all laryngeal cancers (BATSAKIS 1979; BECKER et al. 1998b). It must not be confused with the common form of squamous cell carcinoma as it differs both in structural characteristics and prognosis, which is excellent when adequate treatment is adopted from the beginning. It occurs predominantly in men in their seventies and eighties and presents clinically as a warty, bulky outgrowth with multiple filiform projections usually affecting one vocal cord. Viral infection with the human papilloma virus (HPV) type 16 appears to play an important etiologic role (BRANDSMA et al. 1986). Verrucous carcinoma of the larynx almost never metastasizes to the lymph nodes. Considerable controversy exists as to the correct treatment for this tumor. A recurrence rate of 51–71% after radiation

Table 5.6. Atypical forms of squamous cell carcinoma: characteristic radiologic features. Reproduced with permission from BECKER et al. 1998b

Atypical form	Tumor location	Enhancement pattern, morphology	Lymph node metastases
Undifferentiated carcinoma of nasopharyngeal type	Supraglottis, hypopharynx, submucosal location	Homogeneous enhancement pattern, large tumor mass, no ulceration, no necrosis, no cartilage invasion	Yes
Verrucous carcinoma	Glottis	Inhomogeneous enhancement, exophytic mass with a rugged surface, limited deep infiltration, rarely cartilage invasion	No
Spindle cell carcinoma	Supraglottis	Inhomogeneous enhancement, bulky, ulcerated lesion, thin stalk	Variable
Basaloid cell carcinoma	Piriform sinus and retrocricoarytenoid region	Inhomogeneous, distinct lobulated enhancement on contrast-enhanced T_1-weighted SE images	Yes, extranodal spread

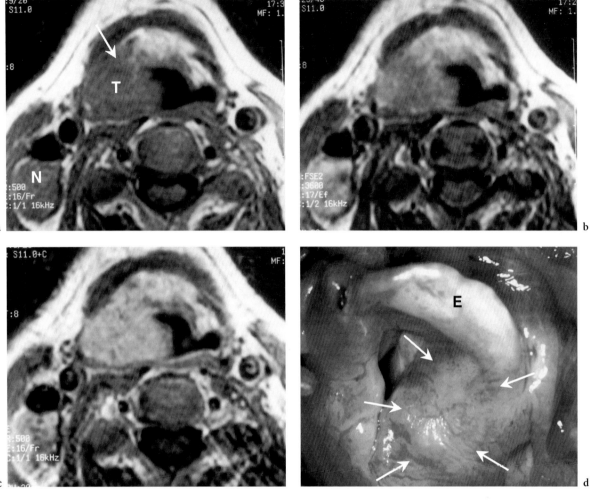

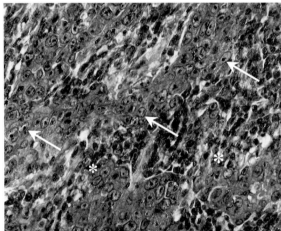

Fig. 5.16a–e. Undifferentiated carcinoma of nasopharyngeal type in a 76-year-old male patient with multiple palpable neck masses: MRI appearance. Endoscopically the right aryepiglottic fold was thicker than the left aryepiglottic fold; the mucosa was, however, intact. **a** Axial T1-weighted SE image. A tumor mass (*T*) with low signal intensity invades the right aryepiglottic fold and the paraglottic fat (*arrow*). Large metastatic lymph node (*N*). **b** Axial T2-weighted FSE image. Slight increase in signal intensity within the tumor mass and within the metastatic lymph node. **c** Contrast-enhanced axial T1-weighted SE image. Moderate homogeneous enhancement without intratumoral necrosis. Deep submucosal biopsy revealed undifferentiated carcinoma of nasopharyngeal type. The patient underwent total laryngectomy and bilateral neck dissection. **d** Gross surgical specimen viewed posteriorly and from above. The large supraglottic tumor (*arrows*) is covered by an intact mucosa (*E* epiglottis). **e** High-power micrograph showing cords of large pale epithelial cells with indistinct boundaries and vesicular nuclei (*arrows*) overrun by small lymphocytes (*asterisks*) characteristic of undifferentiated carcinoma of nasopharyngeal type. Hematoxylin-eosin stain (original magnification +100). The patient was free of recurrence 6 years later. Reproduced with permission from BECKER et al. 1998b

therapy has been reported as opposed to only 7% recurrence rate after surgery. Surgery alone is, therefore, considered in most centers as the treatment of choice (BECKER et al. 1998b; FERLITO and RECHER 1980; GLANZ and KLEINSASSER 1987). Verrucous carcinoma may display a characteristic radiologic aspect: an exophytic mass with a rugged surface and finger-like, deep projections, limited deep tumor infiltration, moderate enhancement after administration of contrast material and absence of lymph node metastases (Table 5.6; Fig. 5.17).

Spindle cell carcinoma is a rare biphasic variant of squamous cell carcinoma in which a pseudosarcomatous component dominates the microscopic appearance. The larynx is the most common site, followed by the oral cavity and esophagus (BATSAKIS 1979; FERLITO 1993). The incidence varies between 0.5% and 1% of all malignant laryngeal neoplasms. Although these tumors have the same age and sex predilection as the common type of squamous cell carcinoma, most spindle cell carcinomas have been reported to have a highly exophytic, polypoid shape. Two-thirds of the tumors present endoscopically as pedunculated masses attached to the mucosa by a stalk, while one-third of the lesions present as sessile or infiltrating masses. As with other atypical forms of squamous cell carcinoma, large biopsies are often necessary to establish the correct diagnosis because superficial biopsies may

lack the characteristic histologic signs (BATSAKIS 1979; BECKER et al. 1998b; KLEINSASSER 1988b). Spindle cell carcinoma may display a characteristic radiologic aspect: large, exophytic, pedunculated, masses arising from the supraglottic region or piriform sinus with inhomogeneous contrast enhancement and a thin stalk (BECKER et al. 1998b) (Table 5.6).

Basaloid squamous cell carcinoma (also called basaloid cell carcinoma) has a mixed basaloid and squamous component (BECKER et al. 1998b; FERLITO 1993). The predilection sites are the supraglottic larynx, hypopharynx and base of the tongue. The prognosis is usually worse than that of the common type of squamous cell carcinoma. The tumor is, therefore, regarded as a high-grade malignancy with a tendency for locally aggressive behavior and early regional and distant metastases (BANKS et al. 1992; BATSAKIS and EL NAGGAR 1989; MCKAY and BILOUS 1989; WAIN et al. 1986). The most common sites of metastatic spread are the cervical lymph nodes followed by the lung, bone and skin. The treatment of choice is surgery followed by radiation therapy. Because of a high incidence of distant metastases some authors have suggested additional adjuvant chemotherapy. The most striking radiologic feature observed in this particular tumor type appears to be a lobulated enhancement pattern (Fig. 5.18), which corresponds histologically to tumor lobules dispersed within and surrounded by a fibrovascular stroma (BECKER et al. 1998b).

5.3
Non-squamous Cell Tumors

A variety of benign and malignant tumors of non-squamous cell origin may affect the larynx and hypopharynx. These tumors are infrequent and comprise less than 5% of all tumors of this region (BANKS et al. 1992; BECKER 1998a; BECKER and KURT 1999; BECKER et al. 1998a). Many of these non-squamous cell tumors are located extramucosally, and the endoscopist may see nothing but an asymmetry or a bulge beneath an intact mucosa. Therefore, the diagnosis of these submucosal tumors is difficult with endoscopy alone, and sampling errors may occur if only traditional superficial biopsies are performed (BECKER and KURT 1999; BECKER et al. 1998a; SALEH et al. 1992). The discrepancy between an intact mucosa at endoscopic examination and an obvious mass at CT or MRI should, therefore, raise the suspicion of a tumor with an unusual histology. Because the treatment of most of the uncommon laryngeal

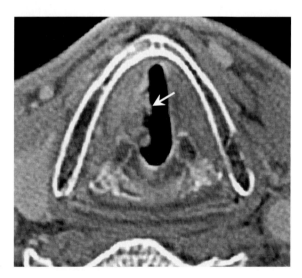

Fig. 5.17. Verrucous carcinoma in a 73-year-old patient with hoarseness. Characteristic CT appearance. Axial CT image (bone window setting) demonstrates a right-sided tumor mass involving the true vocal cord and with a characteristic rugged surface with finger-like projections (*arrow*). The patient underwent endoscopic biopsy which revealed verrucous carcinoma. Reproduced with permission from BECKER et al. 1998b

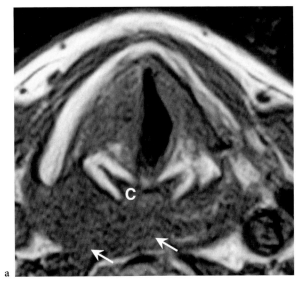

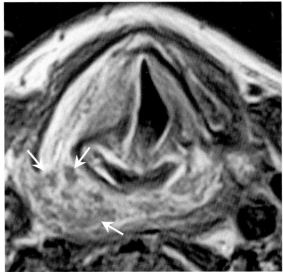

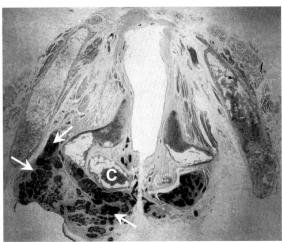

Fig. 5.18a–c. Basaloid cell carcinoma of the hypopharynx in a 64-year-old patient presenting with pain and dysphagia. Characteristic MRI and histologic appearance. a T1-weighted SE image. A tumor mass involves the right piriform sinus and the retrocricoarytenoid region (*arrows*) (*C* cricoid cartilage). b T1-weighted contrast-enhanced SE image. The tumor mass has a distinct lobulated enhancement pattern. The tumor lobules (*arrows*) display a moderate enhancement while the stroma surrounding the tumor lobules is enhanced significantly. The patient underwent total laryngectomy and right-sided neck dissection. c Corresponding axial histologic slice shows the characteristic tumor lobules (*arrows*) which are surrounded by a reactive stroma. Hematoxylin-eosin stain (*C* cricoid cartilage). None of the laryngeal cartilages was invaded histologically. Reproduced with permission from BECKER et al. 1998b

neoplasms differs from the treatment of squamous cell carcinoma, a correct preoperative diagnosis is very important. The role of imaging in unusual laryngeal and hypopharyngeal tumors is to detect or confirm the presence of a submucosal mass, to determine the deep structures involved and to guide the endoscopist to the most appropriate site for obtaining deep aggressive biopsies. Some submucosal masses can be further characterized in terms of their etiology when they display the typical features of chondroid, lipomatous or hypervascularized tissue or those of non-tumoral lesions, such as a cysts or laryngoceles. Benign tumors of the larynx are discussed in Chap. 3.

Chondrosarcoma is the most frequent sarcoma of the larynx. Of laryngeal chondrosarcomas, 50–70% originate from the cricoid cartilage whereas 20–35% originate from the thyroid cartilage (BATSAKIS 1979;

BATSAKIS and EL NAGGAR 1989; BECKER et al. 1998a; FERLITO 1993). The features of chondrogenic tumors are quite characteristic: CT displays a soft tissue mass with coarse or stippled calcifications (Fig. 5.19). On MR imaging, the hyaline tumor matrix has a very high signal intensity on T2-weighted images owing to its low cellularity and high water content. The stippled calcifications are not as visible on MR images as on CT scans but they may appear as areas of low signal intensity on T1- and T2-weighted sequences. Injection of gadolinium chelates may lead to a diffuse central or peripheral enhancement on T1-weighted images. Differentiation between benign chondroma and low-grade chondrosarcoma may be impossible on the basis of imaging studies alone (BECKER et al. 1995b, 1998a).

The differential diagnosis of strongly vascularized laryngeal tumors includes benign lesions such

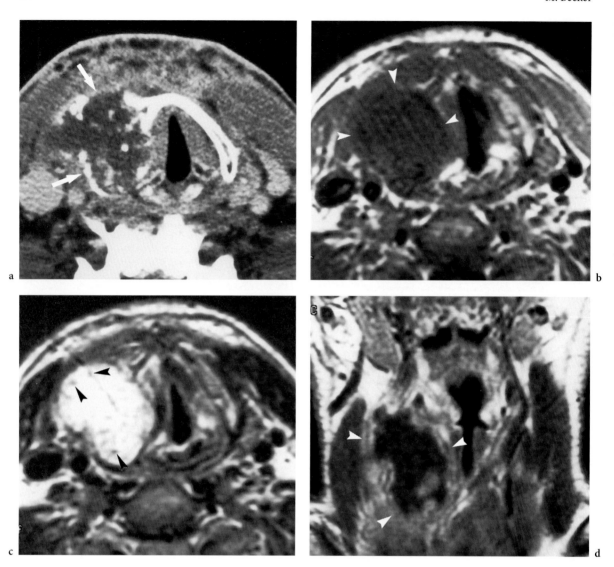

Fig. 5.19a–d. Chondrosarcoma of the thyroid cartilage in a 47-year old male patient presenting with a hard lump in the neck: CT and MRI appearance. **a** Axial contrast-enhanced CT scan shows a large, lobulated mass with coarse and stippled calcifications characteristic of chondrosarcoma (*arrows*). **b** T1-weighted axial MR image shows a lobulated mass with low signal intensity that arises from the right thyroid lamina (*arrowheads*). Note normal aspect of the left thyroid lamina. **c** T2-weighted FSE image. The tumor mass has a very high signal intensity due to a high water content. The hypointense areas within the tumor correspond to intratumoral calcifications (*arrowheads*). **d** T1-weighted contrast-enhanced coronal image. Moderate peripheral enhancement (*arrowheads*). Note extramucosal tumor location. The patient underwent voice-preserving laryngeal resection and was free of recurrence 5 years later. **a** Reproduced with permission from Becker 1998a

as hemangioma and paraganglioma, and malignant lesions, such as Kaposi's sarcoma and hemangiopericytoma. Laryngeal hemangiomas typically occur in the subglottis (infantile type) or in the supraglottis (adult type) (see also Chap. 3). Kaposi's sarcoma is considered an unusual, multifocal, neoplastic disease of the vascular system. It involves the larynx only very rarely. The disease was rare in Europe and the US but has recently become more common in association with the acquired immune defi-

ciency syndrome (AIDS) (Banks et al. 1992; Becker et al. 1998a). Three forms of Kaposi's sarcoma are recognized: classic Kaposi's sarcoma affecting men of Mediterranean origin in their seventh decade, Central African Kaposi's sarcoma, and AIDS-related Kaposi's sarcoma. Currently, the most frequent form of Kaposi's sarcoma is associated with AIDS.

Most patients with laryngeal Kaposi's sarcoma, regardless of whether they are HIV-positive or not, present with multiple classical skin lesions. Involvement of the larynx is, therefore, only to be expected in the late stages when the disease has been diagnosed from the skin lesions. The commonest location of Kaposi's sarcoma in the larynx is the epiglottis. The clinical course of Kaposi's sarcoma is variable. Elderly patients with classical Kaposi's sarcoma may live for many years, and death only rarely occurs as a direct result of the tumor. Complete regression of laryngeal involvement has been recently reported with low doses of alpha 2b interferon. Central African Kaposi's sarcoma involving the larynx is usually rapidly fatal. AIDS-related Kaposi's sarcoma usually affects the larynx at a late stage, when lymph nodes and viscera are already involved. In these patients Kaposi's sarcoma is usually associated with a high incidence of lymphomas. The prognosis is usually very poor.

On CT, hemangioma, paraganglioma and Kaposi's sarcoma appear as well-circumscribed soft tissue masses that display uniform intense contrast enhancement. Phleboliths are, however, pathognomonic for hemangioma (Fig. 5.20). On MRI, laryngeal hemangioma, paraganglioma and Kaposi's sarcoma display a very high signal intensity on T2-weighted sequences and very strong enhancement on T1-weighted images after administration of gadolinium chelates. They may also display multiple curvilinear signal voids on both T1-

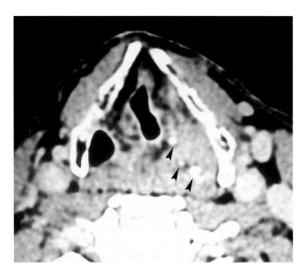

Fig. 5.20. Localized adult hemangioma with phleboliths. Contrast-enhanced CT image at the supraglottic level obtained in a 51-year-old male patient demonstrates a mass involving the left aryepiglottic fold with moderate enhancement after administration of contrast material and with phleboliths (*arrowheads*) characteristic of hemangioma. Note obliteration of the left piriform sinus. Endoscopy and histology confirmed cavernous hemangioma. No treatment was performed. Reproduced with permission from BECKER et al. 1998a

and T2-weighted images, which indicates strongly vascularized tumors (BECKER et al. 1998a). The conspicuousness of these signal-void areas increases with tumor size. Although the radiologic aspect may be nonspecific, the presence of a submucosal laryngeal mass in association with multiple characteristic skin lesions very strongly suggests the diagnosis of Kaposi's sarcoma (BECKER et al. 1998a).

Adenocarcinoma, adenoid cystic carcinoma and mucoepidermoid carcinoma arise from the minor salivary glands. Adenoid cystic carcinoma is typically found in the subglottis of patients without a history of smoking. These tumors can be located beneath a completely intact mucosa and display a characteristic pathway of perineural spread along the recurrent laryngeal nerve. None of these unusual types of carcinoma has any imaging characteristics allowing its distinction from squamous cell carcinoma (BECKER et al. 1995b, 1998a).

Tumors of the lymphoreticular system include Hodgkin's and non-Hodgkin's lymphoma, plasmacytoma, leukemia and pseudolymphoma. Although about 30% of all malignant lymphomas arise in the head and neck (cervical lymph nodes and Waldeyer's ring), lymphomas of the larynx, either in isolation or as a manifestation of generalized disease, are very uncommon. In a series of 55 cases of extranodal non-Hodgkin lymphoma of the head and neck, two patients had laryngeal involvement, presenting as nodular or diffusely infiltrating submucosal masses (HERMANS et al. 1994).

Plasma cell neoplasms are characterized by growth of a single clone of cells forming one of the two immunoglobulin light chains, kappa or lambda. Plasma cell neoplasms may present as multiple myeloma, as solitary plasmacytoma of bone or as extramedullary plasmacytoma (BATSAKIS 1979; BECKER et al. 1995b, 1998a). Extramedullary plasmacytoma is occasionally found in the head and neck, and about 20% of primary plasmacytomas of this region are located in the larynx (BECKER 1998a; BECKER et al. 1998b, 1998c; FERLITO 1993). Plasmacytoma of the larynx occurs predominantly in males between 50 and 70 years and involves the epiglottis, the vocal cords and false cords. Endoscopically, a pedunculated or slightly prominent mass is seen which bleeds easily and the mucosa above the tumor is usually intact. Approximately 40% of extramedullary plasmacytomas terminate in osseous and soft-tissue dissemination. Treatment may consist of surgical excision or radiotherapy in localized disease or of chemotherapy in the case of disseminated disease. On CT and MRI, the tumor presents as a large, smoothly marginated, homogeneous mass without significant contrast-enhancement and without evidence of necrosis or gross ulceration (Becker et al. 1998a) (Fig. 5.21). Because of the nonspecific radiologic aspect, the major role of CT and MRI in the management of patients with plasmacytoma of the larynx is to demonstrate the submucosal extent of the lesion and to follow the patients postoperatively.

Metastases to the larynx are rare, the total number reported to date amounting to approximately 135 cases (Becker et al. 1998a; Ferlito 1993). The most common mechanism of metastatic spread is through the systemic circulation: inferior vena cava, right heart, lungs, left heart, aorta, external carotid artery, upper thyroid artery and upper laryngeal artery. However, when no pulmonary involvement is observed, spread via the retrograde circulation of the paravertebral venous plexus and thoracic duct should be considered. The primary sources of metastatic tumor, in order of decreasing frequency, are: skin (melanoma), kidney, breast, lung, prostate, colon, stomach and ovary. In our own recently published series of non-squamous cell laryngeal tumors, there were three cases of metastases to the larynx (two from skin melanoma and one from renal adenocarcinoma). According to Glanz and Kleinsasser, laryngeal metastases

should be divided into two groups: those metastasizing to the soft tissues, mainly vestibular and aryepiglottic folds, such as melanoma and renal adenocarcinoma, and those metastasizing to the marrow spaces of the ossified thyroid, cricoid and arytenoid cartilages, such as lung and breast carcinoma (Becker et al. 1998a; Ferlito 1993).

Symptoms of metastatic tumors to the larynx vary according to the affected site. Hemoptysis is an important symptom of laryngeal metastases from renal adenocarcinoma because of the abundant vascularization of these tumors. In most cases, radiologic features of laryngeal metastases are nonspecific. However, metastases from renal adenocarcinoma and melanotic melanoma may display typical features at MR imaging. Metastases from renal adenocarcinoma typically display a very strong enhancement after administration of contrast material due to their hypervascularity and flow voids on MR images, therefore suggesting a diagnosis other than squamous cell carcinoma (Becker et al. 1998a). Laryngeal metastases from melanotic melanoma display the signal characteristics of melanotic melanoma elsewhere in the body, namely a high signal intensity on T1-weighted images and an intermediate to low signal intensity on

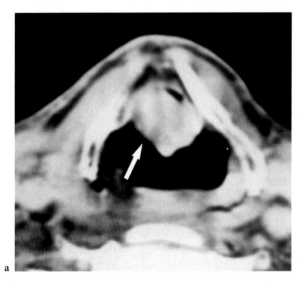

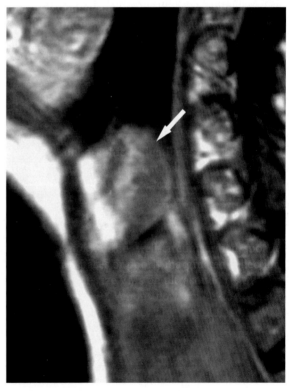

Fig. 5.21a, b. Laryngeal plasmacytoma in a 71-year-old male patient presenting with dyspnea. a Axial contrast-enhanced CT scan shows a large smoothly marginated epiglottic tumor without evidence of ulceration or necrosis (*arrow*). b Contrast-enhanced T1-weighted sagittal image. Moderate slightly inhomogeneous contrast-enhancement of the mass (*arrow*). Endoscopy showed a mass arising from the laryngeal surface of the epiglottis covered by intact mucosa and histology revealed plasmacytoma. The patient underwent endoscopic resection, but 4 years later developed tumor recurrence at the same site. Repeat endoscopic surgery was performed successfully, and the patient was free of recurrence 1 year later. Reproduced with permission from Becker et al. 1998a

T2-weighted images due to the paramagnetic properties of melanin (BECKER et al. 1998a) (Fig. 5.22). Metastases to the larynx have the same histologic features as the primary tumor. In the setting of a known primary tumor, the histologic diagnosis of the laryngeal neoplasm is usually straightforward. The question as to whether a given neoplasm in the larynx is primary or metastatic arises particularly in patients with a solitary nodule. In these instances, a thorough clinical and radiologic evaluation should be performed in order to detect a possible primary neoplasm (Fig. 5.22).

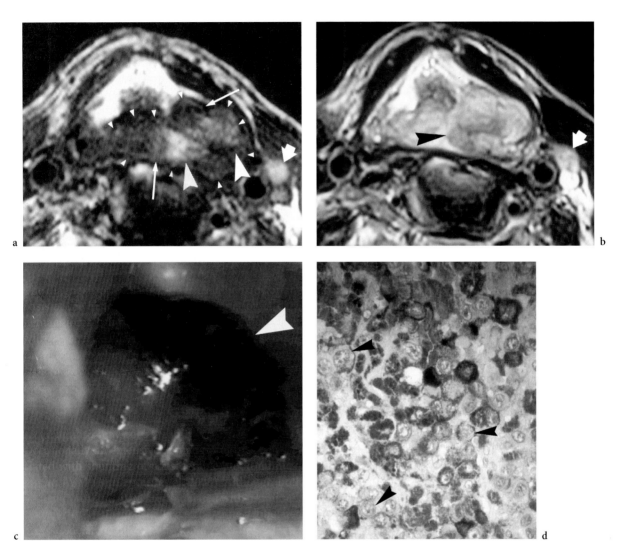

Fig. 5.22a–d. Metastasis from melanotic melanoma in an 81-year-old male with dyspnea and a history of occasional blood in the sputum. **a** Axial unenhanced T1-weighted SE image demonstrates a large mass (*small arrowheads*) involving the left aryepiglottic fold. The mass has areas with low signal intensity (*thin arrows*) and areas with high signal intensity (*large arrowheads*). A lymph node with high signal intensity (*thick arrow*) is seen on the left. **b** In a T2-weighted FSE image at the same level the hyperintense areas on the T1-weighted image have become hypointense (*arrowhead*). The left-sided lymph node maintains a high signal intensity (*thick arrow*). After administration of contrast material moderate enhancement of the tumor mass was observed. The signal characteristics suggested a melanotic melanoma of the supraglottic larynx with lymph node metastasis. **c** Endoscopy shows a darkly stained polypoid supraglottic tumor involving the left aryepiglottic fold (*arrowhead*). **d** High- power micrograph demonstrates the typical appearance of melanotic melanoma: large round cells (*arrowheads*) with hyperchromatic to vesicular nuclei. Large amounts of melanin (*brown to black granularity*) are seen in the cytoplasm of neoplastic cells. Hematoxylin-eosin stain (original magnification +400). The patient stated that he had undergone removal of a small "spot" on the scalp at another institution. Inquiry at this institution revealed the diagnosis of melanotic melanoma of the scalp. The laryngeal tumor and the cervical lymph node metastasis were, therefore, considered metastases of the melanotic melanoma of the scalp. Reproduced with permission from BECKER et al. 1998a

Laryngeal tumors arising from smooth or striated muscle are rare, and include leiomyoma, angioleiomyoma, leiomyosarcoma (Fig. 3.17), extracardiac rhabdomyoma (Fig. 3.12) and rhabdomyosarcoma. The imaging findings are non-characteristic (BECKER et al. 1998a).

5.4
Conclusions

Both CT and MR imaging are very well suited to the evaluation of the submucosal structures of the larynx and hypopharynx complementary to endoscopy. The advantage of MR imaging lies in its ability to provide higher soft tissue contrast than CT. CT, on the other hand, allows faster image acquisition and is less susceptible to artifacts than MR imaging. The most important clinical role of cross-sectional imaging of the larynx and hypopharynx lies in the pretherapeutic workup of patients with squamous cell carcinoma. Adequate interpretation of the CT and MR images requires a thorough knowledge of the patterns of tumor spread within the different regions of the larynx and hypopharynx as well as the predictive value of the diagnostic signs that may indicate neoplastic invasion with each modality. Although non-squamous cell carcinoma and other neoplasms are relatively uncommon, CT and MR imaging usually play a key role in the diagnosis since these lesions are almost always situated submucosally. In addition, their appearance on CT and MR images may be quite typical, e.g., in the case of chondrosarcoma.

References

Banks ER, Frieson HF Jr, Mills SE, et al (1992) Basaloid-squamous cell carcinoma of the head and neck. A clinicopathologic and immunohistochemical study of 40 cases. Am J Surg Pathol 16:939–946

Batsakis JG (1979) Tumors of the head and neck. Clinical and pathologic considerations, 2nd edn. Williams and Wilkins, Baltimore

Batsakis JG, El Naggar A (1989) Basaloid-squamous cell carcinomas of the upper aerodigestive tract. Ann Otol Rhinol Laryngol 98:919–920

Becker M (1998a) Larynx and hypopharynx. Radiol Clin North Am 36:891–920

Becker M (1998b) Diagnose und Stadieneinteilung von Larynxtumoren mittels CT und MRT. Der Radiologe 38:93–100

Becker M (2000) Oral cavity, oropharynx and hypopharynx. Semin Roentgenol 35:21–30

Becker M, Hasso AN (1996) Imaging of malignant neoplasms of the pharynx and larynx. In: Taveras JM, Ferruci JT (eds) Radiology: diagnosis imaging intervention. JB Lippincott, Philadelphia, pp 1–16

Becker M, Kurt AM (1999) Infrahyoid neck: CT and MR imaging versus histopathology. Eur Radiol 9[Suppl 2]:53–68

Becker M, Zbären P, Laeng H, et al (1995a) Neoplastic invasion of the laryngeal cartilage: comparison of MR imaging and CT with histopathologic correlation. Radiology 194:661–669

Becker M, Zbären P, Laeng H (1995b) MRI and CT of unusual laryngeal neoplasms in adults: radiologic-pathologic correlation. Radiographics Supplement (compact disc), Selected Neuroradiology Scientific Exhibits, 15 (part 3), p 1268

Becker M, Schroth G, Zbären P, et al (1997a) Long-term changes induced by high-dose irradiation of the head and neck region: imaging findings. Radiographics 17:5–26

Becker M, Zbären P, Delavelle J, et al (1997b) Neoplastic Invasion of the laryngeal cartilage: reassessment of criteria for diagnosis at CT. Radiology 203:521–532

Becker M, Moulin G, Kurt AM, et al (1998a) Non-squamous cell neoplasms of the larynx: radiologic-pathologic correlation. Radiographics 18:1189–1209

Becker M, Moulin G, Kurt AM, et al (1998b) Atypical squamous cell carcinoma of the larynx and hypopharynx: radiologic features and pathologic correlation. Eur Radiol 8:1541–1551

Becker M, Zbären P, Delavelle J, et al (1998c) Response to Letter to the Editor: Blow-out as a sign of cartilage invasion by laryngeal cancer. Radiology 207:274–275

Bennett A, Carter RL, Stamford IF, et al (1980) Prostaglandin-like material extracted from squamous cell carcinomas of the head and neck. Br J Cancer 41:204–208

Brandsma JL, Steinberg BM, Abramson AL, et al (1986) Presence of human papilloma virus type 16 related sequences in verrucous carcinoma of the larynx. Cancer Res 46:2185–2188

Carter RL, Tanner NSB (1979) Local Invasion by laryngeal carcinoma: importance of focal ossification within laryngeal cartilage. Clin Otolaryngol 4:283–290

Castelijns JA, Gerritsen GJ, Kaiser MC, et al (1987) MRI of normal or cancerous laryngeal cartilages: histopathologic correlation. Laryngoscope 97:1085–1093

Castelijns JA, Gerritsen GJ, Kaiser MC, et al (1988) Invasion of laryngeal cartilage by cancer: comparison of CT and MR imaging. Radiology 167:199–206

Castelijns JA, Becker M, Hermans R (1996a) The impact of cartilage invasion on treatment and prognosis of laryngeal cancer. Eur Radiol 6:156–169

Castelijns JA, van den Brekel MWM, Tobi H, et al (1996b) Laryngeal carcinoma after radiation therapy: correlation of abnormal MR imaging signal patterns in laryngeal cartilage with the risk of recurrence. Radiology 198:151–155

Curtin HD (1989) Imaging of the larynx: current concepts. Radiology 173:1–11

Curtin HD (1995) The importance of imaging demonstration of neoplastic invasion of laryngeal cartilage. Radiology 194:643–644

Curtin HD (1996) Larynx. In: Som PM, Curtin HD (eds) Head and neck imaging, 3rd edn. Mosby Year Book, St. Louis, pp 612–707

Dullerud R, Johansen JG, Dahl T, et al (1992) Influence of CT on tumor classification of laryngeal carcinomas. Acta Radiol 33:314–318

Ferlito A (1993) Neoplasms of the larynx. Churchill Livingstone, Edinburgh London Madrid Melbourne New York Tokyo, pp 1–590

Ferlito A, Recher G (1980) Ackerman's tumor (verrucous carcinoma) of the larynx. A clinicopathologic study of 77 cases. Cancer 46:1617–1630

Gallo A, Mocetti P, De Vincentiis M, et al (1992) Neoplastic infiltration of laryngeal cartilages: histocytochemical study. Laryngoscope 102:891–895

Glanz H, Kleinsasser O (1987) Verrucous carcinoma of the larynx – a misnomer. Arch Otorhinolaryngol 244:108–111

Gregor RT, Hammond K (1987) Framework invasion by laryngeal carcinoma. Am J Surg 154:452–458

Gregor RT, Lloyd GAS, Michels L (1981) Computed tomography of the larynx: a clinical pathologic study. Head Neck Surgery 3:284 – 296

Harrison DFN (1984) Significance and means by which laryngeal cancer invades thyroid cartilage. Ann Otol Rhinol Laryngol 93:293–296

Hermanek P, Henson DE, Hutter RVP, et al (eds) (1993) TNM supplement. A commentary on uniform use, 1st edn. Springer. Berlin Heidelberg New York, pp 19–28

Hermanek P, Hutter RVP, Sobin LH, et al (eds) (1998) TNM atlas: illustrated guide to the TNM/pTNM classification of malignant tumors, 4th edn. Springer, Berlin Heidelberg New York, pp 22–49

Hermans R, Horvath M, De Schrijver T, et al (1994) Extranodal non-Hodgkin lymphoma of the head and neck. J Belge Radiol 77:72–77

Hermans R, Van den Bogaert W, Rijnders A, et al (1999a) Value of computed tomography as outcome predictor of supraglottic squamous cell carcinoma treated by definitive radiation therapy. Int J Radiat Oncol Biol Phys 44:755–765

Hermans R, Van den Bogaert W, Rijnders A, et al (1999b) Predicting the local outcome of glottic squamous cell carcinoma after definitive radiation therapy: value of computed tomography-determined tumor parameters. Radiother Oncol 50:39–46

Hyams VJ, Batsakis JG, Michaels L (1988) Tumors of the upper respiratory tract and ear. In: Hartmann WH, Sobin LH (eds) Atlas of tumor pathology, 2nd series, fasc 25. Armed Forces Institute of Pathology, Washington DC, pp 1–182

Kavanagh KT, Salazar JE, Babin RW (1985) Bone marrow expansion of the thyroid cartilage: a source of confusion with malignant invasion in CT studies. J Comput Assist Tomogr 9:177–179

Kirchner JA (1984) Invasion of the framework by laryngeal cancer. Acta Otolaryngol 97:392–397

Kirchner JA, Carter D (1987) Intralaryngeal barriers to the spread of cancer. Acta Otolaryngol 103:503–513

Kirchner JA, Fischer J (1975) Anterior commissure cancer – a clinical and laboratory study of 39 cases. Can J Otolaryngol 4:637–643

Kleinsasser O (1988a) Epidemiology, etiology and pathogenesis. In: Kleinsasser O (ed) Tumors of the larynx and hypopharynx. Thieme Medical Publishers, New York, pp 2–24

Kleinsasser O (1988b) Other tumors. In: Tumors of the larynx and hypopharynx. ed. Kleinsasser O. Thieme Medical Publishers, Inc. New York, pp 263–341

Kleinsasser O (1988c) Pathology and biology. In: Kleinsasser O (ed) Tumors of the larynx and hypopharynx. Thieme Medical Publishers, New York, pp 25–123

Lehmann W, Raymond L, Faggiano F, et al (1991) Cancer of the endolarynx, epilarynx and hypopharynx in southwestern Europe: assessment of tumoral origin and risk factors. Adv Otorhinolaryngol 46:145 –156

Levi F, Raymond L, Schüler G, et al (1998) Cancer en Suisse. Faits et commentaires. Association suisse des registres des tumeurs. Ligue suisse contre le cancer. Hertig & Co, Bienne, pp 1–60

Loevner LA, Yousem DM, Montone KT, et al (1997) Can radiologists accurately predict preepiglottic space invasion with MR imaging? Am J Roentgenol 169:1681–1687

Mafee MF, Schild JA, Valvassori GE, et al (1983) Computed tomography of the larynx: correlation with anatomic and pathologic studies in cases of laryngeal carcinoma. Radiology 147:123–128

Mafee MF, Schild JA, Michael AS, et al (1984) Cartilage involvement in laryngeal carcinoma: correlation of CT and pathologic macrosection studies. J Comput Assist Tomogr 8:969–973

Mancuso AA (1991) Evaluation and staging of laryngeal and hypopharyngeal cancer by computed tomography and magnetic resonance imaging. In: Silver CE (ed) Laryngeal cancer. Thieme, New York, pp 46–94

Mancuso AA, Hanafee WN (1979) A comparative evaluation of computed tomography and laryngography. Radiology 133:131–138

Mancuso AA, Hanafee WN (1983) Elusive head and neck carcinomas beneath intact mucosa. Laryngoscope 93:133–139

Mancuso AA, Hanafee WN (1985) Larynx and hypopharynx. In: Mancuso AA, Hanafee WN (eds) Computed tomography and magnetic resonance imaging of the head and neck, 2nd edn. Williams and Wilkins, Baltimore, pp 1–503

Mancuso AA, Hanafee WN, Juillard GJF, et al (1977) The role of computed tomography in the management of cancer of the larynx. Radiology 124:243–244

Mancuso AA, Calcaterra TC, Hanafee WN (1978) Computed tomography of the larynx. Radiol Clin North Am 16:195–208

Mancuso AA, Tamakawa Y, Hanafee WN (1980) CT of the fixed vocal cord. Am J Radiol 135:529–534

Mancuso AA, Mukherji SK, Schmalfuss I, et al (1999) Preradiotherapy computed tomography as a predictor of local control in supraglottic carcinoma. J Clin Oncol 17:631–637

Maroldi R, Battaglia G, Nicolai P, et al (1997) CT appearance of the larynx after conservative and radical surgery for carcinomas. Eur Radiol 7:418–431

McKay MJ, Bilous AM (1989) Basaloid-squamous carcinoma of the hypopharynx. Cancer 63:2528–2531

Million RR, Cassisi NJ, Mancuso AA (1994) Larynx. In: Million RR. Cassisi NJ (eds) Management of head and neck cancer. A multidisciplinary approach, 2nd edn. J.B. Lippincott, Philadelphia, pp 431–497

Muñoz A, Ramos A, Ferrando J, et al (1993) Laryngeal carcinoma: sclerotic appearance of the cricoid and arytenoid cartilage – CT-pathologic correlation. Radiology 189:433–437

Pameijer FA, Mancuso AA, Mendenhall WM, et al (1997) Can pretreatment computed tomography predict local control in T3 squamous cell carcinoma of the glottic larynx treated with definitive radiotherapy? Int J Radiat Oncol Biol Phys 37:1011–1021

Pameijer FA, Mancuso AA, Mendenhall WM, et al (1998) Evaluation of pretreatment computed tomography as a predictor of local control in T1/T2 piriform sinus carcinoma treated with definitive radiotherapy. Head Neck 20:159–168

Pameijer FA, Hermans R, Mancuso AA, et al (1999) Pre- and post-radiotherapy computed tomography in laryngeal cancer: imaging-based prediction of local failure. Int J Radiat Oncol Biol Phys 45:359–366

Saleh EM, Mancuso AA, Stringer SP (1992) CT of submucosal and occult laryngeal masses. J Comput Assist Tomogr 16:87–93

Shanmugaratnam K, Chan S, De-The G, et al (1979) Histopathology of nasopharyngeal carcinoma: correlations with epidemiology, survival rates and other biological characteristics. Cancer 44:1029

Silverman PM (1985) Medullary space involvement in laryngeal carcinoma. Arch Otolaryngol 111:541–542

Sulfaro S, Barzan L, Querin F, et al (1989) T-staging of the laryngohypopharyngeal carcinoma; a 7-year multidisciplinary experience. Arch Otolaryngol Head Neck Surg 115:613–620

Thabet HM, Sessions DG, Gado HM, et al (1996) Comparison of clinical evaluations and computed tomographic diagnostic accuracy for tumors of the larynx and hypopharynx. Laryngoscope 106:589–594

Toker C, Peterson DW (1978) Lymphoepithelioma of the vocal cord. Arch Otolaryngol 104:161–162

Tuyns AJ, Esteve J, Raymond L, et al (1988) Cancer of the larynx/hypopharynx, tobacco and alcohol: IARC International Case-Control Study in Turin and Varese (Italy), Zaragoza and Navarra (Spain), Geneva (Switzerland) and Calvados (France). Int J Cancer 41:483–491

Vogl TJ, Heger W, Grevers G, et al (1991) MRI with Gd-DTPA in tumors of the larynx and hypopharynx. Eur Radiol 1:58–64

Wain SL, Kier R, Vollmer RT, et al (1986) Basaloid-squamous carcinoma of the tongue, hypopharynx and larynx: report of 10 cases. Hum Pathol 17:1158–1166

Weissman JL, Holliday RA (1996) Pharynx (section two). In: Som PM, Curtin HD (eds) Head and neck imaging, 3rd edn, Mosby, St. Louis, pp 472–488

Yeager VL. Archer CR (1982) Anatomical routes for cancer invasion of laryngeal cartilages. Laryngoscope 92:449–452

Yousem DM, Hatabu H, Hurst MD, et al (1995) Carotid artery invasion by head and neck masses: prediction with MR imaging. Radiology 195:715–720

Zbären P, Becker M, Laeng H (1996) Pretherapeutic staging of laryngeal cancer: clinical findings, computed tomography and magnetic resonance imaging versus histopathology. Cancer 77:1263–1273

Zbären P, Becker M, Laeng H (1997a) Staging of laryngeal cancer: endoscopy, computed tomography and magnetic resonance imaging versus histopathology. Eur Arch Otolaryngol 254:117–122

Zbären P, Becker M, Laeng H (1997b) Pretherapeutic staging of hypopharyngeal carcinoma: clinical findings, computed tomography, and magnetic resonance imaging compared with histopathologic evaluation. Arch Otolaryngol Head Neck Surg 123:908–913

6 Diagnostic Evaluation of Lymph Node Metastases

ROBERT SIGAL

CONTENTS

6.1
Introduction

Imaging plays an important role in lymph node survey in patients with laryngeal cancer. Imaging can modify the initial clinical staging and therapeutic strategy by detecting clinically inaccessible lymph nodes, or by showing invasion of critical structures such as the common and internal carotid arteries. At the post-therapeutic stage, imaging can detect lymph node relapse which may be difficult to palpate.

6.2
Anatomy

The most used classifications for lymph nodes are the ones of the International Union Against Cancer (UICC 1997) and the American Joint Committee on Cancer (BEAHRS et al. 1988). Since the pioneering

R. SIGAL, MD, PhD
Professor, Department of Radiology, Institut Gustave Roussy, 39, rue C. Desmoulins, 94800 Villejuif, France

work of SHAH et al. (1981), the different areas of cervical lymph nodes are described in terms of *levels* (see also Chap. 1, Fig. 1.7). The widely accepted classification of the American Academy of Otolaryngology, Head and Neck Surgery (ROBBINS et al. 1991) has been recently clarified in order to incorporate clearly defined radiological landmarks (SOM et al. 1999, 2000).

Level I nodes are located above the hyoid bone, below the mylohyoid muscle and anterior to a transverse line drawn through the posterior edge of the submandibular glands. Level IA nodes (previously classified as submental nodes) are located between the medial margins of the anterior bellies of the digastric muscles. Level IB nodes represent the former submandibular nodes. Level II nodes extend from the skull base to the lower body of the hyoid bone. Level IIA nodes are inseparable from the internal jugular vein. Level IIB nodes (previously classified as upper spinal accessory nodes) are located posterior to the internal jugular vein with a fat plane separating the nodes and the vein. Level III nodes lie between the lower body of the hyoid bone and the lower margin of the cricoid cartilage arch. Level IV nodes lie between the lower margin of the cricoid and the clavicle. On an axial plane, a horizontal line drawn though the posterior edge of sternocleidomastoid muscle separates level II and level III from level VA. Level III and level IV are separated from level VI by a vertical line drawn on the medial aspect of the common and internal carotid arteries. Level V nodes extend from the skull base to the clavicle. The lower margin of the cricoid cartilage separates level VA nodes (upper level V) and level VB (lower level V). Level VB nodes are located behind an oblique line through the posterior edge of the sternocleidomastoid muscle and the postero-lateral edge of the anterior scalene muscle. Level VI nodes are located between the hyoid bone and the top of the manubrium and between the medial margins of the carotid arteries. Level VII are located between the top of the manubrium and the innominate vein.

6.3
Lymphatic Spread

The incidence of metastases depends on the location of the primary tumor. In supraglottic carcinomas, nodal metastases are found in over 40% of patients (Bocca 1975; DeSanto et al. 1977; Lindberg 1972; Mendenhall et al. 1994; Schuller and Bier-Laning 1997; Shah and Tollefsen 1974). The incidence of metastases correlates with the T stage, and with the extension to extralaryngeal sites such as the vallecula/base of the tongue, piriform sinus and postcricoid area (Mendenhall et al. 1994; Shah and Tollefsen 1974). However, even T1 lesions harbor a risk of nodal metastases. Because the main structure of the supraglottic larynx, the epiglottis, is in a midline situation, both sides are at risk with over 15% of bilateral nodes positive at the time of diagnosis (Lindberg 1972). Supraglottic spread is associated with nodes to levels II (48%) and III (38%) (Byers et al. 1988). Invasion of level IV (5%) and VI paratracheal (10%) is rare. Levels I and V are not considered at risk.

The glottic region has a sparse lymphatic supply and the metastatic rate approaches zero for lesions confined to the true vocal cord (T1) and is around 5% for T2 lesions (Mendenhall et al. 1994), increasing to about 15% for T3 and T4 lesions (Byers et al. 1988). The nodes are found in level II (55%), level III (27%) and level VI (paratracheal and pretracheal, 18%).

In subglottic carcinoma, positive nodes are found in only 10% of patients, with invasion of levels IV and VI, and of the supraclavicular nodes. In glottic cancer with subglottic extension, positive nodes are found in less than 5% (Sessions et al. 1975).

6.4
Influence of Imaging on Clinical Management

The assessment of the neck remains a difficult challenge. Palpation is not precise as shown by several studies, and presents false-negative and false-positive rates of 15–25% and 30–50%, respectively (Ali et al. 1985; Johnson 1990).

Imaging often influences the decision-making process. In the clinically positive neck, imaging can convert a selective neck dissection into a more comprehensive treatment by showing lymph nodes in areas in which metastases are usually infrequent or in the contralateral neck. Imaging may also modify the

irradiation volume and dose, particularly when displaying clinically inaccessible sites, such as retropharyngeal or paratracheal nodes (Van den Brekel et al. 1994). Imaging can show invasion of vital structures, such as the skull base, thoracic inlet, and the common or internal carotid artery, all features that have a direct impact on prognosis and resectability (Mancuso 1994; Van den Brekel et al. 1998a; Yousem et al. 1995). In the clinically N0 neck, the display of suspicious nodes can transform a wait-and-see policy or an elective neck dissection into a radical neck dissection.

In practice, in treatment planning, most clinicians only consider the unambiguous imaging evidence of neck metastasis and do not attach consequence to negative imaging results because of the low specificity and sensitivity of current imaging techniques (Van den Brekel et al. 1996). Indeed, for clinicians, the most important factor is the sensitivity of the assessment methods which should be at least above 50% so as to show half of occult metastases. In such cases, the risk of occult metastases which is, for example, about 30–40% for supraglottic tumors, would be halved to 15–20%, and this can lead to a wait-and-see decision.

The therapeutic management of the clinically negative (N0) neck remains at the center of many controversies. For most clinicians the decision to treat part or all the neck is taken when the risk of occult metastases is estimated to be more than 15–20% (Baatenburg de Jong et al. 1993). In clinical practice, this applies to patients with carcinomas of the supra- or subglottic larynx which are treated either by elective neck dissection or by limited or wide-field radiotherapy. Overtreatment and additional morbidity are therefore associated with this therapeutic policy. No large prospective studies have yet demonstrated the benefits of this treatment strategy versus a wait-and-see policy with strict follow up (Fakih et al. 1989; Kligerman et al. 1994; VandenBrouck et al. 1980).

6.5
Imaging Techniques

6.5.1
CT

The CT technique is dictated both by the search of lymph nodes and by the evaluation of a laryngeal tumor. In the axial plane, images must be acquired from the skull base down to the thoracic inlet in order to survey completely all head and neck lymph nodes and to detect a second synchronous lesion. With modern spiral CT units, acquisition of this set of images requires less than 3 min, and less than 30 s with multidetector units. At the Institut Gustave Roussy, we prefer a strictly horizontal acquisition plane in order to allow, if indicated, good quality multiplanar reformations and three-dimensional reconstructions. The slice thickness should not exceed 3 mm. Contiguous sections are needed not only to avoid missing a small lesion but also because they allow good quality reformatted views to be obtained. The field of view (10 to 18 cm) and the matrix size (512×512) must be chosen so as to ensure a pixel size below 1 mm. The acquisition is performed either during breath-hold or with quiet breathing. Intravenous injection of contrast material is imperative, and there is no need for a non-contrast study, either for studying the larynx or the lymph nodes.

If a patient presents with a history of severe contrast medium allergy, MR imaging should be considered rather than CT. Iodine injection helps to delineate the tumor extent and to differentiate between lymph nodes and adjacent vessels. It is therefore crucial to get contrast-enhanced views of all vessels (arteries and veins) from the first to the last image of the examination. This can be obtained when rapid scanning of the head and neck is performed synchronously with bolus injection performed via a power injector. The magnification factor should be properly adjusted. At the neck level undermagnification is damaging because the lymph nodes are very small and can be overlooked. Overmagnification of the larynx may exclude level VB lymph nodes, located in the posterior cervical triangles, from the field of view. In practice, the image should include the spinous process. When imaging the thoracic inlet, the zoom factor should be adjusted so that the supraclavicular lymph nodes are included within the field of view.

6.5.2
MR

Dedicated head and neck coils capable of covering the area from the skull base to the thoracic inlet are needed, but this type of coil is not available at all MR sites. MR angiography coils manufactured for imaging the supra-aortic vessels are an excellent option since they completely cover the head and neck region. Claustrophobia and the impossibility of remaining supine (in patients with an obstructed air-

way) account for a low percentage of technical failures. In head and neck imaging, motion artifacts due to swallowing, respiration and blood circulation are especially troublesome. The ability to overcome these by using appropriate "countermeasures" (such as flow compensation, in-plane or out-of-plane saturation, peripheral gating) are the hallmark of high quality MR units and experienced radiographers and radiologists. Education of the patient is also essential. The patient should be instructed to maintain quiet breathing and to minimize swallowing during sequence acquisition.

The selection of the imaging plane and image weighting primarily depends on the choice made for visualizing the primary lesion. The axial plane is always recommended. In the coronal plane, the cervical lymph nodes can be nicely depicted. One should look for lymph nodes on images acquired specifically for imaging of the larynx. However, if MR is the only imaging modality in the therapeutic work-up, it is necessary to perform additional sequences aimed at detecting all head and neck lymph nodes. T1-weighted, fat-suppressed contrast-enhanced images have been described as optimal because the same criteria for central necrosis and extracapsular spread as those used for CT can be applied. However, these data are relatively old (SOM 1992; VAN DEN BREKEL et al. 1990a). In our experience, a T2 nonsaturated fast spin echo technique is the optimal solution in terms of contrast resolution and scan time since the entire neck, from the skull base to the thoracic inlet is covered in less than 10 min.

MRA is not regarded as a useful adjunct in predicting carotid artery invasion by head and neck masses, since standard MR can directly image both the mass and the lumen (YOUSEM et al. 1995).

In general, CT is considered to be slightly superior to MR imaging (CURTIN et al. 1998; YOUSEM et al. 1992), but MR technology is progressing rapidly. Currently, MR is regarded to be as good as CT (SAKAI et al. 2000). In our experience, the real limitation stems from the fact that MR images are less familiar to clinicians than CT images. Education of clinicians will progressively solve this inconvenience, particularly if MR in the future demonstrates better results than CT.

6.5.3
Ultrasound

Ultrasound examinations are done with a high frequency probe (most commonly 7.5 to 10 MHz). Color Doppler and power Doppler sonography identify a true vascular mass (such as a chemodectoma). Not all radiological teams use sonography because the technique has several drawbacks: it does not explore the deep structures, it is operator-dependent, and it does not provide standardized reference images for the clinicians. Its main advantages are low cost, easy accessibility and its easy use in guiding a fine needle aspiration. Several studies, particularly from the Netherlands, have shown the usefulness of ultrasound-guided fine needle aspiration in the diagnosis of lymph node metastasis, with a specificity superior to 95% (Takes et al. 1996; Van den Brekel 1996). The combination of ultrasound-guided fine needle aspiration and lymphoscintigraphy for the identification of sentinel lymph nodes needs further evaluation (Colnot et al. 2001).

6.5.4
Work in Progress

6.5.4.1
PET

Positron emission tomography (PET) is a cross-sectional technique that maps the location and concentration of various radiopharmaceuticals. In cancer evaluation 2-deoxy-2-[18F]fluoro-D-glucose (FDG) has mainly been used. FDG-PET assesses tissue glucose metabolism which increases with tumor growth (McGuirt et al. 1998). Tumor uptake is unrelated to the histological grade. As a metabolic imaging modality, FDG-PET is expected to have an important impact in the management of head and neck malignancies (Anzai et al. 1996; Chisin and Macapinlac 2000; Fischbein et al. 1998). This technique, however, has several drawbacks. The radiopharmaceuticals have a short half-life (110 min for FDG) and must be produced by a cyclotron located close to the imaging site. Investment and running cost are high, and the number of machines is limited. Spatial resolution is equal to 3 mm; this prevents tumoral microdeposits being seen and leads to anatomically poorly defined images. It is likely that the use of a new generation of combined CT-PET scanners will increase the efficacy of this technique, and also the costs (see also Chap. 10).

6.5.4.2
Iron Oxide

The information provided by MR imaging can be modified by the use of contrast agents designed for intravenous MR lymphography (Weissleder et al.

1990). Ultra-small superparamagnetic iron oxide (USPIO) particles with a long plasma circulation time are captured by macrophages in normally functioning lymph nodes. As a result signal intensity reduction is observed in tissue in which the contrast agent accumulates because of the T2 and susceptibility effect of iron oxide. With metastatic tissue invasion, the lymph node will display a high signal intensity. In head and neck lymph nodes, the first results have been promising (Anzai and Prince 1997), and have shown that iron oxide improves the characterization of the cervical lymph node status. However, this improvement still remains limited by technical problems regarding motion and susceptibility artifacts and spatial resolution (Sigal et al. 2001).

6.6
Results

6.6.1
Initial Stage

In the clinically negative neck, CT or MR can detect positive nodes in 7.5% to 19% of cases. The impact of imaging is much higher when it allows a N0 neck to be upstaged, or when lymph nodes are detected outside the planned field of treatment.

The presence of central nodal necrosis with or without peripheral nodal rim enhancement is the most reliable criterion determining the presence of metastatic lymphadenopathy (Dillon 1998; Sakai et al. 2000; van den Brekel 2000; van den Brekel and Castelijns 2000) (Fig. 6.1). The term necrotic is

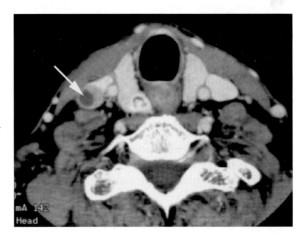

Fig. 6.1. Contrast-enhanced CT. Metastatic lymph node, level IV. Note the central hypodensity which indicates necrosis

a partial misnomer because the nodes contain necrosis as well as keratin pooling, fibrous tissue, interstitial fluid or edema, and viable tumor cells (SAKAI et al. 2000; VAN DEN BREKEL et al. 1998a). At CT, the lower density is easily seen when it is larger than 3 mm. The differential diagnosis includes fatty metaplasia, which is usually located in the hilum and has a lower density than tumor, and intranodal abscess with an eloquent clinical picture. At MR, the gadolinium-enhanced sequence allows the necrosis to be recognized as a low signal intensity area. On T2-weighted images, the necrotic lymph node appears heterogeneous (Fig. 6.2).

Indirect evidence of lymph node metastasis includes shape, nodal size and grouping of three or more nodes in a primary drainage pathway (DILLON 1998) (Fig. 6.3).

The size criterion varies considerably among authors. The size criterion is a compromise between sensitivity and specificity. For many radiologists, a node is described as pathological when it is greater than 15 mm in maximum diameter at level II, or

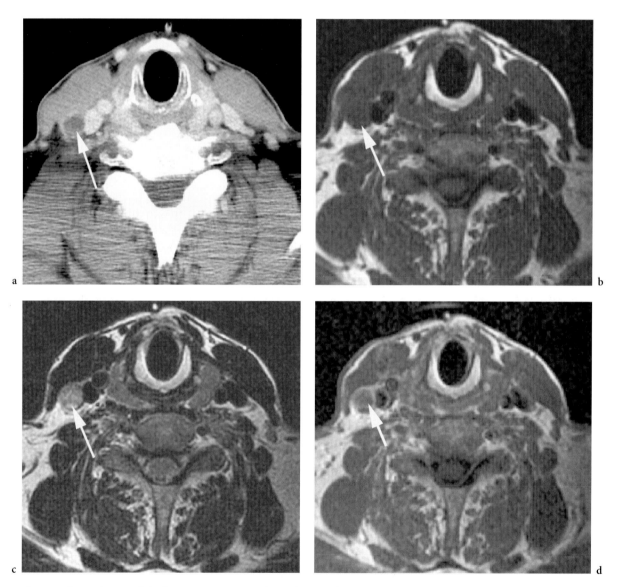

Fig. 6.2a–d. Carcinoma of the larynx. **a** Contrast-enhanced CT. Right necrotic lymph node in level III (*arrow*). **b** MR, T1-weighted sequence. The lymph node (*arrow*) has the same signal intensity as the sternocleidomastoid muscle. **c** MR, T2-weighted sequence. The lymph node (*arrow*) shows higher signal intensity than the sternocleidomastoid muscle. It is slightly heterogeneous. **d** MR, gadolinium-enhanced T1-weighted sequence. The necrotic area within the lymph node is clearly seen (*arrow*)

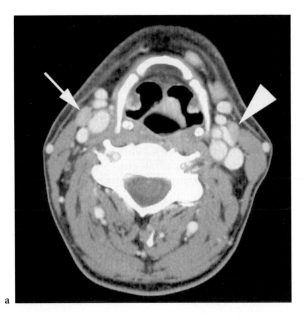 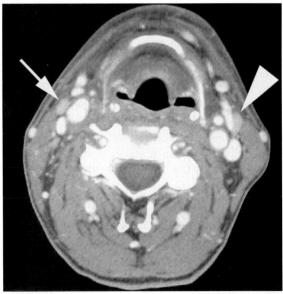

a   b

Fig. 6.3. a Contrast-enhanced CT. Squamous cell carcinoma of the free epiglottic margin. Two lymph nodes are displayed at level II. Because of their size, less than 10 mm, and their ovoid shape, they were not regarded as suspicious. **b** The patient was treated by radiotherapy. On this follow-up study, 3 months after the end of treatment, the left node (*arrowhead*) is unchanged, but the right one (*arrow*) has slightly diminished in size; one can speculate that it was positive

greater then 10 mm at other levels. Van den Brekel et al. (1990b) have proposed the use of a minimal (short) axial diameter of 11 mm for subdigastric nodes (group II) and 10 mm for all other nodes. These criteria, which in their study yielded a sensitivity of 89% and a specificity of 73%, have gained wide acceptance in the radiological community. A recent ultrasound study of van den Brekel et al. (1998b) suggests that a minimal axial diameter of 7 mm in level II nodes and 6 mm for the rest of the neck represent the optimal compromise between specificity and sensitivity in necks without palpable metastases. To our knowledge, the clinical implications of using these criteria has not been evaluated. A grouping of three or more nodes with a maximum diameter of 8 to 15 mm in level II, or 8 to 9 mm in other levels suggests metastatic invasion if they are in the drainage areas of tumors with high rates of nodal metastases.

Normal nodes have an elliptical shape. The ratio of the maximum longitudinal length to the maximum axial length should be greater than 2 for normal nodes. A value of less than 2 suggests nodal metastasis. This criterion is easily applied with ultrasound because the operator can easily rotate the transducer to obtain different planes through the nodes.

Extranodular tumor extension is found at histology in 40% of nodes less than 2 cm in size and in about one-quarter of nodes less than 1 cm (Sakai et al. 2000).

CT is considered the best technique to rule out extracapsular spread (Som 1992; van den Brekel et al. 1996). In a previously untreated patient, extracapsular spread is seen as a thick and irregular enhancing nodal rim (Fig. 6.4). Loss of clear margins and enhancement of adjacent fat or muscles also indicate extracapsular spread. Extracapsular tumor growth can extend to the muscles, carotid arteries, cranial nerves IX to XII and the skull base. Imaging cannot show invasion of the carotid adventitia, but the likelihood of such an event increases with an increasing degree of contact between the tumor and the carotid artery (Yousem et al. 1995). Therefore, it is important to note whether the fatty plane between the arteries and the nodes are preserved and, if not, by how many degrees the tumor encircles the vessel (Fig. 6.5).

One of the key hallmarks of imaging lies in its ability to detect clinically inaccessible lymph nodes. In subglottic cancer, lymph nodes located deep in level VI can be visualized. Retropharyngeal lymph nodes are not expected at the pretherapeutic stage of laryngeal cancer. In the presence of such a finding, the radiologist should carefully look for a concomitant soft palate or nasopharyngeal cancer.

Ultrasound is performed for lymph node assessment only and offers similar or superior accuracy compared to CT and MR imaging (van den Brekel et al. 1998a). A round-to-spherical shape of the

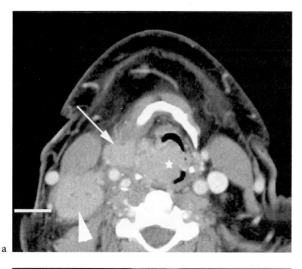

a

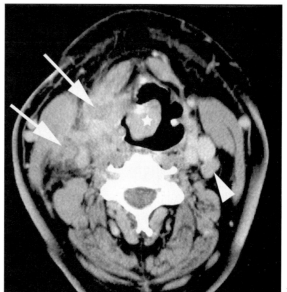

b

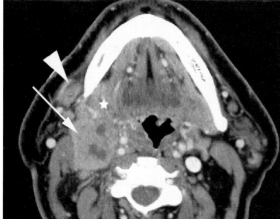

c

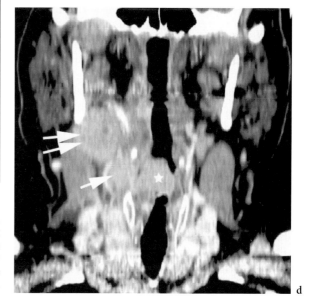

d

Fig. 6.4. a Contrast-enhanced CT. Squamous cell carcinoma
of the left aryepiglottic fold (*star*). There is a metastatic
lymph node in level III (*arrow*) under the hyoid bone; it is
anterior to the common carotid artery and internal jugular
vein, in the superior laryngeal neurovascular bundle. The
continuity between the tumor and the node indicates probable invasion of the thyrohyoid membrane. A second lymph
node (*arrowhead*) is posterior to the vessels. This node
slightly spans into level V since its posterior portion is located posterior to a line drawn through the posterior edge of
the sternocleidomastoid muscle (*line*). **b** Contrast-enhanced
CT. Valsalva's maneuver. The tumor (*star*) is well delineated.
The right metastatic nodes (*arrows*) are not well depicted
because there is no more contrast in the vessels. However, the
diffuse contrast enhancement in the adjacent tissue indicates
extracapsular spread. A contralateral lymph node is seen in
level II (*arrowhead*). **c** Contrast-enhanced CT. A large lymph
node is depicted in level II, showing two areas of necrosis. A
node is also seen in level IB (*arrowhead*) adjacent to the submandibular gland (*star*). **d** Contrast-enhanced CT. Coronal
reformatted view shows the tumor (*star*), the level III node
(*arrow*) and the level II node (*double arrow*). **e** The patient
was treated by radiotherapy. Contrast-enhanced CT shows
the disappearance of the lymph nodes, with nonspecific
nonenhancing residual tissue (*arrow*)

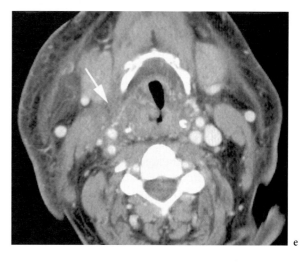

e

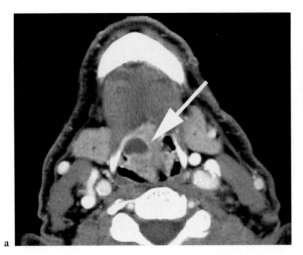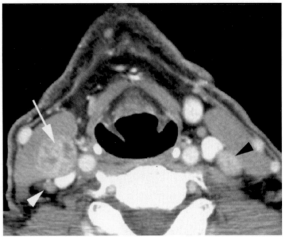

a   b

Fig. 6.5. a Contrast-enhanced CT. Carcinoma of the free epiglottic rim with extension to the vallecula (*arrow*). **b** On the right side, a large lymph node is located in level II (*arrow*), adhering to the carotid artery on less than 1/4th of its surface. A non specific smaller node (*white arrowhead*) is located behind the jugular vein. A left node can be seen (*black arrowhead*), which was also positive at histology

nodes is the best criterion, followed by hypo-echogenicity and loss of hilar definition (Fig. 6.6). In cases of extracapsular spread, the nodal margins are poorly defined. Necrosis creates pseudoliquid areas (KOISCHWITZ and GRITZMANN 2000). On col-or Doppler and power Doppler sonography malig-nant nodes may show increased peripheral perfu-sion, focal absence of perfusion, absence of central vessels, displacement of vessels, or an irregular pat-tern of perfusion. A high variation in the resistance index also indicates metastatic invasion (KOIS-CHWITZ and GRITZMANN 2000) (Figs. 6.7, 6.8). The lack of reliable objective criteria and the overlap-ping patterns in lymphoma, inflammation and nodal metastases should be underlined. Ultrasound combined with ultrasound-guided FNAC (fine nee-dle aspiration cytology) yields a specificity of over 95% and a sensitivity reported between 42% and 98% (BAATENBURG DE JONG et al. 1991; TAKES et al. 1996; VAN DEN BREKEL et al. 1993), but this tech-nique is labor-intensive and operator-dependent and is not available in many centers.

FDG-PET has shown promising results (BRAAMS et al. 1995; LAUBENBACHER et al. 1995), with a 90% sensitivity and a 94% specificity in a recent study (ADAMS et al. 1998) (Fig. 6.9). However, FDG-PET cannot differentiate between malignant nodes and benign reactive nodes. Activated macrophages may cause increased FDG uptake and false-positive re-sults (CHISIN and MACAPINLAC 2000). Post-treat-ment inflammation is also a source of false-positive results.

6.6.2
Post-therapeutic Imaging

6.6.2.1
Normal Aspect: Neck Dissection

In a standard radical neck dissection, all the ipsilateral lymph nodes extending from the mandible down to the clavicle, and from the sternohyoid and contralateral anterior belly of digastric muscle (anteriorly) to the trapezius muscle (posteriorly) are extirpated. This in-cludes levels I–V in the level nomenclature (ROBBINS et al. 1991). This procedure implies the ablation of the following elements: sternocleidomastoid muscle, inter-nal and external jugular veins, spinal accessory nerve and submandibular gland. The result is both a cosmetic deformity and shoulder droop due to denervation of the trapezius muscle, which is partially compensated by hypertrophy of the ipsilateral levator scapulae muscle. The term modified radical neck dissection is used when one or two of the following structures are spared: sternocleidomastoid muscle, internal jugular vein, and spinal accessory nerve. The extended neck dissection is performed when other structures that are invaded or endangered by lymph node spread have to be removed: skin, platysma, strap and paraspinal muscles, thyroid gland, cranial nerve IX and X, and carotid artery. The dissection can also be extended to lymphatic structures not encompassed in the radical neck dissection, such as the retropharyngeal, superior mediastinal (level VII), and paratracheal lymph nodes (level VI) (ROBBINS et al. 1990; SHAH 1996).

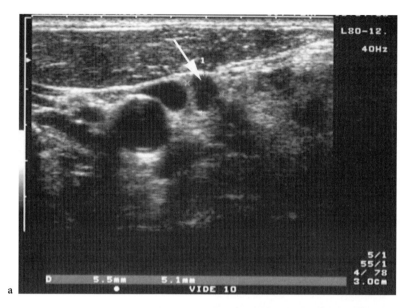

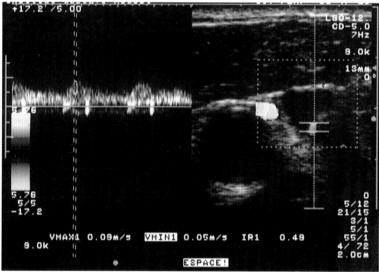

Fig. 6.6. a High frequency ultrasonography shows a small, round-shaped hypoechogenic node (*arrow*) with loss of visibility of the hilum, highly suspicious for nodal metastasis. **b** The low resistance index (<0.50) is characteristic of neovascularization

The concept of selective neck dissection (also called functional or modified, which is a source of confusion with the modified radical neck dissection) stems from the observation that for each primary carcinoma, the pathway of metastatic spread to neck lymph nodes is predictable, and therefore there is no need to remove other groups of nodes which are unlikely to contain metastatic deposits (SOM 1996). Therefore, by removing only the high-risk nodes, it may be possible to spare the sternocleidomastoid muscle, the internal jugular vein, and/or the spinal accessory nerve, hence reducing the cosmetic and functional deficits. Several procedures are described according to the levels which are removed.

At imaging, both radical neck dissection and extended neck dissections are easily identified. The changes associated with a selective neck dissection can be subtle, depending on the type of tissue removed: moderate thickening of the skin, flattening of the neck contour, mild unsharpness of tissue planes (SIGAL 2000; SOM et al. 1993).

6.6.2.2
Relapse

Patients having undergone surgery or irradiation are often difficult to examine clinically due to "woody" thickening of the skin, loss of anatomical landmarks and pain. Furthermore, the information provided by physical examination or by endoscopy is more difficult to interpret than at the initial stage. As a consequence, imaging plays a key role in the management of

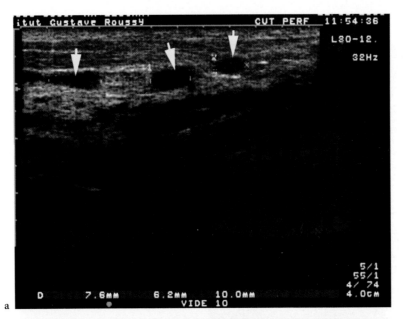

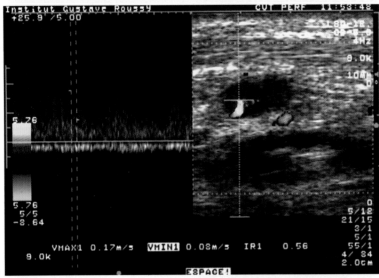

Fig. 6.7. a Ultrasonography shows three infracentimetric nodes (*arrows*). The hypoechogenicity, the round shape and loss of visibility of the hilar region are suspicious for metastatic invasion. b The color Doppler mode shows increased vascularity in the hilar region

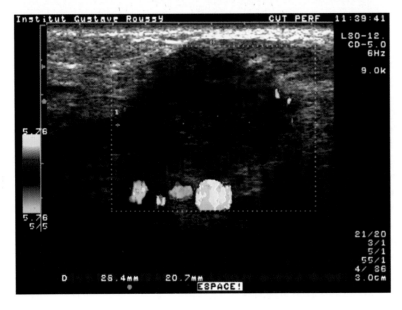

Fig. 6.8. A large subdigastric node is displayed with a heterogeneous echo-structure. The scarcity of vessels is due to central node necrosis

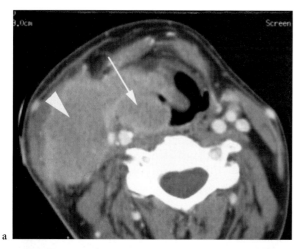

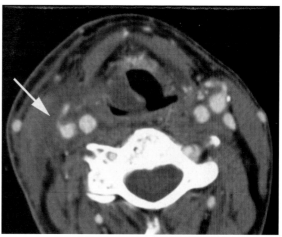

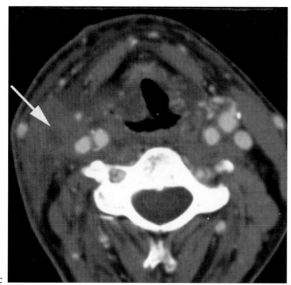

Fig. 6.9. a Patient with a T4 laryngohypopharyngeal cancer (*arrow*) adjacent to a N3 node (*arrowhead*). **b** The patient was treated by radiotherapy. The tumor showed a dramatic response to treatment: 3 months after radiotherapy there was no clinical evidence of tumor. As well as slight asymmetry within the larynx and hypopharynx, CT at this time showed an asymmetric appearance of the fatty tissues in the right neck (*arrow*). **c** After a further 2 months, clinically the neck did show some soft swelling, but not really indicative of malignancy. However, on CT a definite progression was noted, with the appearance of centrally hypodense and peripherally enhancing nodules (*arrow*). **d** A PET scan clearly showed two areas of tracer accumulation in the right neck, corresponding with the findings on the CT scan, and was reported as tumor recurrence. Cytological study after fine needle aspiration was negative. Based on the radiological findings, a radical neck dissection was performed, definitely showing invasive squamous cell carcinoma with extensive necrosis. In addition, faint uptake is visible in the laryngeal region, and some months later the patient also developed a local tumor recurrence (case courtesy of R. Hermans, MD, PhD, Leuven, Belgium)

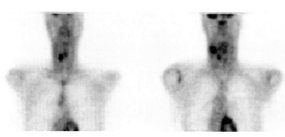

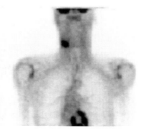

post-treatment patients because it may detect recurrence at an early stage. However, the lack of specificity of imaging should be underlined. This emphasizes the need for clinical information when interpreting imaging data and the value of close communication between clinicians and head and neck radiologists (HUDGINS et al. 1994; MANCUSO 1994; SOM et al. 1993).

Relapses may occur in lymph nodes, with or without relapse at the primary site. The metastatic nodes may show the same pattern as seen at the pretherapeutic stage. However, because of neck dissection and/or irradiation, neck lymph nodes tend to present as poorly marginated, heterogeneous masses. In fact, any mass in the neck, whatever its appearance, should be considered as a nodal relapse, until the contrary has been proven (Fig. 6.10).

Recurrences also occur in the retropharyngeal space, even when the primary was initially located at

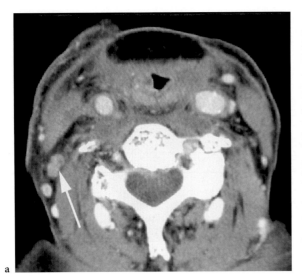
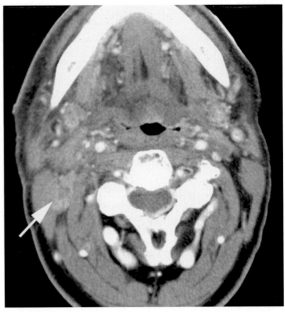

Fig. 6.10. a Contrast-enhanced CT. Lymph node relapse. The patient had been treated by complete pharyngolaryngectomy with a pectoralis major flap and radiotherapy 3 years before. A small enhancing node (*arrow*) is visible at level V. **b** A node is also present at level II. Note that the node (*arrow*) is seen as an ill-defined mass with moderate contrast enhancement

the infrahyoid level, and this justifies the need to scan from the skull base to the clavicles, just as in the initial work-up.

6.6.2.3
Follow-up Policy

The follow-up policy is not specific for the lymph nodes. In the post-treatment period, reference baseline scans are recommended in patients at risk for tumor relapse or when post-treatment edema or pain prevent a good physical examination. Performing a baseline scan for every patient at risk is important because the patterns of post-treatment changes over time are highly variable from one subject to another. The baseline study should be performed no sooner than 3 months after completion of all treatments, at a time when acute and subacute inflammatory changes should have disappeared (MANCUSO 1994), although in some patients, a stable postoperative appearance is not reached until 12–18 months after completion of treatment (SOM et al. 1993). In practice, comparison between successive examinations often provides a clue to diagnosis by showing either a new mass and/or abnormal reappearance of contrast enhancement (HERMANS et al. 2000). Most tumor relapses occur within the first 2 years and the majority of cancer deaths occur within the first 3 years following treatment. It therefore seems logical

to propose two or three systematic follow-up scans during the first 2 years, a 6-month interval for the 3rd year, and an annual examination for at least 2 more years (SOM et al. 1993).

References

Adams S, Baum R, Stuckensen T, et al (1998) Prospective comparison of 18F-FDG PET with conventional imaging modalities (CT, MRI, US) in lymph node staging of head and neck cancer. Eur J Nucl Med 25:1255–1260

Ali S, Tiwari R, Snow G (1985) False positive and false negative neck nodes. Head Neck Surg 8:78–83

Anzai Y, Prince M (1997) Iron oxide-enhanced MR lymphography: the evaluation of cervical lymph node metastases in head and neck cancer. J Magn Reson Imaging 7:75–81

Anzai Y, Carroll W, Quint D, et al (1996) Recurrence of head and neck cancer after surgery or irradiation: prospective comparison of 2-deoxy-2-(F-18) fluoro-D-glucose PET and MR imaging diagnoses. Radiology 200:135–141

Baatenburg de Jong R, Rongen R, Verwoerd C, et al (1991) Ultrasound-guided fine-needle aspiration biopsy of neck nodes. Arch Otolaryngol Head Neck Surg 117:402–404

Baatenburg de Jong R, Knegt P, Verwoerd C (1993) Reduction of the number of neck treatments in patients with head and neck cancer. Cancer 71:2312–2318

Beahrs O, Henson D, Hutter R, et al (1998) American Joint Committee on Cancer manual for staging cancer, 3rd edn. Lippincott, Philadelphia

Bocca E (1975) Supraglottic cancer. Laryngoscope 85:1318–1326

Braams J, Pruim J, Freling N, et al (1995) Detection of lymph node metastases of squamous-cell cancer of the head and neck with FDG-PET and MRI. J Nucl Med 36:211–216

Byers R, Wolf P, Ballantyne A (1988) Rationale for elective modified neck dissection. Head Neck Surg 10:160–167

Chisin R, Macapinlac H (2000) The indications of FDG-PET in neck oncology. Radiol Clin North Am 38:999–1012

Colnot D, Nieuwenhuis E, van den Brekel M, et al (2001) Head and neck squamous cell carcinoma: US-guided fine-needle aspiration of sentinel lymph nodes for improved staging – initial experience. Radiology 218:289–293

Curtin HD, Ishwaran H, Mancuso AA, et al (1998) Comparison of CT and MR imaging in staging of neck metastases. Radiology 207:123–130

DeSanto L, Lillie J, Devine K (1977) Cancers of the larynx: supraglottic cancer. Surg Clin North Am 57:505–514

Dillon W (1998) Cervical nodal metastases: another look at size criteria. AJNR Am J Neuroradiol 19:796–797

Fakih A, Rao R, Borges A, et al (1989) Elective versus therapeutic neck dissection in early carcinoma of the oral tongue. Am J Surg 158:309–313

Fischbein N, Assar O, Caputo G, et al (1998) Clinical utility of positron emission tomography with 18F-fluorodeoxyglucose in detecting residual/recurrent squamous cell carcinoma of the head and neck. AJNR Am J Neuroradiol 19:1189–1196

Hermans R, Pameijer FA, Mancuso AA, et al (2000) Laryngeal or hypopharyngeal squamous cell carcinoma: can follow-up CT after definitive radiotherapy be used to detect local failure earlier than clinical examination alone? Radiology 214:683–687

Hudgins P, Burson J, Gussack G, et al (1994) CT and MR appearance of recurrent malignant head and neck neoplasms after resection and flap reconstruction. AJNR Am J Neuroradiol 15:1689–1694

Johnson J (1990) A surgeon looks at cervical lymph nodes. Radiology 177:607–610

Kligerman J, Lima R, Soares J, et al (1994) Supraomohyoid neck dissection in the treatment of T1/T2 squamous cell carcinoma of oral cavity. Am J Surg 168:391–394

Koischwitz D, Gritzmann N (2000) Ultrasound of the neck. Radiol Clin North Am 38:1029–1045

Laubenbacher C, Saumweber D, Wagner-Manslau C, et al (1995) Comparison of fluorine-18-fluorodeoxyglucose PET, MRI and endoscopy for staging head and neck squamous-cell carcinomas. J Nucl Med 36:1747–1757

Lindberg R (1972) Distribution of cervical lymph node metastases from squamous cell carcinoma of the upper respiratory and digestive tracts. Cancer 29:1446–1449

Mancuso A (1994) Imaging in patients with head and neck cancer. In: Million R, Cassisi N (eds) Management of head and neck cancer. A multidisciplinary approach, 2nd edn. Lippincott, Philadelphia, pp 43–59

McGuirt WF, Greven K, Williams D, et al (1998) PET scanning in head and neck oncology: a review. Head Neck 20:208–215

Mendenhall W, Million R, Mancuso A, et al (1994) Larynx. In: Million RR, Cassisi NJ (eds) Management of head and neck cancer. A multidisciplinary approach, 2nd edn. Lippincott, Philadelphia, pp 443–446

Robbins K, van Sonnenberg E, Casola G, et al (1990) Image-guided needle aspiration of inaccessible head and neck lesions. Arch Otolaryngol Head Neck Surg 116:957–961

Robbins KT, Medina JE, Wolfe GT, et al (1991) Standardizing neck dissection terminology. Official report of the Academy's Committee for Head and Neck Surgery and Oncology. Arch Otolaryngol Head Neck Surg 117:601–605

Sakai O, Curtin H, Romo L, et al (2000) Lymph node pathology. Benign proliferative, lymphoma, and metastatic disease. Radiol Clin North Am 38:979–398

Schuller D, Bier-Laning C (1997) Laryngeal carcinoma nodal metastases and their management. Otolaryngol Clin North Am 30:167–177

Sessions D, Ogura J, Fried M (1975) Carcinoma of the subglottic area. Laryngoscope 85:1417–1423

Shah JP (1996) Reconstructive surgery. In: Shah JP (ed) Head and neck surgery. Mosby-Wolfe, London, pp 559–605

Shah JP, Tollefsen H (1974) Epidermoid carcinoma of the supraglottic larynx. Role of neck dissection in initial surgical treatment. Am J Surg 128:494–499

Shah JP, Strong E, Spiro R, et al (1981) Surgical grand rounds. Neck dissection: current status and future possibilities. Clin Bull 11:25–33

Sigal R (2000) Post-therapeutic imaging of upper aerodigestive tract tumors. Semin Roentgenol 35:101–110

Sigal R, Vogl T, Casselman J, et al (2001) Lymph node metastases from head and neck squamous cell carcinoma. MR imaging with ultrasmall superparamagnetic iron oxide particles (Sinerem MR). Results of a phase III multi center clinical trial. Eur Radiol (in press)

Som P (1992) Detection of metastasis in cervical lymph nodes: CT and MR criteria and differential diagnosis. AJR Am J Roentgenol 158:961–969

Som P (1996) Postoperative neck. In: Som P, Curtin H (eds) Head and neck imaging. Mosby, Baltimore, pp 992–1005

Som P, Urken ML, Biller H, et al (1993) Imaging of the postoperative neck. Radiology 187:593–603

Som P, Curtin H, Mancuso A (1999) An imaging-based classification for the cervical nodes designed as an adjunct to recent clinically based nodal classifications. Arch Otolaryngol Head Neck Surg 125:388–396

Som P, Curtin H, Mancuso A (2000) Imaging-based nodal classification for evaluation of neck metastatic adenopathy. AJR Am J Roentgenol 174:837–844

Takes R, Knegt P, Manni J, et al (1996) Regional metastases in head and neck squamous cell carcinoma: revised value of US with US-guided FNAB. Radiology 198:819–823

UICC (1997) TNM classification of malignant tumours, 5th edn. Springer, Berlin Heidelberg New York

van den Brekel M (1996) US-guided fine-needle aspiration cytology of neck nodes in patients with N0 disease. Radiology 201:580–581

van den Brekel M (2000) Lymph node metastases: CT and MRI. Eur J Radiol 33:230–238

van den Brekel M, Castelijns J (1993) Modern imaging techniques and ultrasound guided aspiration cytology for the assessment of neck node metastases: a prospective comparative study. Eur Arch Otorhinolaryngol 250:11–17

van den Brekel M, Castelijns J (2000) Imaging of lymph nodes in the neck. Semin Roentgenol 35:42–53

van den Brekel M, Castelijns J, Stel H, et al (1990a) Detection and characterization of metastatic cervical adenopathy by MR imaging: comparison of different MR techniques. J Comput Assist Tomogr 14:581–589

van den Brekel M, Stel H, Castelijns J, et al (1990b) Cervical lymph node metastasis: assessment of radiologic criteria. Radiology 177:379–384 van den Brekel M, Bartelink H, Snow G (1994) The value of staging of neck nodes in patients treated with radiotherapy. Radiother Oncol 32:193–196

van den Brekel M, Castelijns J, Snow G (1996) Imaging of cervical lymphadenopathy. Neuroimaging Clin North Am 6:417–434

van den Brekel M, Castelijns J, Snow G (1998a) Diagnostic evaluation of the neck. Otolaryngol Clin North Am 31:601–620

van den Brekel M, Castelijns J, Snow G (1998b) The size of lymph nodes in the neck on sonograms as a radiologic criterion for metastasis: how reliable is it? AJNR Am J Neuroradiol 19:695–700

VandenBrouck C, Sancho-Garnier H, Chassagne D, et al (1980) Elective versus therapeutic radical neck dissection in epidermoid carcinoma of the oral cavity: results of a randomized clinical trial. Cancer 46:386–390

Weissleder R, Elizondo G, Wittenberg J, et al (1990) Ultrasmall superparamagnetic iron oxide: an intravenous contrast agent for assessing lymph nodes with MR imaging. Radiology 175:494–498

Yousem D, Som P, Hackney D, et al (1992) Central nodal necrosis and extracapsular neoplastic spread in cervical lymph nodes: MR imaging versus CT. Radiology 182:753–759

Yousem DM, Hatabu H, Hurst RW, et al (1995) Carotid artery invasion by head and neck masses: prediction with MR imaging. Radiology 195:715–720

7 Predicting the Local Outcome of Irradiated Laryngeal Cancer: Value of Pretreatment Imaging

Robert Hermans and Jonas A. Castelijns

CONTENTS

7.1 Introduction

Concerns have been expressed about the weakness of the T classification for laryngeal cancer, and for cancers at other head and neck sites, as the cure rates reported in the literature vary and prognosis is not sufficiently related to the T values (Bailey 1991; Harrison 1988; Piccirillo 1995). Modern radiologic imaging methods assist in pretreatment planning by defining the extension of infiltrating head and neck tumors better, and, moreover, quantitative evaluation of tumor volume is feasible. In this chapter the use of pretherapeutic imaging in coming to a more refined estimation of the local outcome of laryngeal cancer after radiation treatment is discussed.

R. Hermans, MD, PhD
Professor, Department of Radiology, University Hospitals Leuven, Herestraat 49, 3000 Leuven, Belgium
J.A. Castelijns, MD, PhD
Professor, Department of Radiology, Free University Hospital Amsterdam, P.O. 7057, 1007 MB Amsterdam, The Netherlands

7.2 Impact of Imaging on T Classification

7.2.1 The Use of Imaging in the T Classification of Laryngeal Carcinoma

Laryngeal tumors are classified according to the TNM classification, as defined by the UICC (Union International Contre le Cancer 1997) and AJCC (American Joint Committee on Cancer 1992). These two staging systems are identical with respect to laryngeal tumors. The classification of a tumor aims at providing information about its extension, gives some indication of prognosis and helps in treatment planning. It can also be used in reporting the results of treatment and facilitates exchange of information between different centers.

For the purpose of tumor classification, the larynx is divided in three distinct anatomic regions: the supraglottis, glottis and subglottis. The criteria used in the classification of laryngeal tumors are extent of tumor spread, vocal cord function and cartilage invasion (see Chap. 5).

The validity of any classification is dependent on the diagnostic methods employed (Snow and Gerritsen 1993). It is recognized that clinical classification of laryngeal cancer is insufficient when compared with pathologic classification (Pillsbury and Kirchner 1979). A marked improvement in accuracy can be obtained when the results of CT or MRI are added to the clinical findings (Katsantonis et al. 1986; Silverman et al. 1984; Sulfaro et al. 1989; Zbären et al. 1996). Imaging is mainly of benefit in detecting deep soft tissue extension, such as in the preepiglottic space, the laryngeal cartilages, and the base of tongue. Findings from imaging studies frequently result in an up-classification of the disease.

For categorization of a given laryngeal tumor the UICC and AJCC are not very precise regarding their recommendations for the use of imaging methods such as CT and MRI. The AJCC, for example, states that a variety of imaging procedures are valuable in evaluating the extent of disease, particularly for advanced tumors. These include laryngeal tomograms, CT and MRI studies, but when to use any or all of these imaging methods is not indicated. Without further specification as to the type of imaging, UICC recommends that imaging should be included in the diagnostic workup.

Although the benefit of CT in the classification of laryngeal cancer has been known for a long time, not all patients with clinically advanced cancer are being examined with this tool; the reasons for this are not clear (Barbera et al. 2001; Shah et al. 1997). Actually, one may argue that patients with clinically localized disease would benefit more from such a CT study, as up-classification of the cancer may result in a change of patient management. In The Netherlands, a recently published national guideline states that all patients with a supraglottic carcinoma, and all patients with a glottic carcinoma (except T1 lesions limited to one vocal cord, not involving the anterior commissure) should undergo a high-quality CT or MRI study (Nationale Werkgroep Hoofd-Halstumoren 2000).

7.2.2
The Problem of Stage Migration

The change in stage occurring because of the inclusion of additional diagnostic information is called stage migration. This is typically seen in situations where a new diagnostic test is applied. As the new test may detect previously undetectable disease, more recently examined patients may become classified into a higher stage than patients who did not undergo the new test. Because of the sensitive new test, patients with previously undetectable spread of disease will migrate from a localized stage with a generally good prognosis to a more advanced stage with a generally worse prognosis (Piccirillo and Lacy 2000).

An example is the use of CT or MRI in the evaluation of glottic cancer. A patient may present with a clinically limited tumor of the vocal cord and anterior commissure (classified as a T1 lesion), while imaging additionally shows tumor growth through the thyroid cartilage (hence classified as a T4 lesion). Also in the other laryngeal sites the use of imaging may cause such migration (Fig. 7.1). In a large retrospective study, reassignment of clinical tumor category occurred in 20.2% of the patients based on information provided by CT, and in most cases, classification into a higher T category occurred because of positive CT findings (Barbera et al. 2001).

The migrating patient has more advanced disease than that present overall in the group he or she leaves, but less advanced disease than that present overall in the group he or she enters. If detection of previously undetectable disease does not influence patient management, the effect of including an additional, more-sensitive diagnostic test will be that each tumor category shows an improvement of outcome. However, as there is only movement of patients between tumor categories, the treatment outcome of the entire cohort will be the same as observed in cohorts in which the additional diagnostic test was not applied (Piccirillo and Lacy 2000), and also the outcome for the individual patient will not be changed. It is important to recognize this phenomenon as a potential source of misleading statistics for treatment outcome in cancer (Feinstein et al. 1985).

7.2.3
Impact of Imaging on Treatment Choice and Prognostic Accuracy in Laryngeal Cancer

Very few studies are available on the impact of imaging on treatment choice and the accuracy of predicting treatment outcome in laryngeal cancer. Such an impact depends on the treatment policy of laryngeal cancer in a given center (Barbera et al. 2001). Charlin et al. (1989) studied the impact of CT on management, working in an institution in which at that time all cancers with a small to moderate tumor volume and no sign of deep infiltration were treated by radiotherapy alone, larger cancers and those with signs of deep infiltration by conservative surgery when the local extension allowed it, and tumors with vocal cord fixation, cartilage destruction and other signs of deep major infiltration by total laryngectomy with postoperative radiotherapy. Charlin et al. (1989) observed a change in therapeutic attitude with CT in 10 of 66 consecutive patients (15.1%). In all ten patients radiotherapy was thought to be the best treatment after endoscopic evaluation. This was changed to conservative surgery in seven and total laryngectomy with postoperative irradiation in three patients.

In other centers, nearly all laryngeal cancers are treated by radical radiotherapy, surgery being used as a salvage procedure. In such institutions the impact of laryngeal imaging on initial treatment selec-

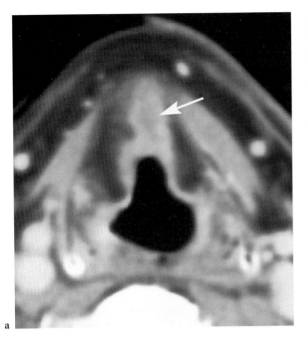
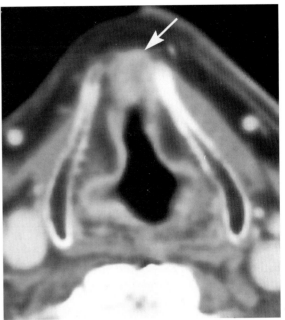

a   b

Fig. 7.1a, b. Contrast-enhanced CT images through the supraglottis. Clinically, the patient has a malignant tumor on the laryngeal side of the epiglottis, classified as T1. The CT study shows a low-volume lesion, but infiltration of the preepiglottic space (**a** *arrow*) and beginning extralaryngeal tumor spread through the thyroid notch (**b** *arrow*) are present. Based on these findings, the cancer was classified as a T4 lesion

tion can be anticipated to be of less importance. However, the radiologic findings may influence the definition of radiation portals, which require an exact knowledge of the local extension of the tumor, the status of the neck lymph nodes, and the location of metastatic neck adenopathies.

In a retrospective multicenter study, the incorporation of CT information did not improve the ability of the T classification to predict local failure or cause-specific survival (BARBERA et al. 2001). However, as noted by these authors, the ability of CT to improve the predictive value of the T classification is constrained by the definitions of the classification, which do not take into account other prognostic information provided by CT.

ARCHER et al. (1984) have proposed a classification system of laryngeal cancer based on CT findings. This classification uses the localization of the tumor mass relative to the arytenoid cartilage, as visible on CT studies. The rationale is that tumors with their plane of maximal size at or below the midbody of the arytenoid cartilage have a much higher likelihood of cartilage invasion. In more than half of their cases such cartilage invasion was only detectable by microscopic study of the resected specimen. This alternative classification system has not been adopted.

7.3
Use of Imaging Parameters Independently from the T Classification

7.3.1
Background

Success in controlling a tumor by radiotherapy depends on killing all clonogenic cells. The probability of cure depends on, among other factors, the initial number of clonogenic cells. In clinical situations, the range of clonogenic cell contents may be large within a certain tumor stage, and is not only dependent on tumor volume but also on other factors such as necrosis or infiltration by normal cells (macrophages, fibrovascular stroma). The number of clonogenic cells also depends on the rate of repopulation during the radiation treatment (WITHERS 1992). Nevertheless, there are indications that the clonogen number increases linearly with tumor volume (JOHNSON et al. 1995). Therefore, tumor volume is an interesting predictor of local outcome.

Although there is a correlation between visible tumor extent and tumor volume, and hence indirectly with the T classification, tumor volume as such is not used in the current TNM classification system. Tumor volume is difficult to determine clinically, especially in the head and neck with its complex regional anatomy and the infiltrating behavior of the tumors occurring in this region. However, volumetric assessment of soft tissue masses is possible with cross-sectional imaging techniques such as CT and MRI.

Apart from tumor volume, other explicit morphologic characteristics, as visible on CT or MR studies, could be considered as prognostic parameters. An example is the depth of neoplastic infiltration within the submucosal laryngeal spaces. Another example is the presence of cartilage abnormalities, such as cartilage sclerosis on CT or intracartilaginous signal changes on MRI, without cancer growing through the cartilage.

7.3.2
Estimating Tumor Extent and Volume on CT and MRI: Intra- and Interobserver Variability

The clinical utility of an imaging study not only depends on the sensitivity, specificity and accuracy obtained, but also on the consistency of interpretation by the same observer on different times or by different observers. Sometimes different opinions exist among observers after independent review of the examinations (BECKER et al. 1995; CASTELIJNS et al. 1995). The choice of therapy may be influenced by subtle imaging findings, which are prone to interpretation differences. Tumor scores reflecting the anatomic tumor extent are increasingly being investigated as possible predictors of local outcome after radiation therapy (LEE et al. 1993; PAMEIJER et al. 1997). Obviously, knowledge about the reproducibility of image interpretations is also of interest in patients considered for surgery, as the decision to operate and which surgical technique to use is influenced by CT or MRI findings.

The intra- and interobserver reproducibility of the interpretation of CT studies for laryngeal carcinoma has recently been evaluated (HERMANS et al. 1997a). Fair to substantial intraobserver reproducibility (kappa=0,29–0,86), and fair to substantial interobserver reproducibility (average kappa=0,26–0,74) were found for most laryngeal structures. On average these kappa-values are in the expected range for clinical diagnostics and imaging studies. Even when multiple choices were possible (e.g., degree of invasion of the paraglottic space), the measured reproducibility in this study remained within acceptable limits. This indicates that concerns about reproducibility should not withhold a trained radiologist from scoring the involvement of a particular laryngeal structure into subcategories.

To determine the volume of a particular structure, its borders are traced onto consecutive images, either manually or using a (semi)automated method. The segmented surface on each image is then calculated. This procedure can be done on the scanner's screen, using a mouse-controlled cursor, or indirectly using a digitizer. The obtained surfaces are then multiplied by the slice interval. The summation of all the volumes obtained represents the total volume of the structure of interest. This technique is called the summation-of-areas technique (BREIMAN et al. 1982).

A very close relationship has been found between CT-determined volume and postoperative weight of enlarged thyroid glands (HERMANS et al. 1997b). As the specific gravity of thyroid tissue is close to 1, this means that the thyroid gland's volume can be accurately estimated based on CT imaging. Although thyroid glands are on average (much) larger than most laryngeal tumors, it is likely that using CT the volume of smaller soft tissue lesions can be measured with comparable accuracy.

A statistically significant effect of the observer has been demonstrated on the variability of the measured laryngeal tumor volumes ($P<0.0001$) (HERMANS et al. 1998). In this study, the most important component of total variability was interobserver variability (89.3%), while intraobserver variability contributed 6.4% to total variability (Fig. 7.2).

Reducing the variability in the measurements as much as possible is necessary to obtain sharp classifications of laryngeal tumors based on their volume. Only measurements with low variability are useful for correlation with local outcome after radiation therapy. This can be achieved by always having the same observer perform the measurements. It has been shown that an observer with experience in head and neck radiology can measure laryngeal tumor volumes with a significantly lower variability than other observers (HERMANS et al. 1998).

Using MRI, the principle of the summation-of-areas technique is applied similarly to estimate the volume of the tumor. In experienced hands, it has been shown to yield a fairly good intra- and interobserver reproducibility (CASTELIJNS et al. 1995). However, considerable operator-computer interaction time is needed to assess each patient. Currently, segmentation (automatic delineation and identification of tumor) cannot be performed due to low contrast between tumor and the surrounding tissue.

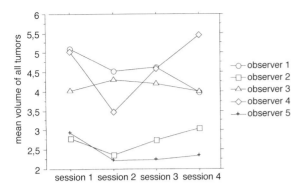

Fig. 7.2. Five observers independently measured the volume of 13 randomly chosen laryngeal tumors on CT images. They repeated these measurements four times. The graph shows the interaction of the mean volume of all tumors (in millili-ters) and the four measurement sessions. Interobserver vari-ability is seen to be the most important component of total variability. By having the volume calculations done by one single observer, measurement variability can be reduced sub-stantially. Observer 3 (head and neck radiologist) obtained the most stable mean tumor volume over all sessions. Three observers obtained less-stable results through the different sessions, while one observer (observer 4) obtained fluctuat-ing mean tumor volumes (the other observers were staff ra-diologists or radiology residents). (Reprinted from Interna-tional Journal of Radiation Oncology Biology Physics, vol 40, Hermans R, Feron M, Bellon E, et al., Laryngeal tumor vol-ume measurements determined with CT: a study on intra-and interobserver variability, pp 553–557, copyright 1998, with permission from Elsevier Science)

7.3.3
Prognostic Significance of Imaging-Defined Parameters

7.3.3.1
Using CT

7.3.3.1.1
Tumor Volume and Deep Tissue Infiltration on CT

A large primary tumor volume has been known for a long time to be a reason for poor local outcome of laryngeal cancer after definitive radiation treatment (FLETCHER and HAMBERGER 1974; FLETCHER et al. 1975). Clinical estimation of tumor volume in vari-ous advanced head and neck cancers treated in a multicenter EORTC trial correlated with survival and locoregional control after radiation treatment (VAN DEN BOGAERT et al. 1995), but the volume class-es defined in that study (<10 ml, 10–30 ml, 30–100 ml, >100 ml) are too rough to be applicable to less-advanced head and neck cancers. OVERGAARD et al. (1986) reported laryngeal tumor diameter (<2 cm, 2–3.9 cm, >4 cm) to be of significant importance to both probability of local control and survival in glot-

tic and supraglottic tumors. However, tumor diame-ters are a rough and potentially inaccurate estima-tion of tumor volume due to invisible deep tumor extension (MARKS et al. 1979; VAN DEN BOGAERT et al. 1983). Using a model of cell population kinetics during irradiation, a 10–20% theoretical difference in local control rate has been calculated for tumors with a similar largest dimension (5 cm) but different width (3 or 5 cm) (HJELM-HANSEN 1980). This indi-cates that correct assessment of tumor volume is an important point.

GILBERT et al. (1987) were the first to report the prognostic value of CT-determined tumor volume for outcome after definitive radiation therapy. Their study included patients with T2-T4 laryngeal cancer (both of glottic and supraglottic origin). The mean tumor volume for patients failing radiotherapy in their study was 21.8 ml, and for patients primarily controlled was 8.86 ml. Tumor volume significantly predicted disease-free interval and outcome after radiotherapy.

Glottic and supraglottic tumors should be consid-ered separately in such studies, as the anatomic situ-ation (and hence extension pattern) is very different for glottic versus supraglottic tumors. Furthermore, the two sites also have their own staging recommen-dations in the AJCC and UICC staging manuals.

FREEMAN et al. (1990) whose study (31 patients) was updated by MANCUSO et al. (1999) (63 patients), were able to identify those patients with T1-T4 supraglottic carcinomas who had a higher likelihood of local control based on pretreatment CT volume-tric analysis (tumors <6 ml had a probability of 89% of local control, while tumors >6 ml had a probabili-ty of only 40%).

LEE et al. (1993), whose study (18 patients) was updated by PAMEIJER et al. (1997) (42 patients), were able to stratify patients with T3 glottic carcinoma in a similar way into groups with different likelihood of local control (tumors of 3.5 ml had a local control probability of 85%, while tumors of >3.5 ml had a probability of only 22%). On the other hand, MUKHERJI et al. (1995), in a study on 28 patients with T2 glottic carcinoma, were not able to distinguish groups with significantly different local control rates using CT-determined tumor volumes. In a more re-cent study, in patients with a T2 laryngeal cancer, a tumor volume of >4 ml predicted a significantly worse local outcome rate (LO et al. 1998).

The results of the studies by HERMANS et al. (1999a, b) provide good corroboration of these pre-vious findings. Both for glottic and supraglottic can-cer, tumor volume was found to be a significant prognostic indicator of local control. In glottic cancer, failure probability analysis showed a clear relationship between larger tumor volume and increasing risk of local failure (Fig. 7.3). A tumor volume of 3,5 ml correlated with a risk of local failure of approximately 50%. From the graph presented by PAMEIJER et al. (1997), an approximately 40% chance of local failure in T3 glottic cancer with a similar tumor volume can be inferred. Also for supraglottic cancer, HERMANS et al. (1999b) found a significant relationship between tumor volume and risk of local failure (Fig. 7.4). Compared to glottic cancer, larger supraglottic tumor volumes were found for similar local control rates; similar results can be inferred from other reports (MANCUSO et al. 1999; PAMEIJER et al. 1998). The reason for the different critical tumor volumes between glottic and supraglottic cancer is not clear; it might be related to a different local environment in the glottic and supraglottic region, but also (and maybe predominantly) to the more exophytic growth pattern exhibited by supraglottic tumors.

In the studies by HERMANS et al. (1999a, b), tumor volume was not found to be an independent predictor of local outcome when a multivariate analysis was applied. In glottic carcinoma, involvement of the paraglottic space at the level of the true vocal cord and involvement of the preepiglottic space were found to be independent predictors of local outcome. In supraglottic carcinoma, involvement of the preepiglottic space and subglottic extension were the strongest independent predictors of local control.

Tumor volume and degree of involvement of the laryngeal deep tissues are correlated to some extent. However, these descriptive CT parameters may also reflect a more aggressive tumoral behavior (ISAACS et al. 1988), which could explain their stronger association with local recurrence. FLETCHER and HAMBERGER (1974) stated that the preepiglottic space is poorly vascularized. They suggested that the anoxic compartment of tumors invading this space must be significant, and thus relatively radioresistant.

PAMEIJER et al. (1997), evaluating pretherapeutic CT studies in patients with T3 glottic carcinomas, found a trend towards decreased local control when the paraglottic space at the true vocal cord level was infiltrated (P=0,14), while infiltration of this space at

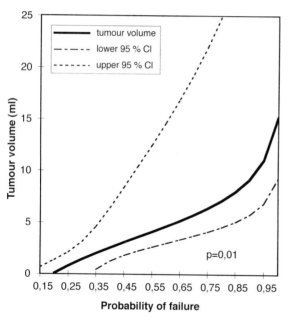

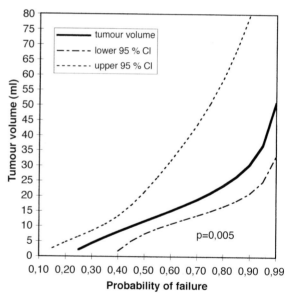

Fig. 7.3. Glottic cancer. Probability of local failure after definitive radiation therapy versus CT-determined primary tumor volume. The local failure rate is significantly higher with larger primary tumor volume. The 95% confidence intervals for tumor volume are indicated. (Reprinted from Radiotherapy and Oncology, vol 50, Hermans R, Van den Bogaert W, Rijnders A, et al., Predicting the local outcome of glottic cancer treated by definitive radiation therapy: value of computed tomography determined tumour parameters. pp 39–46, copyright 1999, with permission from Elsevier Science)

Fig. 7.4. Supraglottic cancer. Probability of local failure after definitive radiation therapy versus CT-determined primary tumor volume. As for glottic cancer, the local failure rate is significantly higher with larger primary tumor volume. The 95% confidence intervals for tumor volume are indicated. (Reprinted from International Journal of Radiation Oncology Biology Physics, vol 44, Hermans R, Van den Bogaert W, Rijnders A, et al., Value of computed tomography determined tumour parameters as outcome predictor of supraglottic cancer treated by definitive radiation therapy. pp 755–765, copyright 1999, with permission from Elsevier Science)

the false cord level was significantly associated with a lower local control rate after definitive radiation therapy ($P=0,01$). However, they did not find that these or other investigated CT parameters provided additional information regarding the probability of local control when considered simultaneously with tumor volume. FREEMAN et al. (1990) reported a "trend" towards decreased post irradiation local control rate with increasing percentage of preepiglottic space involvement in T3 supraglottic cancer ($P=0,384$).

7.3.3.1.2
Laryngeal Cartilage Involvement on CT

Laryngeal cartilage invasion is often considered to predict a low probability of radiation therapy alone controlling the primary tumor site, and to indicate an increased risk of late complications, such as severe edema or necrosis (CASTELIJNS et al. 1990; LLOYD et al. 1981; SILVERMAN 1985).

Before the era of computer-assisted cross-sectional imaging only gross cartilage destruction, usually occurring in large volume laryngeal tumors, could be detected clinically or by conventional radiography. More limited laryngeal cartilage invasion can be detected with modern cross-sectional imaging methods (BECKER et al. 1995). Earlier studies described an association between CT-depicted cartilage involvement in laryngeal carcinoma and poor outcome after radiation therapy (ISAACS et al. 1988; SILVERMAN 1985). However, according to others involvement of laryngeal cartilage is not necessarily associated with a reduced success rate of radiation therapy (MILLION 1989). More recent studies correlating laryngeal cartilage abnormalities, detected on CT, with local outcome after radiotherapy seem to corroborate this last point of view.

The cartilage most often showing abnormalities is the arytenoid cartilage, which usually appears sclerotic. An abnormal appearance of this cartilage was not found to be associated with poorer local control, and may be unimportant in terms of prognosis (HERMANS et al. 1999a; TART et al. 1994). The majority of sclerotic arytenoid cartilages do not contain tumor within ossified bone marrow, which can help to explain why radiation therapy is efficient in a large percentage of patients with isolated arytenoid sclerosis on CT (BECKER et al. 1997).

PAMEIJER et al. (1997) found a lower probability of local control in patients with T3 glottic carcinoma when both the arytenoid and cricoid showed sclerosis. These authors assumed that if both the arytenoid and cricoid cartilage are sclerotic, the probability of microscopic cartilage invasion will increase. HER-MANS et al. (1999b) also found that cricoid cartilage abnormalities in glottic carcinoma yielded a statistically significant lower control rate. Of 13 patients with sclerosis of the cricoid in this study, 10 also had sclerosis of the arytenoid cartilage, corresponding to the "double sclerosis" situation described by PAMEIJER et al. (1997). However, the multivariate analysis performed in the study by HERMANS et al. (1999a) showed that an abnormal appearing cricoid cartilage is not an independent predictor of poor local control in glottic carcinoma: it lost significant when paraglottic and preepiglottic space involvement are included in the statistical model. Even relatively subtle cartilage abnormalities, as detected in this study population (sclerosis of the cartilage being the most frequent alteration seen), seem to be correlated with deep tumor extension. More destructive cartilage changes are associated with very bulky tumors, which are not selected for radiation therapy.

There are only few data available on the correlation between thyroid cartilage abnormalities as seen on CT and local outcome of glottic cancer after definitive radiation therapy. Some studies explicitly excluded patients showing evidence of thyroid cartilage involvement (MUKHERJI et al. 1995; PAMEIJER et al. 1997). In the study by HERMANS et al. (1999a), in which tumor visible on both sides of the cartilage and lysis of ossified cartilage were used as signs of thyroid cartilage invasion, only a limited number of patients with glottic carcinoma had an abnormal appearance of this cartilage. No evidence was found that thyroid cartilage involvement alone as seen on CT is associated with a poorer local outcome after definitive radiation therapy but the number of patients in this study with signs of neoplastic involvement of this cartilage was small.

No conclusions can be drawn concerning cricoid or thyroid cartilage abnormalities on CT in supraglottic carcinoma due to the limited number of patients selected for radiation therapy with abnormalities of these cartilages.

7.3.3.1.3
Involvement of the Anterior and Posterior Commissure on CT; Extralaryngeal extension

Involvement of the posterior commissure as shown by CT has been found to be associated with a poorer local outcome of borderline significance ($P=0,07$) after radiation therapy (HERMANS et al. 1999a, b). Involvement of the posterior commissure occurs most often in relatively large glottic cancers.

Involvement of the anterior commissure as shown by CT in glottic cancer has not been found to be an independent predictor of local recurrence (HER-MANS et al. 1999a). Also in the study on T3 glottic cancer by PAMEIJER et al. (1997), CT evidence of anterior commissure involvement was not related to poorer local outcome after radiotherapy.

Extralaryngeal spread has been found to be associated with a higher recurrence rate in glottic cancer after radiation therapy, but this does not reach significance as only 10/119 patients showed such spread on CT (HERMANS et al. 1999a). In the same study, nearly half of the patients with supraglottic cancer had some evidence of an extralaryngeal abnormality on CT, but this was not associated with poorer local control. This is likely related to the subtle character of the extralaryngeal abnormalities (usually in the valleculae or piriform sinuses) detected with CT in most of these patients. According to the UICC classification extralaryngeal spread should be staged T4; in supraglottic cancer this probably would be an overcalling if based on subtle CT findings.

7.3.3.2
Using MRI

In a retrospective analysis a variety of MRI- and non-MRI-dependent prognostic factors for the success of radiation therapy in laryngeal carcinoma were evaluated (CASTELIJNS et al. 1995). Age, sex, histopathology, invasion of the vocal muscle or preepiglottic space did not influence the risk of tumor recurrence significantly. Cord mobility as seen clinically, and invasion of laryngeal cartilages and tumor volume shown by MRI, appeared to influence the risk of tumor recurrence. That tumor volume is important is not surprising, as it has been demonstrated for many tumor sites and is consistent with established radiobiologic principles. Comparison between statistically significant parameters by logistic regression model revealed three relevant prognostic parameters: cord mobility, tumor volume and cartilage invasion. These findings indicate that information obtained from pretreatment MRI examination can help to predict the rate of local control with irradiation alone.

The false-positive rate of MRI in determining neoplastic cartilage invasion, often due to peritumoral inflammation (BECKER et al. 1995), is a concern. The effect of inflammation on prognosis is unknown. Perhaps this inflammatory tissue must be treated as tumor and one must consider a safe margin as being beyond the edema. The spreading inflammation could carry neoplastic cells, inducing a higher recurrence rate. In this case, the effect of the false-positive rate would be much lower. However, the inflammation may also be less ominous than actual tumor. A method must be found to help differentiate between actual tumor tissue and peritumoral inflammation.

Cartilage involvement in patients with small tumors (under 5 ml) is not correlated with tumor recurrence. An abnormal MR signal pattern in cartilage combined with a large tumor volume (above 5 ml) worsens the prognosis significantly (CASTELIJNS et al. 1996). Consequently, an abnormal MR signal pattern in laryngeal cartilage should not automatically imply laryngectomy, especially in lesions with smaller volumes. It is incorrect to postulate that radiotherapy cannot cure a substantial number of lesions with cartilage involvement. CASTELIJNS et al. agree with MILLION (1989), that minimal cartilage involvement in patients with low-staged tumors does not imply a bad prognosis (CASTELIJNS et al. 1995, 1996).

The thyroid cartilage frequently appears to be involved in the area of the anterior commissure. Abnormal signal intensity in the area of the anterior commissure, as shown at MRI, has a predictive value for tumor recurrence. In the literature it is stated that patients with glottic tumors primarily staged as T1b (tumor in both vocal cords, involving the anterior commissure) have an increased risk of tumor recurrence compared to tumors staged as T1a (tumor limited to one vocal cord) (KIRCHNER 1970; MANTRA-VADI et al. 1983). This may be explained by underlying cartilage invasion. However, in T1b glottic lesions abnormal signal in the thyroid cartilage on MRI in the area of the anterior commissure seems not to explain this increased risk of tumor recurrence: tumor recurred in 2 out of 5 patients in whom MRI showed an abnormal signal intensity in cartilage in the area of the anterior commissure, whereas tumor recurred in both patients in whom no abnormal signal was seen (CASTELIJNS et al. 1996).

Involvement of the lamina of the thyroid cartilage significantly increases the risk of tumor recurrence (CASTELIJNS et al. 1996). It should be noted that this result is based on a limited number of patients showing such involvement, since patients with T3 or T4 lesions in whom CT and/or MRI showed major cartilage involvement of the thyroid cartilage were treated by surgery and consequently were not included in the study. Involvement of cartilages around the cricoarytenoid joint on MRI, seen in a relatively high number of patients, have no clear predictive value for tumor recurrence (CASTELIJNS et al. 1996).

In further studies dealing with the prognostic value of MR parameters glottic and supraglottic tumors should be considered separately, as the anatomic situation (and hence extension pattern) is different for glottic and supraglottic tumors.

7.4
Conclusion

As staging procedures, CT and MRI have important functions in corroborating clinical findings and ruling out more extensive disease. Accurate staging is critical in decision making in oncology (Barbera et al. 2001).

However, to what extent CT or MRI influence treatment decisions in laryngeal cancer is currently not very clear, and likely varies from institute to institute. This influence depends on the treatment policy conducted, more precisely the relative role of radiotherapy and surgery as primary treatment modalities in more advanced laryngeal cancer.

The parameters defined in the T classification are mainly based on clinical examination. The addition of modern imaging methods in staging laryngeal cancer may compromise the prognostic information of the T classification itself (by causing stage migration). Furthermore, if imaging is only used to determine tumor extent according to the T classification, no optimal use is made of the available information. Other imaging-derived parameters, not included in the definitions of the T classification, such as tumor volume and depth of invasion in the deep tissues, are of significant prognostic value, and these imaging-derived parameters are even more strongly related to local outcome than the T categories. It is important to note that this information is available without the need for any additional investigation or new technology.

Controversy remains about the significance of cartilage involvement as visible on CT and MRI. Overall, in studies evaluating CT, cartilage involvement appears to have fewer prognostic implications, whereas MRI findings of cartilage involvement are reported to be more indicative of an increased risk of tumor recurrence. We agree with Million (1989) that the "myth about the radiocurability of bone and/or cartilage" should be replaced by an understanding of the relative rates of control by radiotherapy. The prognostic value of laryngeal cartilage abnormalities in both CT and MRI studies needs to be studied more extensively. This should be done by a separate evaluation of glottic and supraglottic cancer, using a multivariate analysis, taking into account other imaging-derived parameters such as tumor volume and degree of deep tissue invasion.

Pure morphologic criteria cannot entirely explain the biologic behavior of a tumor and its response to treatment. Ongoing research focuses on the evaluation with radiologic methods of tumor microvascularization, perfusion and oxygenation, factors known to be of important prognostic value (see Chap. 11.3).

New classification systems should be conceived, incorporating not only morphologic extent as in the present TNM system, but also including other variables with independent prognostic significance. Piccirillo and Lacy (2000) anticipate that this will be developed as computer software staging packages, not only calculating prognosis, but also estimating the accuracy of this prognosis based on the amount of information used to generate it.

References

American Joint Committee on Cancer (AJCC) (1992) Manual for staging of cancer, 4th edn. Lippincott, Philadelphia

Archer CR, Yeager VL, Herbold DR (1984) Improved diagnostic accuracy in laryngeal cancer using a new classification based on computed tomography. Cancer 53:44–57

Bailey BJ (1991) Beyond the 'new' TNM classification. Editorial. Arch Otolaryngol Head Neck Surg 117:369–370

Barbera L, Groome PA, Mackillop WJ, et al (2001) The role of computed tomography in the T classification of laryngeal carcinoma. Cancer 91:394–407

Becker M, Zbären P, Laeng H, et al (1995) Neoplastic invasion of the laryngeal cartilage: comparison of MR imaging and CT with histopathologic correlation. Radiology 194:661–669

Becker M, Zbären P, Delavelle J, et al (1997) Neoplastic invasion of the laryngeal cartilage: reassessment of criteria for diagnosis at CT. Radiology 203:521–532

Breiman RS, Beck JW, Korobkin M, et al (1982) Volume determinations using computed tomography. AJR Am J Roentgenology 138:329–333

Castelijns JA, Golding RP, van Schaik C, et al (1990) MR findings of laryngeal cartilage invasion by laryngeal cancer: value in predicting outcome of radiation therapy. Radiology 174:669–673

Castelijns JA, van den Brekel MWM, Smit EMT, et al (1995) Predictive value of MR imaging-dependent and non-MR imaging dependent parameters for recurrence of laryngeal cancer after radiation therapy. Radiology 196:735–739

Castelijns JA, van den Brekel MWM, Tobi H, et al (1996) Laryngeal carcinoma after radiation therapy: correlation of abnormal MR imaging signal pattern in laryngeal cartilage with the risk of recurrence. Radiology 198:151–155

Charlin B, Brazeau-Lamontagne L, Guerrier B, et al (1989) Assessment of laryngeal cancer: CT scan versus endoscopy. J Otolaryngol 18:283–288

Feinstein AR, Sosin DM, Wells CK (1985) The Will Rogers phenomenon. Stage migration and new diagnostic techniques as a source of misleading statistics for survival in cancer. N Engl J Med 312:1604–1608

Fletcher GH, Hamberger AD (1974) Causes of failure in irradiation of squamous-cell carcinoma of the supraglottic larynx. Radiology 111:697–700

Fletcher GH, Lindberg RD, Hamberger A, et al (1975) Reasons for irradiation failure in squamous cell carcinoma of the larynx. Laryngoscope 85:987–1003

Freeman DE, Mancuso AA, Parsons JT, et al (1990) Irradiation alone for supraglottic larynx carcinoma: can CT findings predict treatment results? Int J Radiat Oncol Biol Phys 19:485–490

Gilbert RW, Birt D, Shulman H, et al (1987) Correlation of tumor volume with local control in laryngeal carcinoma treated by radiotherapy. Ann Otol Rhinol Laryngol 97:514–518

Harrison DFN (1988) Classification: the great deception. J Otolaryngol 17:12–15

Hermans R, Van der Goten A, Baert AL (1997a) Image interpretation in CT of laryngeal carcinoma: a study on intra- and interobserver reproducibility. Eur Radiol 7:1086–1090

Hermans R, Bouillon R, Laga K, et al (1997b) Estimation of thyroid gland volume by spiral computed tomography. Eur Radiol 7:214–216

Hermans R, Feron M, Bellon E, et al (1998) Laryngeal tumor volume measurements determined with CT: a study on intra- and interobserver variability. Int J Radiat Oncol Biol Phys 40:553–557

Hermans R, Van den Bogaert W, Rijnders A, et al (1999a) Predicting the local outcome of glottic cancer treated by definitive radiation therapy: value of computed tomography determined tumour parameters. Radiother Oncol 50:39–46

Hermans R, Van den Bogaert W, Rijnders A, et al (1999b) Value of computed tomography determined tumour parameters as outcome predictor of supraglottic cancer treated by definitive radiation therapy. Int J Radiat Oncol Biol Phys 44:755–765

Hjelm-Hansen M (1980) Laryngeal carcinoma. IV. Analysis of treatment results using the Cohen model. Acta Radiol Oncol 19:3–12

Isaacs JH, Mancuso AA, Mendenhall WM, et al (1988) Deep spread patterns in CT staging of T2-4 squamous cell laryngeal carcinoma. Otolaryngol Head Neck Surg 99:455–464

Johnson CR, Thames HD, Huang DT, et al (1995) The tumor volume and clonogen number relationship: tumor control predictions based upon tumor volume estimates derived from computed tomography. Int J Radiat Oncol Biol Phys 33:281–287

Katsantonis GP, Archer CR, Rosenblum BN, et al (1986) The degree to which accuracy of preoperative staging of laryngeal carcinoma has been enhanced by computed tomography. Otolaryngol Head Neck Surg 95:52–62

Kirchner JA (1970) Cancer at the anterior commissure of the larynx. Results with radiotherapy. Arch Otolaryngol 91:524–525

Lee WR, Mancuso AA, Saleh EM, et al (1993) Can pretreatment computed tomography findings predict local control in T3 squamous cell carcinoma of the glottic larynx treated with radiotherapy alone? Int J Radiat Oncol Biol Phys 25:683–687

Lloyd GAS, Michaels L, Phelps PD (1981) The demonstration of cartilaginous involvement in laryngeal carcinoma by computerized tomography. Clin Otolaryngol 6:171–177

Lo SM, Venkatesan V, Matthews TW, et al (1998) Tumour volume: implications in T2/T3 glottic/supraglottic squamous cell carcinoma. J Otolaryngol 27:247–251

Mancuso AA, Mukherji SK, Schmalfuss I, et al (1999) Preradiotherapy computed tomography as a predictor of local control in supraglottic carcinoma. J Clin Oncol 17:631–637

Mantravadi RVP, Liebner EJ, Haas RE, et al (1983) Cancer of the glottis: prognostic factors in radiation therapy. Radiology 149:311–314

Marks JE, Freeman RB, Lee F, et al (1979) Carcinoma of the supraglottic larynx. AJR Am J Roentgenol 132:255–260

Million RR (1989) The myth regarding bone or cartilage involvement by cancer and the likelihood of cure by radiotherapy. Head Neck 11:30–40

Mukherji SK, Mancuso AA, Mendenhall W, et al (1995) Can pretreatment CT predict local control of T2 glottic carcinomas treated with radiation therapy alone? AJNR Am J Neuroradiol 16:655–662

Nationale werkgroep hoofd-halstumoren (2000) Richtlijn Larynxcarcinoom. Kwaliteitsinstituut voor de Gezondheidszorg, Utrecht

Overgaard J, Hansen HS, Jørgensen K, et al (1986) Primary radiotherapy of larynx and pharynx carcinoma – an analysis of some factors influencing local control and survival. Int J Radiat Oncol Biol Phys 12:515–521

Pameijer FA, Mancuso AA, Mendenhall WM, et al (1997) Can pretreatment computed tomography predict local control in T3 squamous cell carcinoma of the glottic larynx treated with definitive radiotherapy? Int J Radiat Oncol Biol Phys 37:1011–1021

Pameijer FA, Mancuso AA, Mendenhall WM, et al (1998) Evaluation of pretreatment computed tomography as a predictor of local control in T1/T2 pyriform sinus carcinoma treated with definitive radiotherapy. Head Neck 20:159–168

Piccirillo JF (1995) Purposes, problems, and proposals for progress in cancer staging. Arch Otolaryngol Head Neck Surg 121:145–149

Piccirillo JF, Lacy PD (2000) Classification and staging of laryngeal cancer. In: Ferlito A (ed) Diseases of the larynx. Arnold, London, pp 563–564, 574

Pillsbury HR, Kirchner JA (1979) Clinical vs histopathologic staging in laryngeal cancer. Arch Otolaryngol 105:157–159

Shah JP, Karnell LH, Hoffman HT, et al (1997) Patterns of care for cancer of the larynx in the United States. Arch Otolaryngol Head Neck Surg 123:475–483.

Silverman PM (1985) Medullary space involvement in laryngeal carcinoma. Arch Otolaryngol 111:541–542

Silverman PM, Bossen EH, Fisher SR, et al (1984) Carcinoma of the larynx and hypopharynx: computed tomographic-histopathologic correlations. Radiology 151:697–702

Snow GB, Gerritsen GJ (1993) TNM classification according to the UICC and AJCC. In: Ferlito A (ed) Neoplasms of the larynx. Churchill Livingstone, Edinburgh, pp 425–434

Sulfaro S, Barzan L, Querin F, et al (1989) T staging of the laryngohypopharyngeal carcinoma. Arch Otolaryngol Head Neck Surg 115:613–620

Tart RP, Mukherji SK, Lee WR, Mancuso AA (1994) Value of laryngeal cartilage sclerosis as a predictor of outcome in patients with stage T3 glottic cancer treated with radiation therapy. Radiology 192:567–570

Union International Contre le Cancer (UICC) (1997) TNM classification of malignant tumours, 5th edn. Wiley, New York

Van den Bogaert W, Ostyn F, van der Schueren E (1983) The different clinical presentation, behavior and prognosis of carcinomas originating in the epilarynx and the lower supraglottis. Radiother Oncol 1:117–131

Van den Bogaert W, van der Schueren E, Horiot JC, et al (1995) The EORTC randomized trial on three fractions per day and misonidazole in advanced head and neck cancer: prognostic factors. Radiother Oncol 35:100–106

Withers HR (1992) Biologic basis of radiation therapy. In: Perez CA, Brady LW (eds) Principles and practice of radiation oncology, 2nd edn. Lippincott, Philadelphia, pp 64–96

Zbären P, Becker M, Laeng H (1996) Pretherapeutic staging of laryngeal cancer: clinical findings, computed tomography and magnetic resonance imaging versus histopathology. Cancer 77:1263–1273

8 Imaging After Radiation Treatment of Laryngeal Cancer

Robert Hermans

CONTENTS

8.1 Introduction

After radiation treatment, clinical examination of the larynx is difficult because of the effects of the radiation which alter the mucosa and produce varying degrees of deeper edema and fibrosis. Residual or recurrent tumor, therefore, can be difficult to detect by physical examination. Accurate interpretation of CT or MR studies in patients irradiated for laryngeal cancer requires that the expected radiographic changes due to treatment not be misinterpreted as residual or recurrent tumor (MUKHERJI et al. 1994a; NÖMAYR et al. 2001). Several studies have shown that CT may be useful in the early differentiation of treatment responders from non-responders (HERMANS et al. 2000; MUKHERJI et al. 1994b); in this regard, the value of MRI is less well established.

Other studies have indicated that imaging-based identification of patients at high risk of local failure is possible *before* treatment with definitive radiation treatment (see Chap. 7). In patients triaged to such a high-risk profile, intensive imaging surveillance could be added to the already careful clinical follow-up regimen and possibly lead to earlier salvage surgery in

non-responders. In the good responders and those patients with low-risk profiles, cost reductions could be achieved by limiting or eliminating the imaging surveillance. A recent study (PAMEIJER et al. 1999) has indeed shown that patients irradiated for a laryngeal carcinoma can be stratified into risk groups for primary site recurrence based on a *posttreatment* CT study performed during the first 6 months after radiation treatment.

Definitive radiotherapy for laryngeal cancer may cure the cancer but lead in some cases to severe edema or necrosis of the larynx, requiring removal of the larynx because of pain or threat to airway patency (O'BRIEN 1996). In a number of cases conservative measures may bring such a complication under control and leave the patient with a functional larynx.

The differentiation between recurrent laryngeal cancer after radiation treatment and a significant treatment complication is a difficult clinical problem. Since most necroses and many recurrences occur within 1 year of radiation treatment, time of onset is not helpful in distinguishing the two (PARSONS 1994). As the predictive value of a negative biopsy result is relatively low in patients who have received definitive radiation treatment (KEANE et al. 1993), the presence of tumor may only be confirmed on histological examination of the entire larynx. Imaging can have a role in the evaluation of patients showing severe postradiotherapy laryngeal edema or necrosis, facilitating treatment choices and possibly leading to a better chance of the patient keeping a functional larynx.

8.2 Expected Tissue Changes After Radiation Treatment

8.2.1 Histopathological Changes

During the first 2 weeks after radiotherapy, there is an acute inflammatory reaction in the deep tissues,

R. HERMANS, MD, PhD
Professor, Department of Radiology, University Hospitals Leuven, Herestraat 49, 3000 Leuven, Belgium

with increased permeability and resultant interstitial edema due to detachment of the lining endothelial cells within small blood and lymphatic vessels. After this initial period of a few weeks, during the following months after radiation treatment, progressive thickening of the connective tissue, with deposition of collagenous fibers occurs. Endothelial proliferation, eventually resulting in complete obstruction of the vessels, is also observed. The reduction in venous and lymphatic drainage results in further accumulation of interstitial fluid. The fibrosis becomes progressively more advanced, but after 6–8 months a reduction in interstitial fluid may be seen, due to the formation of collateral capillary and lymphatic channels (ALEXANDER 1963; WARD et al. 1975).

The laryngeal mucous membrane is damaged early during radiotherapy. The clinically seen mucositis corresponds to caking of dead epithelial cells, fibrin and inflammatory cells (PARSONS 1994). In most patients, this mucositis heals within 1 month of completing of therapy.

The laryngeal cartilage is very resistant to irradiation as it has no vascularization of its own. Thus, as long as the laryngeal perichondrium remains intact, large doses can be tolerated. Degeneration of nuclei and infiltration with inflammatory cells have been described in the perichondrium, but without much change in the matrix of the cartilage itself.

8.2.2
Expected Changes on Cross-sectional Imaging Studies

8.2.2.1
Changes Within the Larynx

8.2.2.1.1
Follow-up CT
At the glottic level, there are usually few posttherapeutic changes visible. The paraglottic spaces may show increased density, and sometimes the anterior commissure appears thickened. Less frequently the posterior commissure also appears thickened (Fig. 8.1).

During the first months after radiotherapy, the false vocal cords are always thickened. Very often, the fat of the paraglottic space shows somewhat increased attenuation. The walls of the laryngeal ventricles, visible within the paraglottic spaces, may be thickened. The epiglottis appears thickened in about half of patients. Marked thickening of the aryepiglottic folds may be seen, often one of

the most pronounced findings early after radiotherapy of the larynx. The fat within these aryepiglottic folds also shows increased density. At the subglottic level, a symmetric soft tissue thickening between the cricoid ring and the subglottic air is often seen.

All these changes are most pronounced during the first months after completion of radiotherapy, and have diminished or even resolved completely by 10 to 15 months after irradiation (MUKHERJI et al. 1994a). It is important to know that these expected tissue changes appear symmetric. This means that the primary tumor disappears after successful radiation treatment, the former tumor bed only showing the changes that would be expected in the surrounding soft tissues (see also below).

The laryngeal cartilages do not show changes after irradiation. Reduction in the degree of cartilage sclerosis in the neighborhood of the tumor has been described, and this seems to correlate with local control (MUKHERJI et al. 1994b).

8.2.2.1.2
Follow-up MRI
Overall, the changes seen on MR studies are similar to those observed on CT studies. The better soft tissue contrast resolution with MRI allows edema (increased signal intensity on T2-weighted images) to be detected before thickening of the laryngeal structures is visible. NÖMAYR et al. (2001), using follow-MRI, reported a higher incidence of dose-dependent epiglottic edema than was reported for CT.

8.2.2.2
Generalized Changes Within the Neck

The pharyngeal walls, included within the radiation fields, may appear thickened and show increased enhancement (Fig. 8.1). Atrophy of the lymphoid tissue in Waldeyer's ring may be observed, if these structures are included in the irradiated tissues. Such lymphoid tissue atrophy is also seen in irradiated lymph nodes. The submandibular and parotid salivary glands may show increased enhancement and volume loss, if included in the radiation fields; these changes are caused by radiation sialoadenitis. Retropharyngeal edema, thickening of the platysma muscles and increased attenuation of the subcutaneous fat may be observed. As in the intralaryngeal tissue changes, these generalized tissue changes tend to diminish with time, and may even disappear.

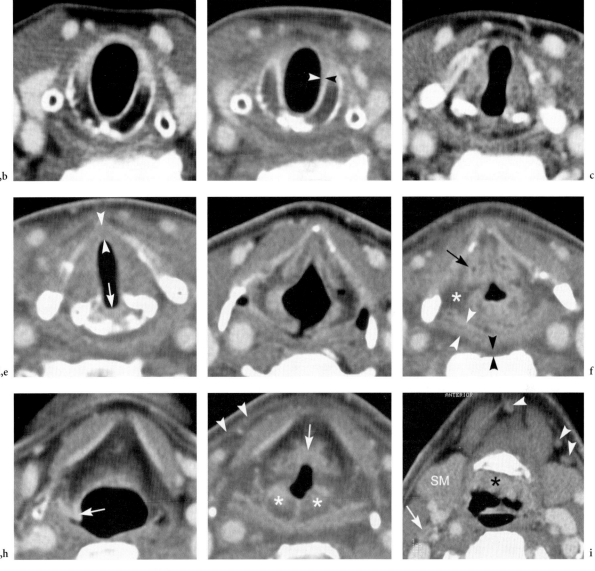

Fig. 8.1a–j. Patient with a right-sided T2 piriform sinus cancer, treated by definitive radiotherapy (RT). Anatomically corresponding axial contrast-enhanced CT images are shown, obtained just before and 6 months after completion of radiation treatment. **a, b** Level of subglottis. Before RT (**a**) air reaches the inner surface of the cricoid cartilage; after RT (**b**) slight circumferential soft tissue thickening can be seen (*between arrowheads*). **c, d** Glottic level. Before RT (**c**); after RT (**d**) slight soft tissue thickening in the anterior commissure can be seen (*between arrowheads*), and more limited also in the posterior commissure (*arrow*). **e, f** Supraglottic level (just above false vocal cords). Before RT (**e**); after RT (**f**) there is considerable soft tissue thickening, with increased density of the paraglottic spaces (*asterisk*). The walls of the laryngeal ventricles (*arrow*) appear thickened. Note also thickening and increased enhancement of the posterior hypopharyngeal wall (*white arrowheads*) and retropharyngeal edema (*black arrowheads*), and increased attenuation of the subcutaneous fat. **g, h** Supraglottic level, 9 mm more cranial than **e** and **f**. Before RT (**g**) the primary cancer can be seen on the right aryepiglottic fold (*arrow*); after RT (**h**) thickening of the infrahyoid epiglottis (*arrow*), as well as pronounced and symmetric thickening and increased attenuation of the aryepiglottic folds can be seen (*asterisks*). Note again the changes in the hypopharyngeal walls and the retropharyngeal edema. Also, slight thickening of the platysma muscles can be seen (*arrowheads*). **i, j** Level of the free epiglottic edge. Before RT (**i**) the lymphoid tissue within the lingual tonsil (*black asterisk*) can be seen (*SM* normal-appearing submandibular salivary glands, *arrow* small parajugular, *arrowheads* submental and submandibular lymph nodes); after RT (**j**) the lingual tonsil has disappeared, and the swollen preepiglottic fat bulges into the valleculae (*white asterisk*). The normal parajugular lymph nodes show volume loss (*arrow*), the submental and submandibular lymph node can no longer be seen. Volume reduction and increased enhancement of the submandibular salivary glands can also be seen (*arrowheads*): radiation sialoadenitis

8.3
Predicting the Local Outcome and Detecting Local Failure Early After Radiation Treatment

As described in Chapter 7, a risk profile for local tumor recurrence can be determined on *pretreatment* CT. A recent study has shown that patients irradiated for a supraglottic carcinoma or T3 glottic carcinoma can also be stratified in different risk groups for primary site failure based on *posttreatment* CT studies

(PAMEIJER et al. 1999). Based on the appearance of the larynx on the postradiotherapy CT studies, the patients were classified according to the following scores: 1, expected postradiotherapy changes, i.e., complete resolution of the tumor at the primary site and symmetrically appearing laryngeal and hypopharyngeal tissues, as described above (Fig. 8.1); 2, focal mass with a maximal diameter of <1 cm and/or asymmetric obliteration of laryngeal tissue planes (Fig. 8.2); 3, focal mass with a maximal diameter of >1 cm, or <50% estimated tumor volume reduction (Fig. 8.3).

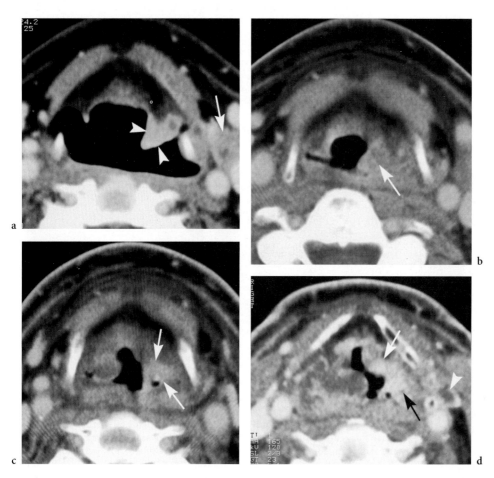

Fig. 8.2. a Pretreatment CT image of patient with T2 supraglottic squamous cell carcinoma shows infiltrating lesion within the left aryepiglottic fold (*arrowheads*). A pathological lymph node can be seen along the left internal jugular vein (*arrow*). **b** Clinical examination 3 months after radiation treatment shows pronounced laryngeal edema but no evidence of tumor. On CT, thickening of the supraglottic soft tissues can be seen, more pronounced in the left aryepiglottic fold (*arrow*); the density within the left aryepiglottic fold is also somewhat higher than in the surrounding tissues. This is a nonspecific finding (score 2) warranting further imaging follow-up. **c** Clinically favorable evolution 9 months after radiation treatment. However, CT shows more pronounced enhancement in the left aryepiglottic fold compared to the previous study (*arrows*). This was reported as suspect for tumor recurrence. Direct laryngoscopy was performed but showed no mucosal abnormalities; biopsies were negative. **d** By 1 year after radiation treatment, apart from increasing generalized laryngeal edema, the enhancing mass in the aryepiglottic fold now extends more anteriorly into the left paraglottic space (*arrows*). Also note the appearance of a small necrotic lymph node in the left neck (*arrowhead*). Direct laryngoscopy, performed after the CT study, revealed caking of necrotic tissue over the left aryepiglottic fold, suspect for tumor recurrence. Biopsy revealed squamous cell carcinoma. The patient died with progressive locoregional disease 7 months later

A CT examination obtained between 1 and 6 months after completion of radiation treatment and classified as a postradiotherapy CT score of 1 was shown to be a very strong predictor of long-term local control (Fig. 8.4). Patients with such findings on postradiotherapy CT will probably not benefit from further follow-up imaging studies, regardless of their pretreatment risk classification.

Patients with a first follow-up examination classified as a postradiotherapy CT score of 3 did very poorly in this study; almost all developed a local failure (Fig. 8.4). Although most patients in this group belonged, as would be expected, to the pretreatment high-risk CT group, some poor responders identified by follow-up CT initially had a low-risk pretreat-

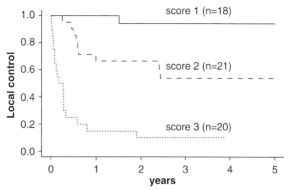

Fig. 8.4. Local control after radiotherapy over time for patients with different post-radiotherapy CT scores (*n*=59). The difference in local control between these three scores is highly significant. (From PAMEIJER et al. 1999, with permission)

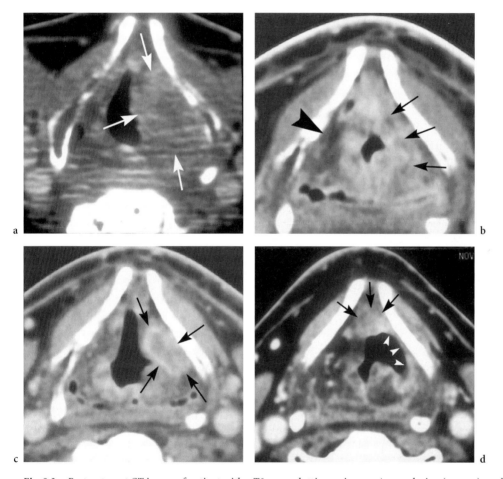

Fig. 8.3. a Pretreatment CT image of patient with a T3 supraglottic carcinoma. A mass lesion (*arrows*) can be seen in the region of the left false cord and paraglottic space. **b** CT image obtained 2.5 months after radiotherapy. The tumor has regressed, but persistent obliteration of the paraglottic fatty tissue (*thin arrows*) at the left side can be seen without a focal mass. CT score 2 (compare with normal-appearing paraglottic fat (*arrowhead*) at right side). Clinically no evidence of disease. **c** A focal mass (*arrows*) with a maximal diameter slightly over 1 cm is present 5 months after radiotherapy in the original tumor bed. CT score 3. Clinically some nonspecific left-sided mucosal irregularities were noted. A wait-and-see policy was adopted. **D.** CT 10 months after radiotherapy shows progressive extension of the mass lesion in the preepiglottic space (*arrows*) and ulceration (*arrowheads*) at the level of the left false vocal cord of the mass lesion. Laryngectomy was performed soon after the last CT study and confirmed the presence of local tumor recurrence. (From HERMANS et al. 2000, with permission)

116 R. Hermans

ment CT profile. The poor response in these patients could have been due to an aggressive tumor biology or a suboptimal tumor-host interaction. The sensitivity, specificity, accuracy, and negative and positive predictive value of a postradiotherapy CT score of 3 for local failure were reported as respectively 83%, 95%, 89%, 88% and 92%. These findings strongly suggest that further exploration in such postradiotherapy CT score 3 patients is warranted, even though deep biopsies could aggravate or initiate necrosis. FDG or thallium imaging may prove to be a useful intermediate step in cases where biopsy is considered too risky, or if a biopsy result is returned as negative. Indeed, the predictive value of a negative biopsy for local control has been reported to be only 70% (KEANE et al. 1993). This is likely due to sampling error, as tumor recurrences initially develop submucosally and can therefore not be accurately targeted. On the other hand, hypervascular scar tissue or limited laryngeal necrosis may mimic the appearance of tumor recurrence on imaging studies.

In cases of contradiction between the clinical findings, CT findings, results of radionuclide studies and/or biopsy, close clinical follow-up and repeat imaging studies are needed. Benign tissue changes will remain unchanged or will reduce in size over time. In some cases of progressive deterioration of the local situation, laryngectomy may have to be performed without histological proof of tumor recurrence despite repeat biopsies with negative result; often, pathological examination of the whole organ will reveal tumor recurrence and/or extensive laryngeal necrosis (Fig. 8.5).

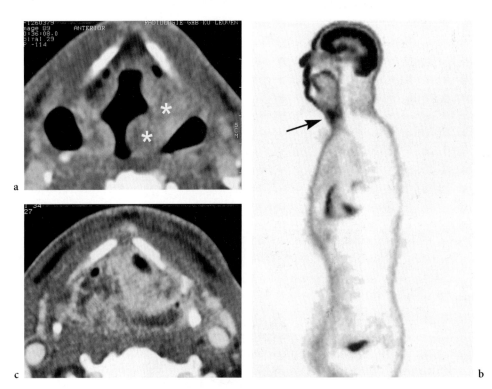

Fig. 8.5a–c. Patient treated by definitive radiotherapy for a left T2 supraglottic cancer. Laryngoscopy 4 months after completion of therapy shows asymmetric swelling of the supraglottic tissues; biopsy only reveals changes after radiotherapy. **a** Contrast-enhanced CT 5 months after radiotherapy. The patient suffered worsening dysphonia, dyspnea and dysphagia. Clinical examination showed a fixed left hemilarynx, very suspect for tumor recurrence. The CT study shows obvious asymmetry in the supraglottic tissues: the left paraglottic space has a higher attenuation, and the left supraglottic tissues appear thicker compared to the right (*asterisks*). The CT appearance is definitely suspect for recurrent tumor. Subsequently, a deep surgical biopsy was obtained from the left paraglottic space. Pathological study showed only changes after radiotherapy and no malignancy. Placement of a tracheostomy clearly diminished the clinical symptoms. **b** FDG-PET study obtained 8 months after radiotherapy. Pronounced laryngeal accumulation of the tracer, very suspect for tumor recurrence. As no histological proof of recurrent cancer was obtained, a wait-and-see policy was adopted. **c** Follow-up CT study obtained 12 months after radiotherapy. The soft tissue thickening of the laryngeal tissues is clearly increased (compare **a**): enhancing mass lesion in the left paraglottic space. Based on the findings of the FDG-PET study, and the disease progression visible on CT studies, total laryngectomy was performed. Pathological examination of the resection specimen revealed squamous cell carcinoma diffusely infiltrating the larynx

The local outcome of patients initially classified as postradiotherapy CT score 2 has been found to be indeterminate (Fig. 8.4). About 60% of the patients in this group belonged to the preradiotherapy high-risk group, and half of them failed locally. About 40% of the patients in the postradiotherapy CT score 2 group were at low risk for local failure based on a preradiotherapy CT study. Most of them (78%) were controlled at the primary site in this study, but this difference in local control between low- and high-risk patients was statistically not significant (PAMEIJER et al. 1999).

Obtaining a follow-up CT study before 4 months after completion of radiotherapy will result in more false-positive results. This is related to more severe normal tissue changes early after radiotherapy, and to the time needed by a sterilized tumor to regress. A similar observation has been made in FDG-positron emission tomography (PET) studies showing that baseline examinations before 4 months after radiation treatment may not accurately reflect outcome, while those done at 4 months and later result in a more accurate prediction of local outcome (GREVEN et al. 1994). Preliminary experience with MRI as follow-up tool also shows more false positive results during the first 6 months after radiation treatment (NÖMAYR et al. 2001).

In about 40% of local failures, follow-up CT has been shown to be able to detect this event earlier than clinical examination alone (HERMANS et al. 2000). In the patients in this study the CT diagnosis of local failure was eventually confirmed with a mean delay of 5.5 months (Figs. 8.2, 8.3). Use of this imaging-based information could lead to more prompt salvage surgery and potentially improve the survival of these patients. Proof of such a survival benefit requires further study.

In a prospective study, an improved survival following surgery for local recurrence has been shown for those cases with less extensive local failure after radiation treatment alone or combined with chemotherapy (KEANE et al. 1993). These patients underwent examination under anesthesia with biopsy of the original primary tumor site 8–12 weeks after completion of radiation treatment. These authors support routine biopsy reassessment 8 to 12 weeks following completion of radiation treatment in an effort to detect recurrence as early as possible. Use of follow-up CT (or MRI) could substantially reduce the number of patients needing a biopsy. Furthermore, imaging could be used to target the biopsy into the radiologically most suspect area, increasing the predictive value of a negative biopsy result.

New or progressive laryngeal cartilage alterations after radiation treatment are often associated with local failure, either due to local tumor recurrence or to laryngeal necrosis (see also below). These cartilage alterations can occur without a focal mass with a diameter of more than 1 cm. Such cartilage changes may be due to limited chondronecrosis, without structural collapse of the laryngeal framework, and are predominantly seen in the arytenoid cartilage. It seems justified to adopt a wait and see policy in patients with progressive arytenoid cartilage changes and minimal soft tissue asymmetry. Close follow-up, both clinically and radiologically, is necessary to detect progressive soft tissue changes, since such progression is associated with tumor recurrence or severe laryngeal necrosis (HERMANS et al. 1998).

Follow-up CT is probably not cost-effective in patients who were irradiated for a small carcinoma of the larynx, as the local control rates for such tumors after radiation therapy are very high. There are strong indications that patients with a higher likelihood of local failure, such as supraglottic cancer, and T3 or T4 glottic cancer do benefit from a baseline follow-up CT study about 4 months after completion of radiation treatment.

In summary, if the baseline CT study shows complete resolution of the tumor at the primary site and symmetrically appearing laryngeal tissues (i.e., expected radiotherapy-related changes), the patient is very likely to be controlled locally and further follow-up CT studies are not necessary. If less than 50% estimated volume reduction or a focal mass with a diameter larger than 1 cm is found, immediate further investigation is warranted, as the likelihood of local failure is high. If the laryngeal tissues appear asymmetric, or a focal mass with a diameter smaller than 1 cm is found, unless local failure is already suspected on clinical examination, further follow-up CT studies are needed. A time interval of 3 to 4 months is recommended, to be continued up to 2 years after completion of radiation treatment. In a substantial number of cases, it seems possible to detect local failure earlier by CT than by clinical examination alone. These patients can then be salvaged at an earlier stage of local recurrence.

8.4
Persisting Edema and Laryngeal Necrosis

8.4.1
Definition, Incidence and Pathogenesis

As discussed above, acute changes occur in the laryngeal tissues during and immediately following radiation treatment, and are clinically most apparent in the mucosa (O'BRIEN 1996). Edema occurs acutely, but usually does not persist beyond 6 months after radiotherapy.

There is quite a degree of interclinician variability in the definition as to which postradiotherapy changes should be considered as "significant" (such as the degree of edema) and what should be regarded as a complication of radiation treatment. Terms such as "edema" and "necrosis" are sometimes interchanged or used simultaneously. "Necrosis" itself is often not clearly defined, and may represent a spectrum of clinical scenarios, including soft tissue necrosis or chondronecrosis, or both. Also terms such as "chondritis" or "perichondritis" are sometimes encountered, without exact definitions of their meaning.

Laryngeal necrosis can be defined as a situation in which the larynx is not able to maintain its structural integrity, without evidence of persisting or recurrent tumor. Laryngeal soft tissue necrosis will lead to ulceration, and necrosis of the laryngeal framework may lead to collapse of the upper airway.

Laryngeal necrosis is a condition whose frequency is affected by the institutional treatment policy of large laryngeal cancers and the irradiation technique applied. Large tumors require higher total doses and larger treatment volumes than small tumors. The daily fraction size and time interval between fractions are also important factors in the pathogenesis of late injury such as laryngeal necrosis (PARSONS 1994).

Persisting severe edema and radionecrosis of the larynx are uncommon treatment complications, with an incidence of about 1% (PARSONS 1994). The occurrence of laryngeal necrosis peaks during the 12 months following treatment, which is more or less contemporaneous with the peak incidence of tumor recurrence. However, cases of laryngeal necrosis occurring more than 10 years after radiation treatment have been described (O'BRIEN 1996). Recurrent tumor is not a concern after such a long delay, but one has to be aware that rarely second primary tumors may originate from an irradiated larynx (ERKAL et al. 2001).

These late effects after radiation treatment are largely due to impaired vascular and lymphatic flow caused by endothelial damage and fibrosis (ALEXANDER 1963). Certain risk factors for the development of laryngeal necrosis after radiation treatment have been described, including diabetes mellitus, arterial hypertension, and continued smoking.

Cartilage itself is resistant to the effects of radiation (see above). Cartilage changes usually occur when the perichondrium is breached by trauma or tumor, exposing the underlying irradiated cartilage to microorganisms in the airway (KEENE et al. 1982). This may lead to infectious perichondritis, which may result in necrosis and laryngeal collapse. Many patients developing thyroid cartilage necrosis had a tumor reaching to or involving this cartilage, as visible on pretreatment imaging studies, suggesting a relationship between the two events. Most of these patients also had a large pretherapeutic tumor volume, requiring the use of larger irradiation portals.

The laryngeal cartilages show progressive ossification in adults, developing a blood supply, and this may play a role in the pathogenesis of laryngeal cartilage necrosis. In the concept of MARX (1983), osteoradionecrosis is a problem of tissue homeostasis and wound healing, not of infection. Irradiation produces a hypoxic, hypocellular and hypovascular tissue, which is not able to maintain its normal tissue turnover. Traumatic events or infections create a demand for tissue repair which is beyond the capabilities of the irradiated bone, and this accelerates its breakdown.

The arytenoid and cricoid cartilages are known to ossify more completely than the thyroid cartilage. The pathogenesis of necrosis in the arytenoid and cricoid cartilages, rather resembling bone necrosis, may be different from that in the thyroid cartilage (HERMANS et al. 1998; MARX 1983). Laryngeal trauma, such as that caused by endotracheal intubation or biopsy, may accelerate the breakdown of the cricoarytenoidal structures.

8.4.2
Symptoms and Imaging Findings

Patients with laryngeal necrosis often have neck and/or ear pain, some degree of dysphagia, and anterior neck swelling. Hoarseness and dyspnea are caused by increasing edema with impairment of vocal cord mobility, resulting in cord fixation. Inflammatory changes in the overlying skin, or cutaneous fistulae may be present. Palpation of the laryngeal region is usually painful.

On imaging studies, a variable degree of laryngeal soft-tissue swelling can be seen (HERMANS et al. 1998). These soft tissue changes surrounding the necrotic cartilage can be very pronounced and may be the only visible abnormality, making differentiation from recurrent tumor very difficult (Fig. 8.6). Furthermore, laryngeal necrosis and tumor recurrence may occur simultaneously. In laryngeal necrosis,

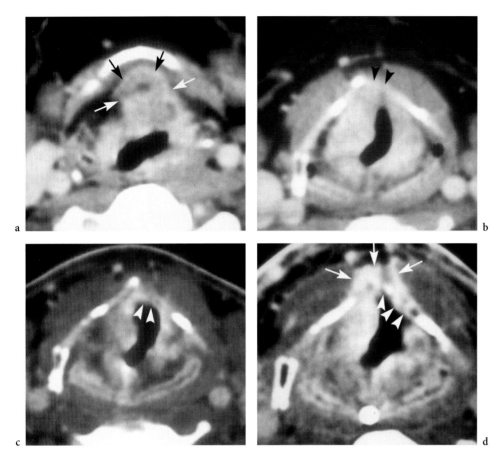

Fig. 8.6. a, b Pretreatment CT study in a patient with a T3N1 supraglottic carcinoma (**b** was obtained 5 mm below **a**). Tumor can be seen growing into the preepiglottic space (*arrows*) over the upper margin of the thyroid cartilage notch (*arrowheads*). **c** Posttreatment CT study obtained 1 month after radiotherapy. Thickening of the false cords with tissue loss at the anterior side of the left false cord (*arrowheads*) reaching close to the thyroid cartilage. **d** CT study obtained 3 months after radiotherapy. Progression of the soft tissue thickening around notch of thyroid cartilage (*arrows*). The thyroid cartilage appears denuded at the anterior side of the left false cord (*arrowheads*). Total laryngectomy was performed 3 months later because of pain and aspiration. Pathological examination revealed severe soft tissue inflammation and chondritis. (From HERMANS et al. 1998, with permission)

some fluid may be seen surrounding the cartilages; the precise nature of this fluid is unknown.

Cartilaginous abnormalities are often visible, but in some patients they may only become apparent on follow-up CT studies. Necrosis of the thyroid cartilage may cause fragmentation and collapse of this cartilage with or without gas bubbles visible adjacent to it (Fig. 8.7). Patients with arytenoid cartilage necrosis may show anterior dislocation of this cartilage, possibly due to cricoarytenoidal joint effusion, secondary to inflammation or infection. Septic arthritis of the cricoarytenoidal joint after irradiation for laryngeal cancer has been described (KEENE et al. 1982). Progressive lysis of the arytenoid, during which it shows a crumbly aspect evolving to complete disappearance, is possible (DE VUYSERE et al. 1999). Sloughing of the

arytenoid cartilage into the airway has also been described (HERMANS et al. 1998) (Fig. 8.8). The adjacent part of the cricoid cartilage may appear sclerotic. Cricoidal sclerosis may also be seen in association with lysis of the thyroid cartilage.

On MR studies, laryngeal necrosis may appear as focal swelling of the laryngeal soft tissues, loss of the normal high signal in the medullary space of ossified laryngeal cartilage on T1-weighted images, and enhancement of the affected cartilage after injection of gadolinium (BOUSSON et al. 1995).

In some cases, the imaging findings allow better differentiation between tumor recurrence and chondronecrosis than clinical examination alone. Recent studies on postradiotherapy surveillance of laryngeal and hypopharyngeal cancer (MUKHERJI et al. 1994b;

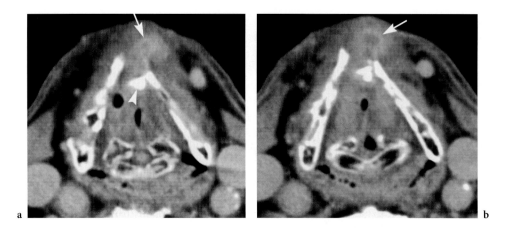

Fig. 8.7a, b. Patient presenting with hoarseness, dyspnea and pain in the laryngeal region 14 years after radiotherapy for laryngeal cancer. The CT images (**b** was obtained 5 mm below **a**) show fragmentation of the anterior part of the thyroid cartilage (*arrowhead*), intra- and extralaryngeal soft tissue thickening including a small prelaryngeal enhancing area with central fluid density possibly corresponding to a small abscess (*arrow*). This study was reported as suggestive for laryngeal necrosis. A FDG-PET study at that time was negative. Conservative treatment was started, with gradual improvement of the symptoms; this evolution corroborates the hypothesis of (limited) laryngeal necrosis

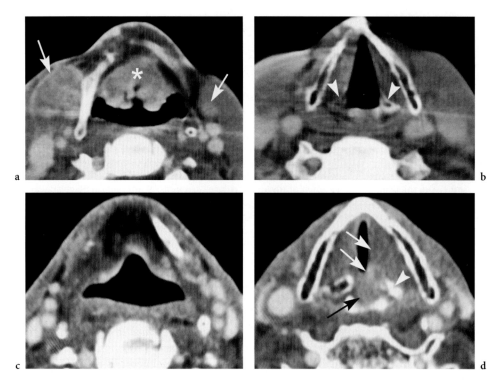

Fig. 8.8. a, b Pretreatment CT images of patient with a T4N3 supraglottic cancer. A bulky mass can be seen in the supraglottis (*asterisk*). Adenopathies can be seen on both sides of the neck (*arrows*). Note the intact appearance of the arytenoid cartilages (*arrowheads*). The tumor responded to radiation treatment. **c, d** CT images obtained 8 years after radiotherapy. At that time, the patient presented with hoarseness. Indirect laryngoscopy revealed slight thickening and reduced mobility of the left vocal cord. At the supraglottic level, only expected changes after radiotherapy can be seen (**c**). At the glottic level, the left arytenoid (*arrowhead*) appears sclerotic, shows irregular borders and is surrounded by thickened and slightly enhancing tissue without an obvious mass lesion (*arrows*). This was reported as suggestive for late-onset limited laryngeal necrosis. The soft tissue swelling resolved with conservative treatment

PAMEIJER et al. 1999) have shown that progressive cartilage alterations on postradiotherapy CT studies predict a poor local outcome, either due to tumor recurrence or chondroradionecrosis. In these studies gas bubbles in the vicinity of cartilage and cartilage collapse were not observed in cases of tumor recurrence. Such findings can be regarded as suggestive of radionecrosis. Nevertheless, a coexistent tumor recurrence may be difficult to exclude, depending on the associated tissue alterations (Fig. 8.9).

In the differential diagnosis, albeit very rare, laryngeal actinomycosis may be considered. The laryngeal environment after radiation treatment may permit the growth of *Actinomyces*, an anaerobic organism. Both laryngeal necrosis and actinomycosis of the larynx may present as chronic edema, with superim-

posed episodes of fulminant inflammation. Biopsy will yield the diagnosis of actinomycotic infection. A rapid and complete response to antibiotic therapy has been reported (NELSON and TYBOR 1992).

In summary, the imaging findings in laryngeal necrosis are nonspecific, but the diagnosis can be strongly suggested in cases of sloughing of the arytenoid cartilage, fragmentation and collapse of the thyroid cartilage, and/or in the presence of soft tissue thickening with gas bubbles surrounding the laryngeal cartilage(s).

In the absence of frank necrosis, conservative treatment is indicated, consisting of steroids and antibiotics. Temporary tracheostomy may be needed. In some cases, such measures may control this complication and leave the patient with a function-

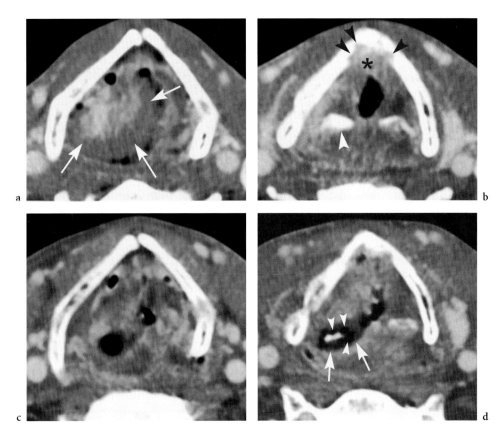

Fig. 8.9. a, b Pretreatment CT images in a patient with a T3 supraglottic cancer. A large, exophytic soft tissue mass (*arrows*) can be seen arising from the right aryepiglottic fold. The lesion extends into the right paraglottic space and the true vocal cord, and into the anterior commissure (*asterisk*). Sclerosis of the right arytenoid cartilage can be seen (*white arrowhead*), and an irregular appearance of the inner margin of the thyroid cartilage, possibly corresponding to early neoplastic invasion (*black arrowheads*). **c, d** The patient suffered from increasing dysphonia and dyspnea 6 months after completion of radiation treatment. The findings during indirect laryngoscopy are suspect for tumor recurrence. The CT images show severe supraglottic (**c**) and glottic (**d**) soft tissue thickening, and particularly at the glottic level, the tissue thickening is asymmetric, being more pronounced and showing more contrast enhancement on the right. A deep soft tissue ulcer (*arrows*) filled with debris extends around the irregular appearing right arytenoid cartilage, and pericartilaginous gas bubbles (*arrowheads*) are apparent. This was reported as suggestive for tumor recurrence, possibly combined with laryngeal radionecrosis. Total laryngectomy was performed. Pathological examination revealed inflammation and scar-like tissue, but no residual cancer

al larynx. Recent studies showed that even in advanced cases of laryngeal necrosis a functional larynx can be retained after intensive treatment with hyperbaric oxygen therapy (FELDMEIER et al. 1993; FERGUSON et al. 1987). The major problem in these cases is to exclude the coexistence of local tumor recurrence. Ongoing studies suggest that radionuclide imaging may detect local recurrences with a higher accuracy than purely anatomically based methods, such as CT and MR (LAPELA et al. 1995). FDG-PET scanning may also be helpful in the distinction of laryngeal necrosis from local tumor recurrence (MCGUIRT et al. 1998).

If there is no response to medical treatment, surgical intervention with removal of necrotic tissues is indicated (BALM et al. 1993; MCGUIRT 1997). If possible, the larynx is spared. The resultant wound is reconstructed with healthy, non-irradiated, well-vascularized tissue, improving the vascularization of the larynx. A pedicled pectoralis muscle is well suited for this purpose.

Advanced cases of radionecrosis, leaving the patient with a dysfunctional larynx (airway obstruction, intractable pain, loss of airway protection with aspiration), may need to be treated by total laryngectomy.

References

Alexander FW (1963) Micropathology of radiation reaction in the larynx. Ann Otol Rhinol Laryngol 72:831–841

Balm AJ, Hilgers FJ, Baris G, et al (1993) Pectoralis major muscle transposition: an adjunct to laryngeal preservation in severe chondroradionecrosis. J Laryngol Otol 107:748–751

Bousson V, Marsot-Dupuch K, Lashiver X, et al (1995) Nécrose post-radique du cartilage cricoïde: un cas inhabituel. J Radiol 76:517–520

De Vuysere S, Hermans R, Delaere P, et al (1999) CT findings in laryngeal chondroradionecrosis. J Belge Radiol 82:16–18

Erkal HS, Mendenhall WM, Amdur RJ, et al (2001) Synchronous and metachronous squamous cell carcinoma of the head and neck mucosal sites. J Clin Oncol 19:1358–1362

Feldmeier JJ, Heimbach RD, Davolt DA, et al (1993) Hyperbaric oxygen as an adjunctive treatment for severe laryngeal necrosis: a report of nine consecutive cases. Undersea Hyperb Med 20:329–335

Ferguson BJ, Hudson WR, Farmer JC Jr (1987) Hyperbaric oxygen therapy for laryngeal radionecrosis. Ann Otol Rhinol Laryngol 96:1–6

Greven KM, Williams DW III, Keyes JW, et al (1994) Positron emission tomography of patients with head and neck carcinoma before and after high dose irradiation. Cancer 74:1355–1359

Hermans R, Pameijer FA, Mancuso AA, et al (1998) Computed tomography findings in chondroradionecrosis of the larynx. AJNR Am J Neuroradiol 19:711–718

Hermans R, Pameijer FA, Mancuso AA, et al (2000) Laryngeal or hypopharyngeal squamous cell carcinoma: can follow-up CT after definitive radiotherapy be used to detect local failure earlier than clinical examination alone? Radiology 214:683–687

Keane TJ, Cummings BJ, O'Sullivan B, et al (1993) A randomized trial of radiation therapy compared to split course radiation therapy combined with mitomycin C and 5 fluorouracil as initial treatment for advanced laryngeal and hypopharyngeal squamous carcinoma. Int J Radiat Oncol Biol Phys 25:613–618

Keene M, Harwood AR, Bryce DP, et al (1982) Histopathological study of radionecrosis in laryngeal carcinoma. Laryngoscope 92:173–180

Lapela M, Grénman R, Kurki T, et al (1995) Head and neck cancer: detection of recurrence with PET and 2-[F-18]fluoro-2-deoxy-D-glucose. Radiology 197:205–211

Marx RE (1983) Osteoradionecrosis: a new concept of its pathophysiology. J Oral Maxillofac Surg 41:283–288

McGuirt WF (1997) Laryngeal radionecrosis versus recurrent cancer. Otolaryngol Clin North Am 30:243–250

McGuirt WF, Greven KM, Williams DW III, et al (1998) Laryngeal radionecrosis versus recurrent cancer: a clinical approach. Ann Otol Rhinol Laryngol 107:293–296

Mukherji SK, Mancuso AA, Kotzur IM, et al (1994a) Radiologic appearance of the irradiated larynx, part I. Expected changes. Radiology 193:141–148

Mukherji SK, Mancuso AA, Kotzur IM, et al (1994b) Radiologic appearance of the irradiated larynx, part II. Primary site response. Radiology 193:149–154

Nelson EG, Tybor AG (1992) Actinomycosis of the larynx. Ear Nose Throat J 71:356–358

Nömayr A, Lell M, Sweeney R, et al (2001) MRI appearance of radiation-induced changes of normal cervical tissues. Eur Radiol 11:1807–1817

O'Brien P (1996) Tumour recurrence or treatment sequelae following radiotherapy for larynx cancer. J Surg Oncol 63:130–135

Pameijer FA, Hermans R, Mancuso AA, et al (1999) Pre- and post-radiotherapy computed tomography in laryngeal cancer: imaging-based prediction of local failure. Int J Radiat Oncol Biol Phys 45:359–366

Parsons JT (1994) The effect of radiation on normal tissues of the head and neck. In: Million RR, Cassisi NJ (eds) Management of head and neck cancer: a multidisciplinary approach. Lippincott, Philadelphia, pp 245–289

Ward PH, Calcaterra TC, Kagan AR (1975) The enigma of post-radiation edema and recurrent or residual carcinoma of the larynx. Laryngoscope 85:522–529

9 Imaging After Laryngeal Surgery

Roberto Maroldi, Davide Farina, Guiseppe Battaglia, Laura Palvarini, and Patrizia Maculotti

CONTENTS

9.1
Introduction

When compared to primary tumor assessment, the effectiveness of CT is somewhat limited in the follow-up of laryngeal carcinomas treated by conservative or total surgery. This is due to the fact that endoscopic examination is relatively easy and yields a high degree of accuracy in detecting recurrent neoplasms. Moreover, the incidence of local relapses is quite low. The combination of the two elements explains why CT is used only in selected cases.

Even the extent of the primary lesion does not predict the probability of developing a relapse.

R. Maroldi, MD
Professor, Department of Radiology, University of Brescia, Piazza Spedali Civili 1, 25 123 Brescia, Italy
D. Farina, MD
Department of Radiology, University of Brescia, Piazza Spedali Civili 1, 25 123 Brescia, Italy
G. Battaglia, MD
Department of Radiology, University of Brescia, Piazza Spedali Civili 1, 25 123 Brescia, Italy
L. Palvarini, MD
Department of Radiology, University of Brescia, Piazza Spedali Civili 1, 25 123 Brescia, Italy
P. Maculotti, MD
Department of Radiology, University of Brescia, Piazza Spedali Civili 1, 25 123 Brescia, Italy

Therefore CT is not justified in the follow-up program. For example, the recurrence rate is lower – 2–5% – for "advanced" supraglottic neoplasms treated by open surgery (Laccourreye et al. 1998) than for early glottic carcinomas (close to 14%) resected endoscopically (Eckel 2001). One may argue that the greater tissue resection and the more adequate exposure should account for such a difference in the local control. Moreover, although the overall rate of recurrences after conservative surgery is limited, it is higher than for patients treated by total laryngectomy. This is an indication of the great challenge to conservative surgery, i.e., the effort to combine the goal of patient survival with organ preservation.

Actually, the presence of lymph node metastases, rather than local recurrent tumor, represents the most important predictive factor for survival (Shah et al. 1997). Furthermore, several reports underline the fact that few (up to 30%) early local relapses are asymptomatic and are rarely undetectable at endoscopy. Therefore, the main role of cross-sectional imaging after surgery is to determine the precise submucosal extent of recurrences or to differentiate relapsing tumors from submucosal complications, rather than the early detection of recurrences.

Essential requirements for a proper CT evaluation of the postoperative larynx include knowledge of the initial tumor location, its extent, and the type of resection and reconstruction. Additionally, it is necessary to know the normal CT findings for that specific surgical approach, the most frequent sites of recurrences and the pattern of growth (Maroldi 2000). Of course, interpretation of CT studies after conservative or total surgery is made challenging by the altered anatomy and the absence or the rearrangement of normally symmetric landmarks. Moreover, radiation therapy causes additional changes to the normal aspect of the soft tissues of the neck. Therefore, it is necessary to know the key aspects of conservative and total surgical techniques and the relative imaging findings.

9.2
Conservative Surgery: a Conceptual Understanding

Conservative surgical techniques have been developed with the aim of combining radical tumor resection with preservation of organ function. This means that, in most conservative approaches, tumor ablation has to be followed by the reconstruction of a neolarynx obtained either by using local spared tissue or by the use of free flaps. Laser excision and open-surgical conservative laryngectomy differ not only in the extent of the resection but also in the reconstruction. In fact, in all open-surgical procedures, restoration of laryngeal function needs an accurate rearrangement of both soft tissues and cartilages to achieve the goals of organ sparing.

The postoperative CT appearance of the reconstructed larynx largely depends on the changes to both the cartilaginous framework and the soft tissues. Normal postoperative imaging findings will range from minimal alterations – usually observed after laser resections – to the complex appearance of the neolarynx after open surgery. CT changes of morphology, density and contrast enhancement of laryngeal soft tissues are rather unpredictable, as they depend upon the specific surgical technique performed – including particular variations needed for the resection – and the variability in healing, edema and scarring among patients. Conversely, modifications of the laryngeal framework (partial or complete resection of some cartilages and changes of their location in relation to the hyoid bone) represent specific landmarks, and therefore play a key role in interpreting postoperative CT findings (Table 9.1).

Three essential conditions are required to preserve laryngeal function: the continuity and patency of the upper airway has to be maintained (breathing); an effective separation between airway and digestive tract has to be provided (deglutition); and a glottis has to be spared or reconstructed (phonation). From an anatomical and functional perspective, these requirements involve the sparing, respectively, of the cricoid ring, a portion of the base of the tongue and/or epiglottis, and at least one cricoarytenoid unit (superior and recurrent laryngeal nerves, arytenoid cartilage, cricoarytenoid musculature).

Although the different conservative surgical techniques may be described according to the site of origin of the tumor (supraglottis vs glottis/subglottis) or to the neoplastic local extent (T classification), they are listed in relation to the width of tissue resected. The "conservative surgical" options accordingly include laser excision (small glottic and, less frequently, supraglottic lesions), horizontal supraglottic laryngectomy (advanced supraglottic lesions), vertical hemilaryngectomy (some glottic lesions), supracricoid partial laryngectomy (advanced glottic or supraglottic lesions), and selected complex procedures, among which hemicricohemilaryngectomy (advanced unilateral laryngeal lesions or selected piriform sinus neoplasms), and this approach is attracting a lot of interest.

9.2.1
Transoral Laser Excision

Transoral laser excision (TLE) is the least-invasive surgical option. It bears a low risk of complications

Table 9.1. CT landmarks after conservative laryngeal open surgery: cartilages and hyoid bone (*HSL* horizontal supraglottic laryngectomy, *VH* vertical hemilaryngectomy, *SCPL with CHP* supracricoid laryngectomy with cricohyoidopexy, *SCPL with CHEP* supracricoid laryngectomy with cricohyoidoepiglottopexy, *HCH* hemicricohemilaryngectomy)

Surgery	Hyoid bone	Cartilage Epiglottis	Thyroid	Cricoid	Arytenoid (ipsilateral)	Arytenoid (contralateral)
HSL	Present (resected)	Resected	Upper third resected	Not modified	Present (resected)	Present
VH	Present	Present	Ipsilateral ala resected	Not modified	Resected	Present
SCPL with CHP	Present	Resected	Resected	Shifted and closer to hyoid bone	Resected (present)	Present
SCPL with CHEP	Present	Present suprahyoid	Resected	Shifted and closer to hyoid bone	Resected (present)	Present
HCH	Present	Present	Half resected	Half resected	Resected	Present

and provides a good voice quality (PERETTI et al. 2000a; ECKEL 2001). At present, this is the most frequent surgical treatment for glottic carcinoma. As a consequence, a significant decrease in open-surgical approaches, such as cordectomy and vertical hemilaryngectomy, has been reported (PERETTI et al. 1994). Even though in recent years the indications for TLE have been extended, this treatment is suggested only for "limited" tumors – i.e., Tis, T1 and T2 mainly arising in the glottic region. In the supraglottis, laser resections are usually performed only in small (T1) neoplasms of the suprahyoid epiglottis, false vocal cords or aryepiglottic folds (ECKEL 1997).

TLE consists of the laser ablation of the tumor and the adjacent soft tissues without relevant modifications of the cartilaginous framework, because the deepest extension of the resection encompasses the inner perichondrium. The width of the resection varies according to the depth of tumor extension and is classified into five different levels (Table 9.2).

TLE offers various advantages compared to RT and open surgery. In particular, it requires shorter hospitalization, and has lower morbidity and fewer side effects resulting in an overall better cost effectiveness. One of the main disadvantages of this approach relates to the correct assessment of the actual depth of the neoplastic extent, particularly when the lesion involves the anterior commissure. More than 30% of local failures of TLE occur at this level (ECKEL 2001).

A new approach, that of combining TLE and open surgery, has recently been proposed for the treatment of lesions invading the anterior commissure. With this technique, the reconstruction is accomplished by the placement of muscular flaps through a small window of the thyroid cartilage (REBEIZ et al. 2000).

It must be emphasized that local recurrences after TLE can be treated by conservative salvage techniques in more than 40% of cases (ECKEL 2001). Of course, early detection of relapsing lesions requires a meticulous and strict follow-up. The rate of local control obtained by TLE in early glottic carcinomas (T1, T2a) ranges from 86% to 92% (PERETTI et al. 2000a; ECKEL 2001).

Regardless of the type of resection performed, soft tissue loss is limited. Therefore, normal CT findings after TLE range from the absence of changes to a focal tissue defect or to the complete replacement of the cord – and paralaryngeal fat tissue – by scar (Fig. 9.1). This fibrotic tissue appears quite homogeneous, denser than vocal muscle and with a straighter inner shape. Of course, the most crucial point is to differentiate the scar from a relapse. The detection of a plaque-like lesion with no contrast enhancement points the diagnosis towards a scar. Nevertheless, in all cases in which endoscopic findings are also doubtful, biopsy is recommended. An additional CT finding after TLE is the presence of a sclerotic thyroid lamina. This may be observed after resection of perichondrium, and is probably related to a chronic inflammatory reaction.

9.2.2
Horizontal Supraglottic Laryngectomy

Supraglottic carcinomas not extending into the ventricle and with normal vocal cord motility can be removed by resecting the whole supraglottis through a horizontal cut passing a few millimeters up to the true vocal cord level. This surgical technique removes, therefore, the upper half of the larynx, including the upper third of the thyroid cartilage, the preepiglottic space, the epiglottis, the aryepiglottic folds, and the false vocal cords. The inferior border of the resection corresponds to the floor of the ventricle (Fig. 9.2).

As the epiglottis is resected, a new solution is necessary to prevent aspiration during deglutition. That is accomplished by the active opposition of the residual arytenoid cartilages – plus the surrounding mucosa – to the base of the tongue. Consequently, the distance between the base of the tongue and the mucosa covering the arytenoid(s) should be reduced to obtain an adequate contact. Due to the resection of the supraglottis, a significant shortening is obtained, permitting the residual larynx to lie very close to the base of the tongue. Swallowing is the only function to be restored after horizontal supraglottic laryngectomy (HSL), as both the continuity of the upper airway and the normal activity of the glottis are preserved.

HSL may also be extended to include resection of part of the tongue base, one arytenoid, or the piri-

Table 9.2. Classification of laser excisions

Class	Excision type	Depth of excision
I	Mucosectomy	Superficial layer of lamina propria
II	Superficial cordectomy	Superficial portion of vocalis muscle
III	Partial cordectomy	Medial portion of vocalis muscle
IV	Total cordectomy	Inner perichondrium of thyroid lamina
V	Extended cordectomy	Surrounding laryngeal subsites

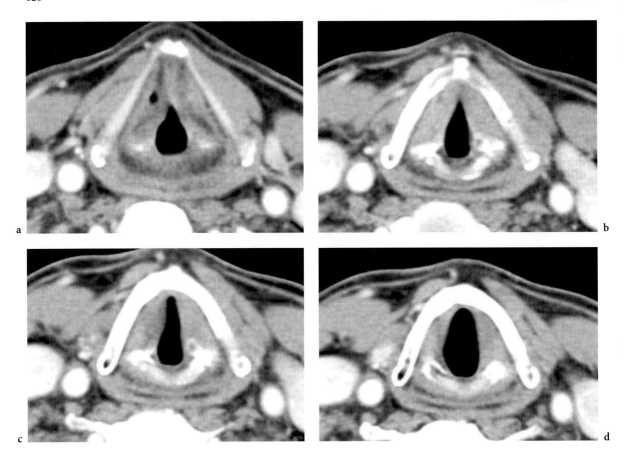

Fig. 9.1a–d. CT of the larynx after laser excision: normal findings. The patient has been operated on for a T1 carcinoma of the left true vocal cord (type 2 resection). No significant change in density or morphology of the cord can be appreciated

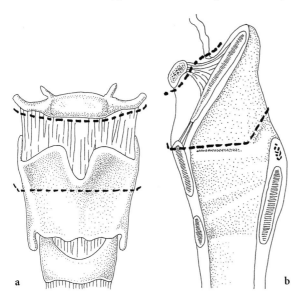

Fig. 9.2a, b. Supraglottic horizontal laryngectomy. The supraglottis is resected along a horizontal cut that removes the upper part of the thyroid cartilage (**a**) passing a few millimeters up to the glottic level (**b**). A second cut through the thyrohyoid membrane spares the hyoid bone and reaches the border of the base of the tongue (**b**)

form sinus, unless the apex is invaded. HSL is not feasible when a tumor infiltrates both arytenoids, the posterior commissure, the postcricoid area, the glottis (via the anterior commissure, the ventricle, or the paraglottic space) or the thyroid cartilage. Preepiglottic space invasion (T3) is not a contraindication for the procedure as this subsite is entirely resected.

Partial resection of the thyroid cartilage associated with removal of the whole supraglottis and preservation of the glottis are the landmarks of HSL. The residual thyroid cartilage is shifted upwards and sutured to the hyoid bone (thyrohyoidopexy).

At CT the hyoid bone and the residual thyroid cartilage appear close together. Their edges may appear sclerotic and irregular in up to 70% of cases. As a consequence of the supraglottic resection, only a few millimeters separate the base of the tongue from the arytenoids (neovestibule). An additional typical finding is the hypertrophy of the mucosa overlying the apex of the arytenoid cartilage, redundant in about 40% of patients (Fig. 9.3). At CT its density appears homogeneous, and the edges are smooth (MAROLDI et al. 1997). This hypertrophied mucosa can

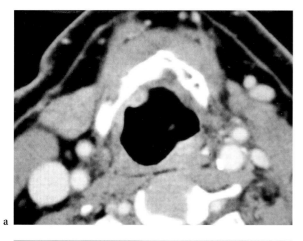

a

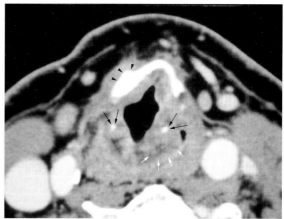

b

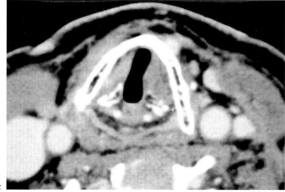

c

Fig. 9.3a–c. CT of the larynx after HSL: normal findings. At the level of the hyoid bone (a) the lumen appears quite irregular, its shape is rather smooth. b The apices of both arytenoids (*arrows*) are imaged close to the hyoid level. Due to the surgical cut, the right thyroid lamina appears irregular (*arrowheads*). The arytenoids are surrounded by abundant residual mucosa (*white arrows*). c Normal orientation and shape of the glottic level. Asymmetry of soft tissues is related to a previous supraomohyoid neck dissection on left side

"fill" the whole neovestibule. In most cases, it extends upwards to the level of the hyoid bone because of the shortening of the larynx. Although some asymmetry of the neovestibule is common, the long axes of both the neovestibule and the glottis are still orientated in the anteroposterior direction (Fig. 9.4). Usually, no changes at the level of the glottis and subglottis are detected in uncomplicated cases.

The postoperative CT appearance of extended HSL may consist of a more pronounced asymmetry of both the neovestibule and the glottis, when one arytenoid cartilage is removed. Conversely, no significant changes are noticeable in the case of marginal excision of the base of the tongue or of the piriform sinus.

9.2.3
Vertical Hemilaryngectomy (VH)

Glottic neoplasms with more or less posterior spread towards the arytenoid may be treated by vertical laryngectomy (BILLER and SOM 1977). Several technical variations exist, all sharing the same access, namely the partial excision of a vertical segment of the ipsilateral thyroid lamina as far as the neoplasm. Through the defect, the true vocal cord, the anterior commissure and if necessary the anterior third of the contralateral true vocal cord are removed (Fig. 9.5). The vertical partial laryngectomy with epiglottic reconstruction (SCHRODER et al. 1997) is a technique particularly suitable for neoplasms arising from or extending to the anterior commissure. It allows the resection of the ventricle, the false vocal cord and the vocal process of the arytenoid cartilage (BILLER and SOM 1977).

Total resection of the arytenoid is feasible (extended vertical partial laryngectomy). However, it predisposes the patient to postoperative aspiration, since adequate laryngeal closure during swallowing cannot be obtained. Reconstruction is achieved by using a local, mucosally based corniculate-cuneiform flap (PERSKY and DAMIANO 1998).

Vertical laryngectomy is challenged by laser excision (a less-invasive technique) and supracricoid partial laryngectomy (see below), as the latter yields

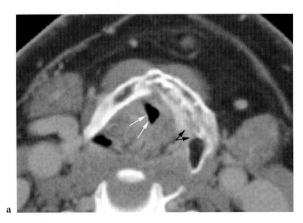 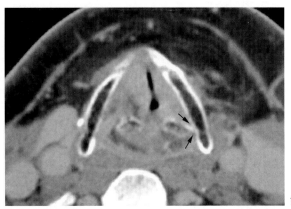

Fig. 9.4a, b. CT of the larynx after HSL. The patient, operated on for a supraglottic carcinoma 7 years before, complained of worsening dyspnea. Endoscopy detected hypomotility of the left vocal cord; the right appeared fixed. a CT shows a stenotic neovestibule (*white arrows*), probably due to chronic edema. Irregular outlines of the left thyroid lamina are present (*arrows*). b Fat within the paraglottic space is not detectable on the left side, along with a reduced distance between the arytenoid cartilage and the thyroid lamina (*arrows*). The latter finding suggests fibrotic changes. A biopsy of the right true vocal cord was negative

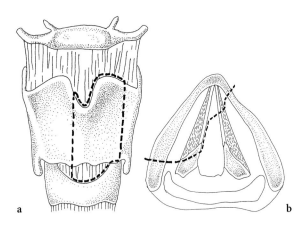

Fig. 9.5a, b. Vertical hemilaryngectomy. A window is obtained by resecting a vertical fragment of the thyroid cartilage (a). This approach allows the ipsilateral true vocal cord, the anterior aspect of the ipsilateral arytenoid cartilage and the anterior third of the contralateral true vocal cord to be removed (b)

a better local control rate (LACCOURREYE et al. 2000).

Even though its use is decreasing, the indications for vertical surgery include T1-T2 anterior glottic cancers arising from the anterior commissure or true vocal cords without impairment of cord mobility or subglottic/supraglottic neoplastic spread [except for the ventricle, entirely removed during vertical hemilaryngectomy (VH)]. Paraglottic space or thyroid cartilage invasion is a contraindication.

The postoperative CT landmarks consist of a vertical defect of the thyroid cartilage, with sclerotic but sharp edges, and an asymmetric appearance of the glottic level (Fig. 9.6). Usually, the reconstructed neocord shows an irregular and convex outline. As it is composed of dense scar tissue, which extends from the thyroid lamina defect to the arytenoid, it appears denser than the contralateral cord and it shows reduced or absent enhancement (DiSANTIS et al. 1984a) (Fig. 9.7). An asymmetric shape of the supraglottis is observed only when the false vocal cord has been included in the resection.

9.2.4
Supracricoid Partial Laryngectomy

Advanced supraglottic or glottic neoplasms not invading the cricoid or the cricoarytenoid joint and not extending deep into the subglottis may be resected by supracricoid partial laryngectomy (SCPL). A subtotal resection of both supraglottis and glottis is obtained by this technique. The true and false vocal cords, the paraglottic spaces, the whole thyroid cartilage, as well as the preepiglottic space are resected. The cricoid cartilage, the hyoid bone, and at least one arytenoid cartilage are preserved (Fig. 9.8a). The epiglottis is totally removed when supraglottic carcinomas are treated, whereas its suprahyoid part is spared in glottic carcinomas.

In both variations the substantial shortening of the larynx has to be managed by moving the cervicomediastinal trachea upwards, pulling together the cricoid cartilage and the hyoid bone either with the spared epiglottis (cricohyoidoepiglottopexy, CHEP; Fig. 9.8b) or without it (cricohyoidopexy, CHP; Fig. 9.8c). To assist with swallowing, cricoid and

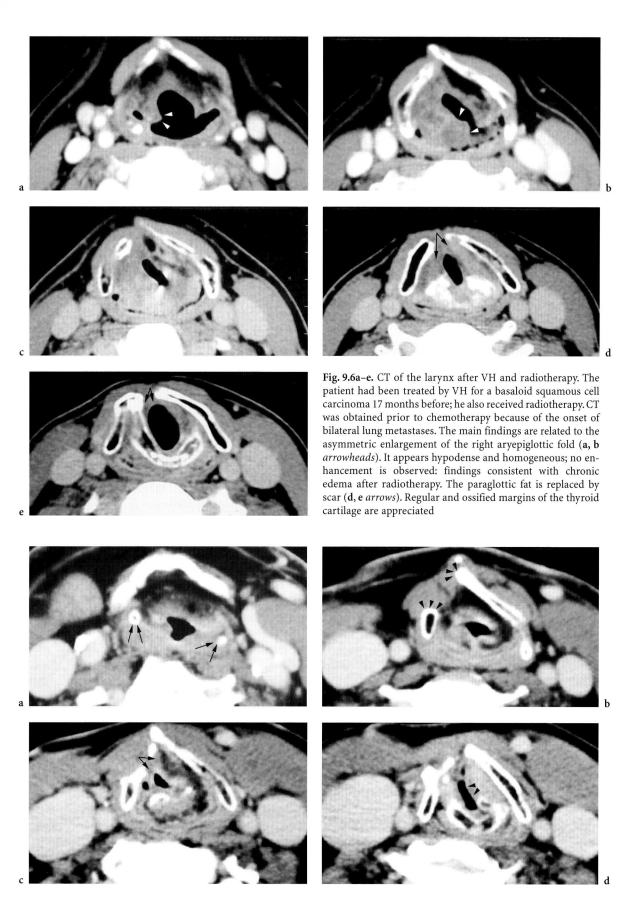

Fig. 9.6a–e. CT of the larynx after VH and radiotherapy. The patient had been treated by VH for a basaloid squamous cell carcinoma 17 months before; he also received radiotherapy. CT was obtained prior to chemotherapy because of the onset of bilateral lung metastases. The main findings are related to the asymmetric enlargement of the right aryepiglottic fold (**a, b** *arrowheads*). It appears hypodense and homogeneous; no enhancement is observed: findings consistent with chronic edema after radiotherapy. The paraglottic fat is replaced by scar (**d, e** *arrows*). Regular and ossified margins of the thyroid cartilage are appreciated

Fig. 9.7a–d. CT of the larynx after VH: normal findings. The patient, operated on for a right T2 true vocal cord (TVC) carcinoma 13 months before, complained of worsening dysphonia. **a** Asymmetric position of the upper cornua of the thyroid cartilage (*arrows*) because of rotation. **b, c** Part of the right thyroid lamina was resected; its margins are regular and ossified (*arrowheads*). **c** Scar tissue replaces the paraglottic fat (*arrows*). **d** Due to surgical resection of the TVC, scar is detected also in front of the cricoarytenoid joint. The left TVC appears more convex than normal (*arrowheads*) to compensate for the absence of the right TVC

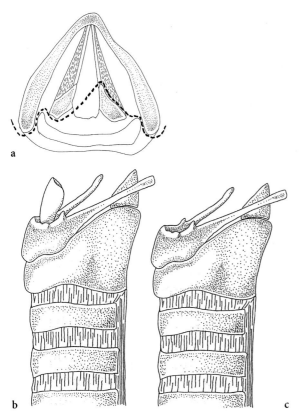

Fig. 9.8a–c. Supracricoid partial laryngectomy. **a** Anterior to the resection line, several structures are resected: both true vocal cords and paraglottic spaces, one arytenoid cartilage, and most of the thyroid cartilage. Depending on the site of the tumor, the upper part of the epiglottic cartilage may be preserved (SCPL with cricoepiglottohyoidopexy) (**b**) or resected (SCPL with cricohyoidopexy) (**c**)

hyoid are carefully aligned, sutured in close contact with their opposite midline surfaces and tightly fixed. As with HSL, recovery of the sphincteric function is achieved by the active opposition of the arytenoid cartilage with the base of the tongue.

The key to preserving voice and glottic sphincteric function relies on the maintenance of a functional cricoarytenoid unit – superior and recurrent laryngeal nerves, arytenoid cartilage, cricoarytenoid musculature – and the sparing of mucosal sensitivity (MONZIOLS et al. 1995). A residual arytenoid cartilage with its surrounding muscles is essential for a functional outcome. The scar tissue and the healed mucosa in front of the arytenoid create a neocord that vibrates, providing speech.

SCPL with CHP is suitable for advanced supraglottic carcinomas not amenable to a HSL. Indications are neoplasms extending to the ventricle, invading the glottis and the anterior commissure with

or without impaired mobility of the true vocal cord. Advanced glottic carcinomas invading the supraglottis are the indications for SCPL with CHEP. In selected cases, either supraglottic or glottic tumors with limited thyroid cartilage invasion (LACCOURR-EYE et al. 1990) (T4) can be treated by SCPL.

Contraindications are mainly related to the involvement of the cricoid cartilage. They include arytenoid cartilage fixation, posterior commissure invasion, subglottic extension greater than 10 mm anteriorly and 5 mm posteriorly, cricoid cartilage invasion, and extralaryngeal spread of the lesion. The involvement of the hyoid bone, rather than the massive spread into preepiglottic space, is an additional contraindication (LACCOURREYE et al. 1998).

The extended resection results in a significant shortening of the larynx with the hyoid bone and the anterior part of the cricoid ring touching in the midline. One arytenoid cartilage and the ipsilateral inferior cornu of the thyroid cartilage are still present. This residual part of the cartilage has to be spared to preserve the recurrent laryngeal nerve, essential for the functionality of the cricoarytenoid unit.

As the cricoid cartilage and the hyoid bone are tightly sutured, they may show some misalignment on both the axial (rotation) and coronal (tilting) planes. Changes of the cartilaginous framework are reflected in the intraluminal soft tissue CT appearance (Figs. 9.9 and 9.10). The subtotal resection of the thyroid cartilage causes a discrepancy in size between the residual larynx and the hypopharynx. As a consequence, the lateral edges of the hypopharynx come into a more anterior position. This anterior "recess" may be dilated by air or fluid, thereby mimicking a pharyngocele (Fig. 9.9).

Excessive residual hypopharyngeal mucosa on the top of the arytenoid, besides causing asymmetry of the short neovestibule, may be so large as to entirely fill the lumen. This thickened mucosa (and submucosa) typically shows a smooth and regular lining and a homogeneous hypodensity, deep to the surface (Figs. 9.11, 9.12).

A key finding, the most challenging for the radiologist, is the presence of a quite variable scar in front of the residual arytenoid. Covered by healed mucosa, this scar acts as a neocord, vibrating according to the arytenoid movements. The dense tissue extends downward with asymmetric thickening of the mucosa lining the subglottis (Figs. 9.9 and 9.10). Marked asymmetry and transverse orientation of the long axis of the neoglottis have been noted (MAROLDI et al. 1997).

It has been reported that the fibrous scar may cause the late development of an iatrogenic laryngo-

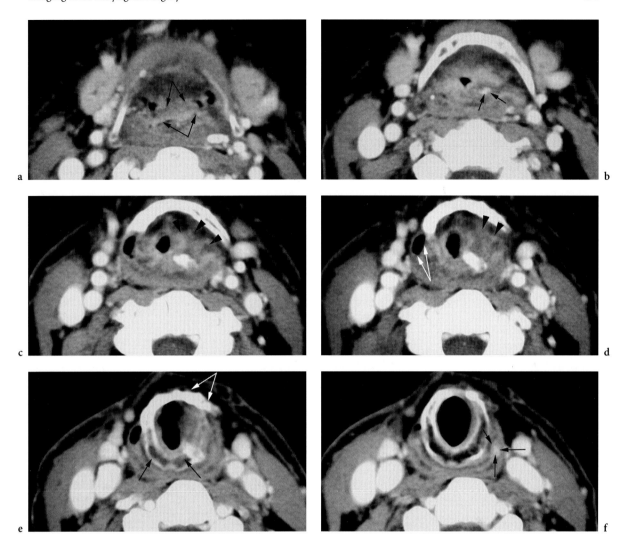

Fig. 9.9a–f. CT of the larynx after SCPL with CHEP: normal findings. The patient had been treated for a T2 right glottic tumor 5 years before. Follow-up CT after endoscopic resection of a mucosal flap causing stenosis of the neovestibule. **a** The spared epiglottis is detected at the level of the base of the tongue (*arrows*). **b** The spared arytenoid (*arrows*) is imaged at the same level as the hyoid bone, due to shortening of the larynx. **c, d** In front of the vocal process of the spared arytenoid typical aspect of the scar is demonstrated (*arrowheads*). An anterior "recess" dilated by air is detected close to the cricoid, mimicking a pharyngocele (*white arrows*). **e** Due to cricohyoidopexy the bone (*white arrows*) and the cartilage (*arrows*) appear in the same slice. Thyroid cartilage has been removed. The discrepancy in size between the hypopharynx and the residual larynx explains why the latter is partially surrounded by the pharynx. **f** The left inferior cornu of thyroid cartilage was spared to preserve one cricoarytenoid unit (*arrows*)

cele or laryngomucocele after supracricoid partial laryngectomy (up to 2%). This may be related to incomplete resection of a preexisting saccule or laryngocele. In this scenario, blockage of the saccule orifice may result in a flap-valve mechanism, thereby producing a laryngocele (MAROLDI et al. 1997; CARRAT et al. 1998).

CT findings of SCPL with CHEP do not significantly differ from SCPL with CHP, except for the presence of the residual suprahyoid epiglottis, usual-ly detectable at the same level as the cricoid due to major shortening of the larynx.

9.2.5
Extended Surgical Techniques

A third group of complex surgical procedures is suitable for either glottic cancers extending into the subglottis (BARTUAL and ROQUETTE 1978) (glottosub-

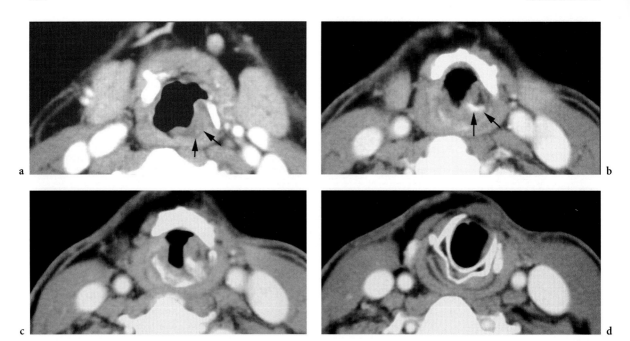

Fig. 9.10a–d. CT of the larynx after SCPL with CHP: normal findings. The patient, operated on for a supraglottic carcinoma 5 years before, showed worsening of dysphonia and dyspnea. Findings are similar to those in SCPL with CHEP except for the absence of the spared epiglottis. A significant amount of tissue surrounds the left (residual) arytenoid cartilage (*arrows*). In this patient, excessive clockwise rotation of the cricoid in respect to the hyoid is present (**c, d**)

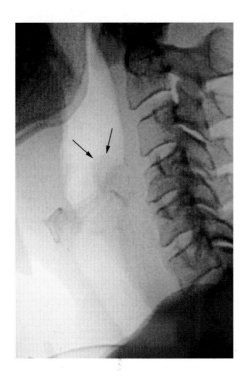

Fig. 9.11. SCPL with CHP. Increased thickening of the mucosa surrounding the spared arytenoid cartilage (*arrows*) helps closure of the airway during swallowing

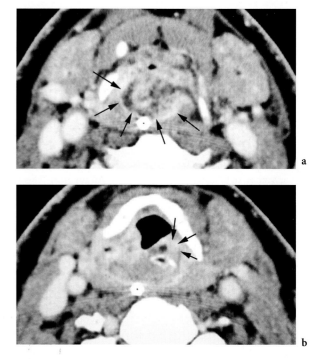

Fig. 9.12a, b. CT of the larynx after SCPL with CHEP. **a** The neovestibule is entirely filled by excess residual mucosa covering the arytenoid apex (*arrows*). Deep to the enhancing mucosa, the homogeneous hypodensity of the connective tissue suggests the absence of recurrence. **b** The scar in front of the arytenoid is demonstrated (*arrows*)

glottic laryngectomy) or transglottic lesions with subglottic invasion (PEARSON 1981) (near total laryngectomy). Both techniques allow partial removal of the cricoid cartilage and some tracheal rings. Near total laryngectomy is an extension of conservative surgery techniques beyond the limits of a reconstructed glottic lumen sufficient for oral respiration. Although this technique keeps a mild quality phonation, it requires permanent tracheostomy.

An interesting recently developed surgical technique enables the removal of unilateral T3 glottic tumors with subglottic extension and/or arytenoid cartilage fixation or selected piriform sinus tumors extending into the apex. The hemicricohemilaryngectomy developed by DELAERE et al. (1998) consists of a two-step procedure. The first step encompasses the transformation of a segment of the tracheal tube (four tracheal rings) into a potential patch by enfolding the tracheal segment in a free flap obtained from the forearm. In the second phase, performed about 2 weeks later, the tumor is resected with a hemilaryngectomy extending to the subglottis and including the ipsilateral hemicricoid cartilage. The tracheal segment (in the meantime revascularized by vessels from the free flap) will be resected, adapted and transposed to cover the laryngeal defect.

This technique is a further development of conservative surgery as it also allows the treatment of unilateral glottic tumors with arytenoid cartilage fixation and subglottic tumor extension reaching the upper border of the cricoid cartilage, two major contraindications for all classical conservation procedures. It is a functional reconstruction, allowing the patient to breath and speak through the larynx, and swallow without aspiration; no tracheostomy is needed (DELAERE et al. 1998, 2000; Cox et al. 2000).

After hemicricohemilaryngectomy, the CT appearance consists of a quite normal residual hemilarynx facing a new laryngeal half-wall. This is composed of the rigid framework of the "opened" tracheal rings wrapped into the flap (tracheal autotransplantation). At CT, the axial section of the glottis/subglottis is no longer round, but it appears as a half circle with the residual cord adducted toward a rigid buttress. This technical solution mimics what happens with a unilateral vocal cord paralysis. Extensive changes of the soft tissues surrounding the autotransplanted trachea are related to the presence of the flap (hypodense fascial envelope) and to the neck dissection (Fig. 9.13).

How to manage a low-malignancy (non-squamous cell carcinoma) neoplasm, i.e., a cartilaginous tumor (chondroma or chondrosarcoma) arising from the cricoid cartilage, is a challenging issue in several conditions. Two elements, the indolent growth rate coupled with infrequent metastasization, permit an incomplete removal of the lesion (piecemeal resection). In fact, the goal of organ sparing justifies the risk of residual disease. Interestingly, surgical techniques developed to treat laryngeal stenoses, for example terminoterminal cricothyrotracheal anastomosis, can be adapted and used to manage these non-aggressive neoplasms. In selected chondrosarcomas of the cricoid it is feasible to remove the caudal part of the cartilage (along with the lesion) and four tracheal rings (Fig. 9.14). An anastomosis between the trachea and the residual cricoid (with its preserved cricoarytenoid joints) restores the continuity of the airways (PERETTI et al. 2000b). In selected cases, the above-described hemicricohemilaryngectomy technique may be an interesting alternative, as it allows the removal of half of the cricoid without compromising the laryngeal function.

9.3
Total Laryngectomy

Organ-sparing treatments, particularly radiation therapy and laser excision, have been used increasingly during the last years as they provide excellent control of early tumors. Moreover, the indications for open surgical conservative techniques have been extended, thereby accounting for the decrease in total laryngectomy in the treatment of primary neoplasms. Of course, salvage surgery for failures of conservative treatment is still an important indication for total laryngectomy.

The hyoid bone, the entire strap muscles and the median part of the thyroid gland are removed together with the whole larynx and the piriform fossae. The pharyngeal defect is closed in layers (hypopharyngeal mucosa and inferior constrictor musculature) forming a conical neopharynx from the base of the tongue to the cervical esophagus. Tracheostomy is, of course, necessary.

On CT, the tubular structure of the neopharynx may be partly collapsed. Its walls show variable enhancement of the lining mucosa, deep to the less-dense muscular and adventitial planes. Usually, the wall shows symmetric thickness with a sharp outer lining. On the transverse plane, the morphology of the neopharynx is oval (more often close to the base of the tongue) or round (near the esophagus) (DISANTIS et al. 1984b; MAROLDI et al. 1997) (Fig. 9.15). The nor-

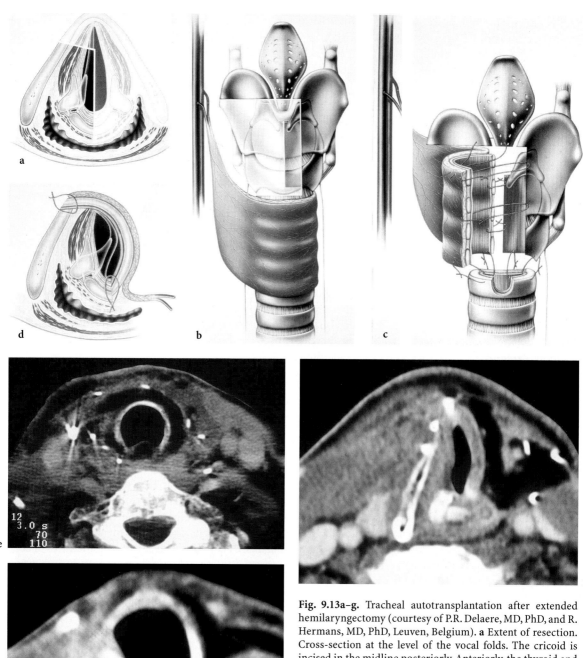

Fig. 9.13a–g. Tracheal autotransplantation after extended hemilaryngectomy (courtesy of P.R. Delaere, MD, PhD, and R. Hermans, MD, PhD, Leuven, Belgium). **a** Extent of resection. Cross-section at the level of the vocal folds. The cricoid is incised in the midline posteriorly. Anteriorly, the thyroid and cricoid cartilages are incised with inclusion of the anterior commissure. The remaining larynx consists of one functional arytenoid with a remnant of vocal fold. **b** First operation: orthotopic revascularization of the trachea. The cervical trachea is wrapped by a radial forearm fascial flap. The vascular pedicle of the flap is reanastomosed to the neck vessels on the same side as the laryngeal tumor. The extent of the right hemilaryngectomy is indicated. **c** Second operation (2 weeks after first operation): autotransplantation of the trachea to extended laryngeal defect. Reconstruction with tracheal patch pedicled on the radial forearm flap. The patch is displaced upward towards the laryngeal defect. **d** Cross-section at the level of the vocal folds after transplantation. Optimal paramedian patch placement with the transplant serving as a buttress of apposition for the remaining mobile arytenoid and vocal fold remnant. **e** CT image, after first operation, at the level of the trachea with its hypodense fascial envelope. **f** CT image, after second operation, at the glottic level with the tracheal patch in a paramedian position. **g** CT image, after second operation, at the subglottic level. The tracheal transplant restores the subglottic airway

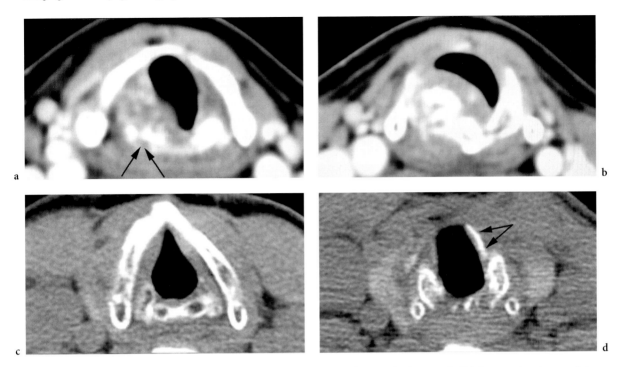

Fig. 9.14a–d. CT of the larynx after cricotracheal resection with cricothyrotrachealpexy. **a, b** CT shows a chondroma of the cricoid cartilage with minimal derangement of the right cricoarytenoid joint (*arrows*). **c** Six months after surgery, the glottic level does not show any abnormality. **d** The resected cricoid ring is replaced by the tracheal rings (*arrows*) anastomosed with the residual cricoid

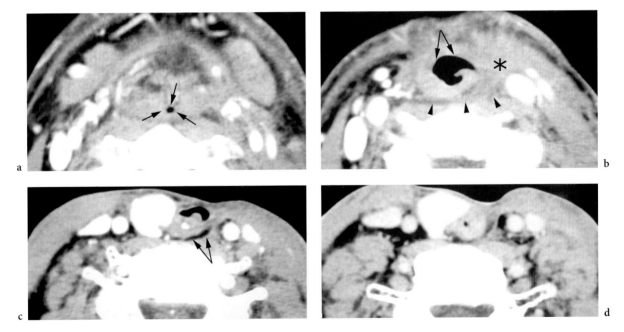

Fig. 9.15a–d. CT of the larynx after total laryngectomy and radiotherapy. **a** The size of the oropharynx is reduced because of chronic edema related to radiotherapy (*arrows*). **b** The neopharynx ranges from an ovoid shape close to the oropharynx (*arrows*) to a more round appearance close to the esophagus (**c, d**). The walls of the neopharynx are smooth and surrounded by soft tissue. This appears solid on the lateral aspects (particularly on the left side) (**b** *asterisk*) due to a previous hemorrhage after modified left neck dissection. The hypodense stripe posterior to the pharynx correlates with radiotherapy changes (chronic edema) (*arrowheads*)

mal tracheostome shows smooth, thin and regular walls (Fig. 9.16).

During total laryngectomy, manipulation of the thyroid parenchyma and surrounding tissues may result in changes of shape of the gland because of the damage to the connective fasciae covering the surface of the gland (WEISSMAN et al. 1998).

Ultrasound has been suggested for the follow-up of total laryngectomy. The absence of interposing cartilages allows easy evaluation of the neopharynx. High-resolution probes enable identification of the different layers and interfaces that make up the pharyngeal wall (LEE et al. 2000).

9.4
Abnormal Postoperative Findings

Statistically most recurrences are expected within the first 24 months after treatment. During this period a strict clinical follow-up is recommended. Although recurrences are observed more frequently after laser resection than conservative laryngectomy, in the former case more lesions are suitable for a subsequent conservative treatment. Two main reasons can be identified. After laser excision most relapsing neoplasms are detected when still superfi-

cial, thereby enabling further laser treatment. Moreover, laser resection spares a large portion of the larynx, allowing a subsequent conservative laryngectomy (Fig. 9.17). Conversely, after open conservative laryngectomy recurrences tend to be larger and show an early deep invasion. This is probably related to the removal of membranes (thyrohyoid) and cartilages (particularly the thyroid) that act as a barrier preventing invasion of extralaryngeal tissues. In addition, reconstruction after open surgery carries the risk of transposing islets of mucosa deep to the superficial lining.

Very few recurrences are missed by endoscopy, particularly among patients treated by laser excision. Although few studies have analyzed the effectiveness of postoperative imaging, data currently available do not justify the use of CT as a screening examination in asymptomatic patients treated by conservative or total surgery (MAROLDI et al. 1997). Therefore, cross-sectional imaging is mainly indicated to assess submucosal masses (iatrogenic laryngoceles have been demonstrated in about 2% of supracricoid laryngectomies) or to determine the full extent of endoscopically proven recurrences.

In a retrospective study of the postoperative CT findings in 52 patients treated by conservative surgery, 19 relapses were examined (9 after laser excision, 7 after HSL), with only one missed by endosco-

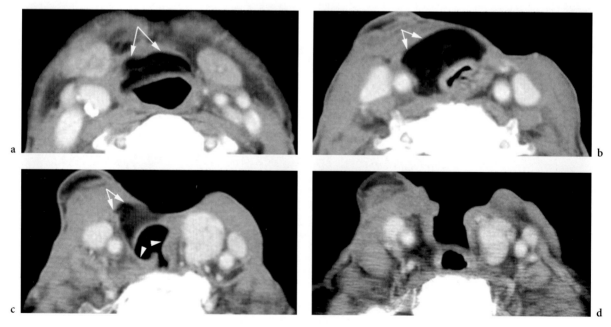

Fig. 9.16a–d. CT of the larynx after total laryngectomy extended to the prelaryngeal muscles and right thyroid lobe. Reconstruction with a flap (pectoralis major muscle). **a–c** The fat density of the flap runs along the anterolateral aspect of the corresponding neopharynx (*white arrows*). At this level, the neopharyngeal wall is formed by the skin; it presents a smooth surface and symmetric thickness. **c, d** The obliquely arranged stoma (*arrowheads*) is imaged on several planes

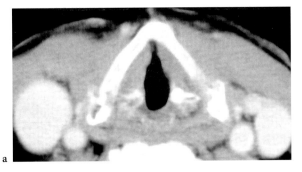
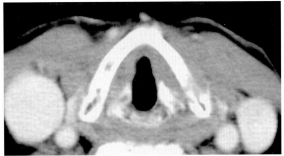

a   b

Fig. 9.17a, b. Bilateral recurrent carcinoma after transoral laser excision (TLE). The patient had been treated with a bilateral TLE type-1 4 years before. The lesions were located on the anterior/central third of the true vocal cord (right) and the anterior third of true vocal cord (left). Two years later bilateral recurrences required a second (type-4 on right, type-3 on left) TLE. The lesions recurred again 4 years after primary TLE. This time CT shows only minimal irregularity of the inner aspect of the cords and sclerotic changes of the left arytenoid joints. A bilateral type-5 TLE was necessary

py. CT signs of a recurrent neoplasm were related to its infiltrative pattern of growth: destruction of spared cartilages (9/19, 47.3%), and the presence of a mass larger than 10 mm (detected in more than 60% of cases) spreading beyond the laryngeal limits (52.9%) (Fig. 9.18). Patchy sclerotic areas within spared cartilages, asymmetry of the laryngeal lumen and obliteration of fat planes of the paraglottic space are relatively common and do not indicate a recurrent tumor.

In the analysis of 15 recurrences after SCPL detected by endoscopy, LACCOURREYE et al. (1998) found five asymptomatic patients, two of whom had a laryngeal mass destroying the cricoid cartilage demonstrated by CT (Fig. 9.19). Among the remaining ten symptomatic patients, CT showed cricoid cartilage invasion in seven due to a mass extending also into prelaryngeal soft tissues (in three), spreading submucosally into the subglottis (in three) or into the piriform sinus (in two) (Fig. 9.20). Overall, after open-surgery procedures, such as HSL or SCPL, recurrences tend to be advanced, with cartilage invaded in approximately 50–60% of cases at diagnosis.

After total laryngectomy, recurrent carcinoma appears at CT as a soft tissue mass with asymmetric thickening of the neopharyngeal walls and irregular narrowing of the lumen (DISANTIS et al. 1984b; WEISSMAN et al. 1998) (Fig. 9.21). Generally, local recurrences after total laryngectomy are expected to arise from two different sites. Those located close to the anastomotic area with the oropharynx may be due to residual, missed, disease, and thus an insufficient partial pharyngectomy. Partial or complete effacement of fat planes adjacent to the neopharynx may be noted in most cases.

At the lower side of the neck, peristomal recurrences are observed. They account for approximately

4% of total laryngectomies, more frequently occurring in tumors invading the subglottis. In spite of advances in laryngeal surgery and modern reconstructive techniques, stomal recurrence is still a major cause of death in patients with laryngeal cancer (MARTIN VILLARES et al. 2000). Stomal recurrences arising from the superior part of the stoma are usually favorable. They require a mediastinal node dissection and the transfer of a myocutaneous flap. Conversely, lesions developing from the inferior aspect of the stoma or invading the esophagus or extending into the mediastinum bear a severe prognosis (SISSON 1985).

CT may be useful not only to assess the actual extent of recurrent disease but also in the evaluation of late complications after surgery (Fig. 9.22). It has no role in the management of early complications (mostly fistulas) that require conventional radiographic studies.

After partial laryngectomy, stenoses and submucosal lesions require CT evaluation to assess, respectively, the clinically inaccessible parts of the larynx and identify the cause (neoplastic or not) of mucosal bulging. The reduction in size of the lumen may be caused by an excessive amount of tissue on top of the arytenoid(s), or by a retracting scar involving the laryngeal walls. In the first case, CT shows the homogeneous hypodense aspect of the submucosal connective tissue that surrounds the apex of the arytenoid(s), lined by enhancing thin mucosa. Scar appears as a dense, non-enhancing, tissue with non-regular margins, quite difficult to differentiate from recurrent disease. Effacement of residual fat spaces is frequent. Although the absence of cartilage erosion should be consistent with scar, a biopsy is recommended.

These complications may be so significant as to impair the functionality of the residual larynx, and

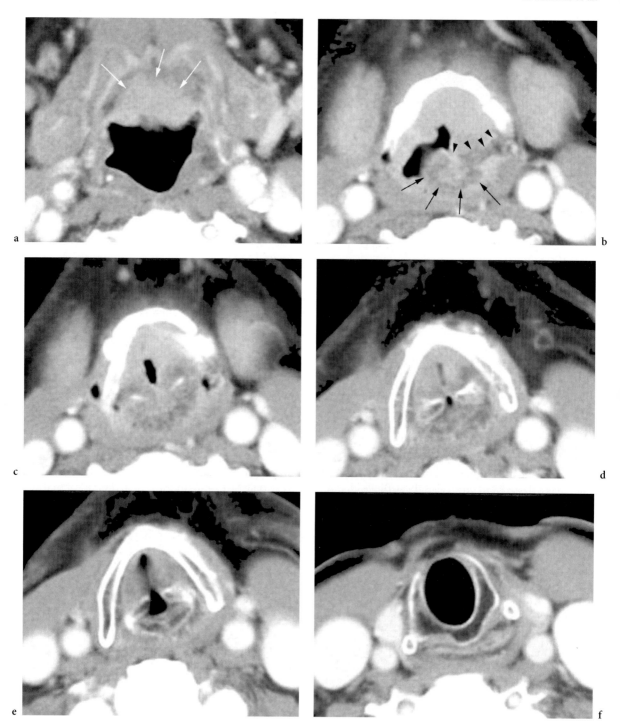

Fig. 9.18a–f. Recurrent carcinoma after HSL. The patient had been operated on for a supraglottic carcinoma (horseshoe pattern of growth) 8 months before. Because of dysphagia, endoscopy and CT were obtained. **a, b** CT demonstrates a recurrent solid lesion at the base of tongue. The fat within the base of the tongue appears subtotally replaced (*white arrows*). There is a significant difference between the relapsing lesion (solid, *arrowheads*) and the excess tissue surrounding the left arytenoid (hypodense deep to the mucosal surface, *arrows*). **c, d** The lesion projects into the lumen growing down towards (but not reaching) the glottis. **e, f** The glottis and subglottis are normal

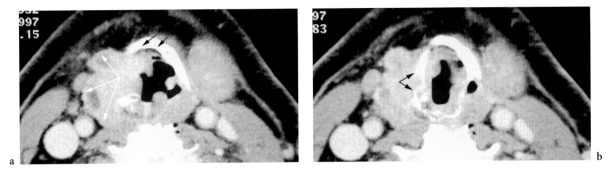

Fig. 9.19a, b. Recurrent carcinoma after SCPL with CHP. Eight months after surgery, endoscopic follow-up showed edema of the right hypopharyngeal wall. **a** A submucosal recurrence extends from the neocord area into the adjacent inferior constrictor muscle (*white arrows*). The hyoid bone is normal (*arrows*). **b** The cricoid cartilage appears destroyed (*arrows*)

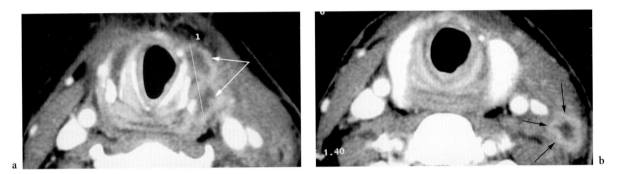

Fig. 9.20a, b. Recurrent carcinoma after SCPL with CHP and radiotherapy. The onset of neck pain and dysphagia 7 months after surgery prompted a CT examination. **a** A recurrent lesion extending along the left hypopharyngeal wall is detectable (*white arrows*). **b** An irregular mass with rim enhancement can be appreciated behind the left sternocleidomastoid muscle (*arrows*). As all the nodes on that side of the neck had been removed by modified radical neck dissection, the lesion can be considered an extranodal-extracapsular recurrence

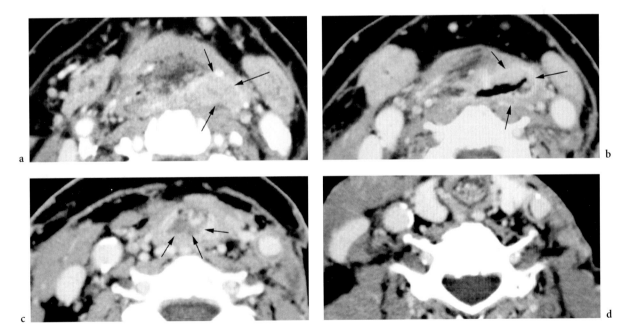

Fig. 9.21a–d. Recurrent carcinoma after total laryngectomy and radiotherapy. The patient complained of left otalgia 4 years after surgery. **a, b** CT shows a soft tissue mass developing at the interface between the oropharynx and neopharynx (hypopharyngeal mucosa) (*arrows*). The lesion invades the left lateral wall and extends into adjacent walls. **c** A second lesion fills the lumen distally (*arrows*). **d** The normal aspect of the esophagus can be appreciated

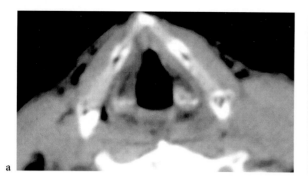
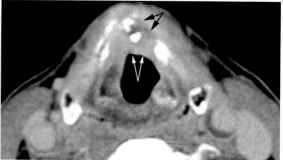

Fig. 9.22a, b. Complication after laser excision. **a** The patient had been treated for a glottic carcinoma extended to the anterior commissure 4 months before. He received local application of an antineoplastic drug (mitomycin) in order to prevent granuloma formation. Because of worsening of dysphonia a new endoscopic examination was obtained. A recurrence was suspected. **b** CT demonstrates fragments of thyroid cartilage surrounding a small fluid collection (chondronecrosis) (*arrows*). Significant thickening of the anterior commissure is present (*white arrows*)

thus lead to failure to achieve the goals of conservative surgical techniques. In some cases a total laryngectomy is indicated, mainly in order to resolve dyspnea and aspiration.

When a submucosal mass is detected by endoscopy, CT may totally resolve the diagnostic question by demonstrating a fluid or gas-filled lesion such as a laryngocele or a laryngomucocele (Fig. 9.23). In the case of a solid lesion without cartilage erosion, CT confirms the need for pathologic assessment. This can be obtained by percutaneous aspiration cytology guided by ultrasound or CT.

Finally, it has to be emphasized that in several patients surgery is associated with radiation treatment. The effects of this therapy may add to the changes produced by surgery and healing, increasing the difficulty of the CT interpretation. One of the most severe complications associated with irradiation is the

avascular necrosis of cartilages or the hyoid bone (see also Chap. 8).

Failure to achieve satisfactory laryngeal function after conservative surgery may be related not only to severe morphologic changes of the lumen (stenosis) but also to impaired coordination in swallowing. The analysis of the different phases of swallowing requires a very fast diagnostic tool (videofluoroscopy or videofluorography) able to obtain a rapid sequence of frames (25–100/s) of the movements of the oropharyngeal and residual laryngeal structures. Videofluoroscopy (or videofluorography) allows the detection of swallowing function disorders as well as structural changes such as strictures, fistulas and mass lesions.

Functional disorders after surgery can be expected to differ according to the type of surgical procedure. For example, aspiration will complicate conser-

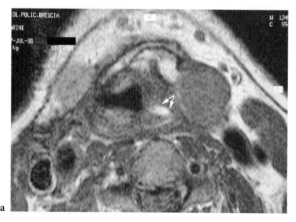
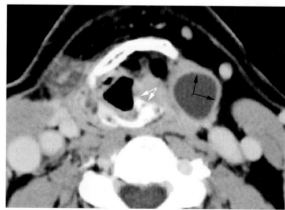

Fig. 9.23a, b. Complication after SCPL with CHEP. The patient developed a tender soft tissue mass on the left side of the neck 1 year after surgery. MR (**a**) and CT (**b**), obtained during the same period, show a lesion with sharp and regular margins. The hypointense signal on MR reveals fluid. The walls show enhancement on CT (*arrows*). The lesion was external to the previous glottic level (the spared arytenoid and the neocord are demonstrated by both techniques; *white arrows*). Surgery confirmed a laryngomucocele

vative laryngectomy whereas bolus retention or de-layed passage will be more typical of total laryngec-tomy.

Information provided by imaging permits the planning of rehabilitation and whether a surgical correction or a total laryngectomy are indicated.

Aspiration, the most frequent complication after conservative open surgery, is the passage of the bolus into the upper airways that may happen before, dur-ing, or after swallowing (Fig. 9.24). It has been ob-served after HSL in approximately 50–76%, more frequently during the late intra- or post-deglutitive phases. This rate is more than 90% among patients complaining of dysphagia. Penetration addresses the passage of bolus into the larynx but is confined to the glottis. Bolus retention may be due to a disorder of the oral phase, i.e., related to a failure of lingual propulsion or to a pharyngeal stenosis.

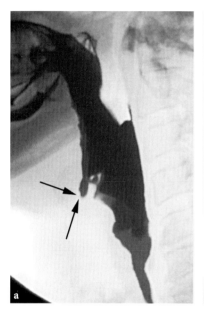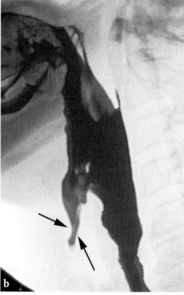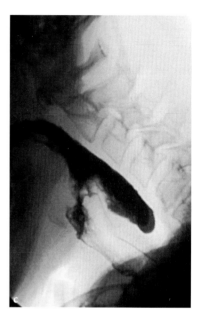

Fig. 9.24a–c. Swallowing impairment after SCPL with CHP. **a, b** Significant intradeglutitive aspiration (*arrows*) while patient swallows in a neutral position. **c** Improvement in aspiration is obtained after the neck is anteriorly flexed

References

Bartual J, Roquette J (1978) Infravestibular horizontal partial laryngectomy. A new surgical method. Arch Otorhino-laryngol 220:213–220

Biller HF, Som ML (1977) Vertical partial laryngectomy for glottic carcinoma with posterior subglottic extension. Ann Otol Rhinol Laryngol 86:715–718

Carrat X, Francois JM, Carles D, et al (1998) Laryngomuco-cele as an unusual late complication of subtotal laryngec-tomy. Case report. Ann Otol Rhinol Laryngol 107:703–707

Cox GJ, Goodacre TE, Corbridge R (2000) Vertical extended hemi crico-laryngectomy and reconstruction with a pre-fabricated tracheal free flap – initial results. Rev Laryngol Otol Rhinol 121:41–43

Delaere PR, Vander Poorten V, Goeleven A, et al (1998) Tra-cheal autotransplantation: a reliable reconstructive tech-nique for extended hemilaryngectomy defects. Laryngo-scope 108:929–934

Delaere PR, Vander Poorten V, Vanclooster C, et al (2000) Results of larynx preservation surgery for advanced la-ryngeal cancer through tracheal autotransplantation. Arch Otolaryngol Head Neck Surg 126:1207–1215

DiSantis DJ, Balfe DM, Hayden R, et al (1984a) The neck after vertical hemilaryngectomy: computed tomographic study. Radiology 151:683–687

DiSantis DJ, Balfe DM, Hayden RÉ, et al (1984b) The neck after total laryngectomy: CT study. Radiology 153:713–717

Eckel HE (1997) Endoscopic laser resection of supraglottic carcinoma. Otolaryngol Head Neck Surg 117:681–687

Eckel HE (2001) Local recurrences following transoral laser surgery for early glottic carcinoma: frequency, manage-ment, and outcome. Ann Otol Rhinol Laryngol 110:7–15

Laccourreye H, Laccourreye O, Weinstein G, et al (1990) Supracricoid laryngectomy with cricohyoidoepiglottopexy: a partial laryngeal procedure for glottic carcinoma. Ann Otol Rhinol Laryngol 99:421–426

Laccourreye O, Laccourreye L, Muscatello L, et al (1998) Local failure after supracricoid partial laryngectomy: symptoms, management, and outcome. Laryngoscope 108:339–344

Laccourreye O, Laccourreye L, Garcia D, et al (2000) Vertical partial laryngectomy versus supracricoid partial laryn-gectomy for selected carcinomas of the true vocal cord classified as T2N0. Ann Otol Rhinol Laryngol 109:965–971

Lee JH, Sohn JE, Choe DH, et al (2000) Sonographic findings of the neopharynx after total laryngectomy: comparison with CT. AJNR Am J Neuroradiol 21:823–827

Maroldi R (2000) Imaging of postoperative larynx and neck. Semin Roentgenol 35:84–100

Maroldi R, Battaglia G, Nicolai P, et al (1997) CT appearance of the larynx after conservative and radical surgery for carcinomas. Eur Radiol 7:418–431

Martin Villares C, Perez Carretero M, Ortega Medina L, et al (2000) Stomal recurrence after laryngectomy. An inevitable late complication. Acta Otorrinolaringol Esp 51:501–505

Monziols F, Verhulst J, Lenoir JL, et al (1995) Prise en charge postoperatoire des pharyngo-laryngectomies partielles ou reconstructives. Rev Laryngol Otol Rhinol 116:277–281

Pearson BW (1981) Subtotal laryngectomy. Laryngoscope 91:1904–1912

Peretti G, Cappiello J, Nicolai P, et al (1994) Endoscopic laser excisional biopsy for selected glottic carcinomas. Laryngoscope 104:1276–1279

Peretti G, Nicolai P, Redaelli De Zinis LO, et al (2000a) Endoscopic CO_2 laser excision for Tis, T1, and T2 glottic carcinomas: cure rate and prognostic factors. Otolaryngol Head Neck Surg 123:124–131

Peretti G, Piazza C, Berlucchi M, et al (2000b) Pleomorphic adenoma: a case treated by laryngotracheal resection and reconstruction. Acta Otorhinolaryngol Ital 20:54–61

Persky MS, Damiano A (1998) Corniculate-cuneiform flap for reconstruction in the extended vertical partial laryngectomy. Ann Otol Rhinol Laryngol 107:297–300

Rebeiz EE, Wang Z, Annino DJ, et al (2000) Preliminary clinical results of window partial laryngectomy: a combined endoscopic and open technique. Ann Otol Rhinol Laryngol 109:123–127

Schroder U, Eckel HE, Jungehulsing M, et al (1997) Indications, technique and results following Sedlacek-Kambic-Tucker reconstructive partial resection of the larynx. HNO 45:915–922

Shah JP, Karnell LH, Hoffman HT, et al (1997) Patterns of care for cancer of the larynx in the United States. Arch Otolaryngol Head Neck Surg 123:475–483

Sisson GA (1985) Mediastinal dissection-resectability and curability of stomal recurrence after total laryngectomy. Auris Nasus Larynx 12:S61–66

Weissman JL, Curtin HD, Johnson JT (1998) Thyroid gland after total laryngectomy: CT appearance. Radiology 207:405–409

10 Positron Emission Tomography in Head and Neck Squamous Cell Carcinoma

PATRICK FLAMEN

CONTENTS

10.1 Introduction

10.1.1 Structural Versus Metabolic Imaging

The technological revolution in medical imaging during the last decades is certainly one of the cornerstones of progress in modern oncology. Recent developments in radiographic imaging have resulted in highly sensitive cross-sectional imaging, providing ever increasing accuracy in detection and defining the extent of tumours. Importantly, it must be born in mind that the diagnosis provided by these techniques entirely depends on the structural and morphometric characteristics of the tumour. Therefore,

P. FLAMEN, MD, PhD
Department of Nuclear Medicine, University Hospitals Leuven, Herestraat 49, 3000 Leuven, Belgium

the accuracy of these so-called structure-based techniques is severely hampered by the fact that structural information alone does not always allow straightforward differentiation between malignant and benign lesions. An example is the use of the lesion diameter as a criterion to diagnose tumoral lymph node involvement by computed tomography (CT) or ultrasound. Lymph node size greater than 10 mm is a major criterion for malignant involvement used in CT and MRI. Using such a criterion results in limitations of sensitivity because normal-sized lymph nodes can harbour neoplastic cells. Indeed, in histopathological studies, EICHHORN et al. (1987) have shown that more than 40% of all lymph node metastases of head and neck squamous cell carcinoma (SCCa) are localized in nodes smaller than 10 mm. On the other hand these criteria also affect the specificity as it is well known that reactive, inflammatory lymph nodes are often enlarged.

Therefore, a strong need exists for sensitive non-invasive imaging techniques which provide information on tissue metabolism. These metabolic imaging techniques can indicate the probable presence or absence of malignancy on the basis of observed differences in biological activity. These examinations yield data independently from associated structural characteristics, and therefore allow the detection or monitoring of specific biochemical perturbations which are not associated with or precede the anatomical changes.

10.1.2 Positron Emission Tomography

Positron emission tomography (PET) is the most sensitive and specific technique for in vivo imaging of metabolic pathways and receptor-ligand interactions in the tissues of humans (JONES 1996). PET uses radio-isotopes of natural elements, oxygen-15, carbon-11, nitrogen-13, and fluorine-18. These radioisotopes allow the synthesis of numerous positron-emitting radiopharmaceuticals. Depending on the selected radiopharmaceutical, PET imaging can provide quantitative information regarding blood flow ($H_2^{15}O$), hypoxia (^{18}F-misonidazole), DNA metabolism (^{11}C-thymidine), glucose metabolism (^{18}F-FDG), protein synthesis rate (^{11}C-tyrosine), amino acid metabolism (^{11}C-methionine), and receptor status.

PET is destined to provide a unique contribution in the translation of molecular biology discoveries to measurements at a regional tissue level in human diseases and during their treatments. The biodistribution of the positron-emitting tracers is measured using a dedicated tomographic imaging device. A positron traverses a few millimetres through the tissue until it combines with an electron in the surrounding medium. This generates a pair of photons which travel in nearly opposite directions (180° apart) with an energy of 511 keV each. These opposed photons can be detected by detector pairs installed in a ring-shaped configuration. Photons that simultaneously (i.e. within a predefined time window) interact with these detectors are registered as decay events. Based on these registrations, tomographic images of the regional radioactivity distribution are reconstructed (emission images).

10.1.3
Biochemical Foundations for the Use of ^{18}F-FDG as a Marker in Malignancy

The tracer most commonly used worldwide is fluorine-18-labeled 2-fluoro-2-deoxy-D-glucose (FDG). This is a D-glucose molecule in which a hydroxyl group in the 2 position is replaced by an ^{18}F-label. The use of FDG for in vivo cancer imaging is based upon the higher rate of glucose metabolism in cancer cells, a feature which was first described several decades ago (WARBURG 1956).

After malignant transformation, cells demonstrate an increased expression of epithelial glucose transporter proteins and an increase in the activity of the principal enzymes of the glycolytic pathway. After intravenous administration, FDG competes with plasma glucose for the glucose transporters in the cell membrane. Figure 10.1 illustrates the molecular basis underlying the use of FDG for imaging cancer. Because FDG lacks a hydroxyl group at the 2 position, its first metabolite, FDG-6-phosphate, is not a substrate for glucose phosphate isomerase, and therefore cannot be converted to the fructose analogue. As most tumours have a low phosphatase activity, the negatively charged FDG-6-phosphate will accumulate intracellularly, resulting in so-called

"metabolic trapping" (PAUWELS et al. 1998). Under steady-state conditions, the amount of FDG-6-phosphate accumulated is proportional to the rate of glucose utilization.

10.1.4
Intratumoral Distribution of FDG at the Cellular Level

Viable cancer cells have an increased accumulation of FDG. In vitro studies have shown that malignant transformation of normal cells by oncogenic viruses or chemical carcinogens leads within hours to an increase in glucose uptake by a factor five (FLIER et al. 1987). In most tumours, this constitutes the major origin of the measured radioactivity. It has been shown that increased tumoral FDG uptake, although a function of proliferative activity, is mainly related to the number of viable tumour cells. This was demonstrated by HIGASHI et al. (1993) who studied the relationship between ^3H-FDG uptake and the rate of proliferation of a human ovarian adenocarcinoma cell line in vitro. It was shown that FDG uptake is strongly related to the number of viable cancer cells, but not clearly associated with the proliferative rate of the cells as determined by ^3H-thymidine uptake or DNA flow cytometry.

When interpreting data on intensity of FDG accumulation in tumours, it has to be kept in mind that other intratumoral non-malignant cells present may significantly contribute to the total radioactivity. It is well known that a variable fraction of a tumour mass consists of non-neoplastic cells, such as stimulated leucocytes, macrophages and proliferating fibroblasts, which appear in association with growth or necrosis of tumour (Fig. 10.2).

FDG, as a non-cancer-specific tracer, also accumulates in these hypermetabolic cells, to a degree often even more marked than neoplastic cells (KUBOTA et al. 1992). Because the viable non-neoplastic part can constitute a large percentage of the total tumour mass, the total amount of radioactivity measured by PET in the tumour is correspondingly increased. The advantage of this phenomenon is an increase of the overall diagnostic sensitivity of FDG-PET for detecting small tumoral foci due to the resulting signal amplification. The disadvantage is that specifically tumoral metabolism cannot be precisely assessed due to this contamination. This is a problem mainly in the field of therapy monitoring. The post-therapeutic FDG signal is then the resultant of several intratumoral changes. On one hand, death of tumour cells leads to a decreased FDG

Normal cell   Neoplastic cell

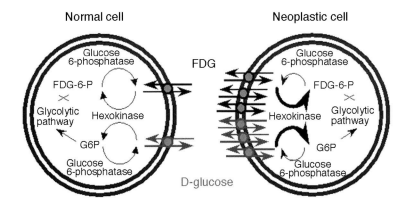

Fig. 10.1. Molecular basis of the use of FDG as a tumour imaging agent

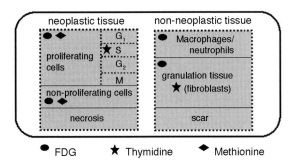

Fig. 10.2. Cellular components of a tumour mass and their uptake of FDG (marker of glucose metabolism), thymidine (marker of proliferation), and methionine (marker of amino acid uptake)

accumulation. On the other hand, however, inflammatory immune and scavenging reactions may be induced by the success of the therapy, and the invasion of the tumour by the inflammatory cells may increase the overall FDG uptake. The latter phenomenon may thus cause underestimation of the effectiveness of treatment (HABERKORN et al. 1997). To avoid this, the use of more tumour-specific radiotracers (^{11}C-methionine; ^{11}C-thymidine) has been proposed, tracers which should be less sensitive to inflammatory contaminants.

10.1.5
Technical Aspects of Whole-body FDG-PET

A typical whole-body PET scan is started 60 min after the intravenous administration of a 10-mCi dose of ^{18}F-FDG. The axial field of view of the PET system (10 to 15 cm) is extended by imaging in multiple bed positions so as to cover the whole body (DAHLBOM et al. 1992). An acquisition time of 4–6 minutes per bed position after a 10 to 15-mCi injection of FDG produces images of good resolution and

contrast, in a total imaging time of 30 to 40 min. Current PET systems allow correction for soft-tissue attenuation (Fig. 10.3).

To achieve this, a set of corresponding images is acquired with an external source of radiation. This can be performed prior to injection of the tracer ("cold transmission") or afterwards ("hot transmission"). At the present time, however, it is still debatable whether, for diagnostic and staging purposes, attenuation correction is of any benefit in clinical whole-body FDG-PET imaging. If, however, semi- or fully quantitative assessment of FDG metabolism is needed, e.g. for the assessment of the metabolic response to an antineoplastic treatment, correction for attenuation is crucial. The most widely used semiquantitative index of FDG uptake is the standardized uptake value (SUV). For this, the measured tumour radiotracer concentration (Q) is normalized to the injected activity (Q_{inj}) and to the body weight (W) of the patient:

$$SUV=(Q+W)/Q_{inj}$$

More complex procedures, using kinetic modelling, are necessary to calculate the metabolic rate for glucose (MR_{gluc}; micromoles per minute per millilitre). For this, the delivery of the FDG at the tumour site (the input curve) has to be known. This is derived from a dynamic PET acquisition (providing the time-course of the radioactivity) together with an arterial blood sampling following the FDG injection. Monitoring of the arterial FDG plasma concentration can be a burden to both the operator and patient. Various approaches have been proposed to provide a surrogate for this, including arterialized-venous sampling, measuring the arterial radiotracer concentration using the left ventricle (if it is in the imaging field-of-view) and a population estimate of the input function shape using a single or small number of blood samples (YOUNG et al. 1999).

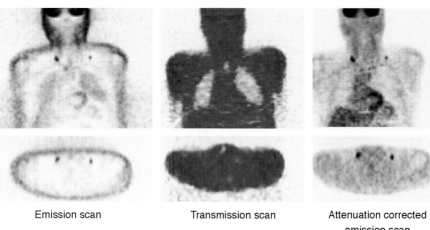

Emission scan   Transmission scan   Attenuation corrected
                                                                 emission scan

Fig. 10.3. FDG-PET images of a patients with bilateral lymph node metastases. The transmission images (*centre*) are used for correcting the emission images (*left*) for tissue attenuation

10.1.6
Clinical Applications of Metabolic Imaging Using FDG and PET

The applications of imaging in oncology can generally be assigned to three major domains: staging disease at the initial diagnosis, staging recurrent disease, and assessment of response to treatment. The relative "weights" of the structural and metabolic aspects of imaging strongly differ according to the specific diagnostic category. In general, the added value of the metabolic information to diagnosis compared to the information provided by the structural modalities is higher in the follow-up of patients (i.e. after initial treatment) than in the initial, pretreatment phase. Indeed, after surgery or radiochemotherapy, the normal anatomical planes are severely disrupted, and the normal structural characteristics of organs and tissues are often changed due to treatment-induced inflammatory and scavenging processes, thereby rendering structure-based diagnosis less accurate. The efficacy of metabolic imaging, on the other hand, is not significantly reduced under these circumstances. The area in which metabolic imaging constitutes by far the major part of diagnostic information is in the early monitoring of therapy. Preliminary results from several in vitro and in vivo experiments in different tumour models have recently shown that the change in FDG accumulation early after chemo- or radiotherapy, before any structural effects have occurred, can predict the responsiveness of the tumour to the treatment (YOUNG et al. 1999). The unique contribution of PET in this indication will certainly constitute a major cornerstone of the future widespread implementation of PET in oncology. Several extensive overviews of the increasing number of clinical oncological applications of FDG-PET for cancer diagnosis, staging and therapy follow-up have recently been published (CONTI et al. 1996; RIGO et al. 1996; SCHIEPERS and HOH 1998; WEBER et al. 1999).

10.1.7
General Considerations on the Use of FDG-PET in Head and Neck Cancer

10.1.7.1
Diagnostic Sensitivity

A major limitation of PET is the limited spatial resolution of the imaging tool. For current PET instrumentations it is approximately 5 to 8 mm. Due to the partial volume effect, tracer activity in all lesions smaller than twice the spatial resolution of the imaging apparatus is underestimated. Below a threshold lesion diameter (depending on the intensity of tracer accumulation), the tracer uptake will no longer be distinguishable from the background activity, leading to false-negative PET results. It is clear that future technological innovations that optimize the spatial resolution of the imaging method, thus reducing the false negativity of small lesions, will significantly increase the additional diagnostic value of PET imaging in staging head and neck cancer. However, even with the maximal achievable spatial resolution of PET (around 2–3 mm), micrometastases will ever remain underdiagnosed.

10.1.7.2
Diagnostic Specificity

FDG is not a very tumour-specific substance, in as much as the leucocytes and macrophages of inflammatory processes also accumulate the tracer. This is a major source of false-positive diagnoses in the application of FDG-PET in oncology (STRAUSS 1996). In order to reduce the potentially negative impact of occasional false-positive FDG-PET results on patient management, it is mandatory to carefully select the candidates for an FDG-PET scan, excluding those with known inflammatory or infectious conditions, to closely correlate the FDG-PET images with data from conventional imaging methods, and to carefully confirm by other means the additional FDG-PET lesions that significantly alter patient management. Therefore, it is our believe that implementation of PET in patient care requires a multidisciplinary approach, with close interactions between radiologists, nuclear medicine physicians and referring oncologists or surgeons.

The interpretation of FDG-PET images of the head and neck is particularly difficult because of the presence of multiple sites showing a certain degree of physiological FDG accumulation, such as the salivary glands and the lymphoid tissues (see below). In some patients, atypical presentations of these physiological uptake sites can lead to confusion with malignancy. Careful correlation of the PET and CT images, preferably using image fusion algorithms, is therefore mandatory to increase diagnostic accuracy.

Another pitfall in the interpretation of the PET images in the head and neck region is physiological FDG uptake by the muscles. The presence of muscular tension following the injection of the tracer can often lead to disturbing hyperactive spots or bilateral lines in the neck. This can both mimic and hide activity present in hypermetabolic, metastatic lymph nodes. To avoid this, all patients with head and neck cancers undergoing FDG-PET in our department receive 5 to 10 mg diazepam 30 min before the FDG injection, which results in sufficient myorelaxation.

Tumour uptake of FDG continues to increase even up to 2.5 h after tracer administration, resulting in an increasing contrast to normal background and inflamed tissues. Therefore, imaging is generally performed at least 60 min after tracer injection, and longer waiting periods (90 or even 120 min) should be considered.

10.2
Clinical Applications

10.2.1
FDG Uptake Distribution in the Head and Neck Region

Familiarity with the complex anatomy of the head and neck is essential for an accurate interpretation of FDG-PET images. The normal uptake of FDG in the extracranial head and neck region was first described by JABOUR et al. (1993) using correlation with MRI. Marked physiological FDG activity is seen in the lymphoid tissue of the adenoids and Waldeyer's ring (palatine and lingual tonsils). The uptake in these areas probably reflects the high metabolic activity necessary for mitosis of lymphocytes. Moderate activity is seen in the parotids, submandibular and sublingual salivary glands. Saliva itself has been found to have negligible activity when measured in a test tube with a gamma well counter. Other areas of mild to moderate uptake of FDG are seen in the nasal turbinates, the mucosa of the hard and soft palate, and gingiva. Importantly, the normal distribution patterns of FDG can be used as internal markers for the coregistration of PET and MRI or CT (UEMATSU et al. 1998).

10.2.2
FDG Uptake and Grading, Proliferative Activity and Prognosis

DI CHIRO et al. (1982) have reported that glucose metabolic studies may provide an independent measure of the aggressiveness of brain tumours and may supplement pathological grading. A positive correlation between the intensity of FDG accumulation and tumour grade has also been reported in non-Hodgkin's lymphoma (LESKINEN-KALLIO et al. 1991) and sarcoma (GRIFFETH et al. 1992). In head and neck SCCa a trend to higher FDG uptake associated with decreasing cell differentiation has been demonstrated (HABERKORN et al. 1991; LAUBENBACHER et al. 1995). However, in both studies, a statistically significant correlation was not observed, probably due to the small patient populations.

MINN et al. (1988) have demonstrated a strong correlation between the proportion of cells in the $S+G_2/M$ (proliferative) phases of the cell cycle and the intensity of FDG uptake. However, other factors certainly contribute to the intensity of the FDG signal. This has been suggested by HABERKORN et al. (1991) who confirmed the correlation, but also discovered two distinct groups on the basis of PET FDG activity in 42 patients with head and neck SCCa. Although these two groups had a comparable proliferative activity as measured by DNA flow cytometry, one group had higher FDG activity. In another study by SLEVIN et al. (1999) pretreatment uptake of FDG using the tumour-to-cerebellum ratio was also found to be significantly related to the histological grade of squamous cancer (P=0.04).

The most important work in this field has been performed by MINN et al. (1997) who carried out a prospective study in 37 patients with SCCa of the head and neck using quantitative FDG-PET. It was found that a high FDG uptake in the primary tumour was associated with a higher mitotic count, absence of keratinization, low or moderate histological grade of differentiation and advanced stage, but not with Ki-67 expression. In a monovariate analysis, the overall survival was related to the FDG uptake intensity. However, in a multivariate analysis the only independent predictors of survival were the mitotic count and stage.

In conclusion, although preliminary reports indicate that FDG-PET provides a non-invasive means of predicting histological grade, it remains to be seen whether therapeutic management, such as the radiotherapy fractionation regimen, should be altered to take account of this in terms of achieving a therapeutic gain in all cases.

10.2.3
Staging the Primary Tumour

Primary tumour staging with FDG-PET will probably contribute little over conventional staging (CT/panendoscopy/clinical examination) in most patients. MR imaging and CT may occasionally fail to delineate a primary tumour that is submucosal or superficial. In a prospective controlled study, DI MARTINO et al. (2000) compared FDG-PET to CT, ultrasound and panendoscopy for visualization of the primary tumour in 37 patients with suspected primary head and neck cancer. It was found that FDG-PET had a superior sensitivity (95%) and specificity (92%) compared to CT (68% and 69%, respectively) and colour-coded duplex sonography (74% and 75%, respectively, in the accessible regions). While sensitivity of panendoscopy was equal to that of PET (95%), its specificity was lower (85%). LOWE et al. (1999) evaluated the effectiveness of FDG-PET

in more challenging conditions: visualization of early-stage (T1-T2) laryngeal cancer. The prospective study included 12 patients, all with histopathological evidence of early-stage cancer. PET detected 11/12 (92%) primary tumour sites. Nine of these patients underwent CT, and the results in the larynx were normal in seven and abnormal in two. Specificity of PET was not assessed because all patients had tumours. These data demonstrate the very high sensitivity of PET for the detection of small tumours, often not visualized using structural imaging modalities. These results are important because they provide the rationale for using PET for the early detection of tumour recurrence in the follow-up of treated patients (see below).

PET might play a role in patients presenting with a malignant cervical lymph node and an occult primary tumour. PET may identify the unknown primary in approximately 20% to 50% of cases as reported by several authors (LOWE and STACK 2001).

10.2.4
Lymph Node Staging

The most important factor in patient assessment, treatment planning, and survival prognosis is accurate staging of the lymph node metastases (SCHULLER et al. 1980). Numerous reports have been published on the utility of FDG-PET in this regard. LAUBENBACHER et al. (1995) compared the use of FDG-PET and MRI for staging lymph node metastases in a prospective study including 22 patients with SCCa of the head and neck. The gold standard consisted of histology obtained through neck dissection. Based on individual lymph nodes, PET correctly identified 75 of 83 (sensitivity 90%) histologically proven malignant lymph nodes. False-negative PET results were found in small lymph nodes (<10 mm) and lymph nodes with only partial tumoral infiltration (micrometastases). False-positive FDG-PET findings were found in 19 benign lymph nodes containing inflammatory cells (specificity 96%). In this study PET compared favourably with MRI which had a sensitivity and specificity of 78% and 71%, respectively. The false-positive MRI lymph nodes were misinterpreted as malignant because of a reactive, inflammatory enlargement. On a "neck side" basis, the sensitivity and specificity of PET was 89% and 100%, compared with 72% and 56%, respectively, for MRI.

In another study (WONG et al. 1997) a sensitivity of 67% and a specificity of 100% was found for PET in 16 patients who underwent neck dissection compared with 58% sensitivity and 75% specificity for clinical examination and 67% sensitivity and 25% specificity for CT and/or MRI.

In another prospective study performed in a routine clinical setting by KAU et al. (1999) static non-attenuation-corrected PET performed on 70 patients in two bed positions was compared with the results of structural imaging modalities (CT and MRI). The diagnostic accuracy of PET for detecting "neck sides" with malignant involvement was superior to CT and MRI, with a sensitivity and specificity of 84% and 94%, respectively, compared with CT (65% and 47%) and MRI (88% and 41%). PET scans in this study produced four false-positive neck sides. Two of these four patients had unsuspected reactive changes probably due to biopsies of these lymph node shortly before PET imaging, and two had a histologically proven sinus histiocytosis.

BENCHAOU et al. (1996) reported a sensitivity of 72% and a specificity of 99% for PET, which was comparable to a sensitivity of 67% and a specificity of 97% for CT in a study of 48 patients who underwent neck dissection. The therapeutic management was changed in only two patients (4%) in whom PET demonstrated contralateral metastatic lymph nodes not suspected by clinical examination and CT. FDG-PET missed 15 metastatic lymph node groups: 2 cases of micrometastases, 1 case of carcinomatous lymphangitis, one pseudocystic metastasis, and 11 cases of small positive lymph nodes.

In one study the role of FDG-PET imaging was evaluated in patients with head and neck SCCa without clinical findings of cervical metastases (N_0). MYERS et al. (1999) studied 14 such patients. In 7 of them 13 neck dissections revealed pathological evidence of lymph node involvement. On a patient basis, PET was found to have an overall sensitivity and specificity of 78% and 100%, respectively. In this study, PET showed a trend to increased accuracy over CT (57% and 90%, respectively; $P=0.11$). These promising preliminary results certainly indicate that further research in this patient subset is warranted.

False-positive findings remain the major drawback of the use of PET in head and neck cancer because in these type of patients, inflammatory lesions are not infrequent in this region. Several authors have studied whether quantification techniques could be useful in the differentiation of true from false positivity. It has been found, however, that quantification of the nodal FDG uptake, expressed as SUV, is not useful for differentiating malignant from reactively inflamed but benign lymph nodes (BRAAMS et al. 1995; KAO et al. 2000). Of special in-terest are the often highly intense lesions found on PET in the parotid gland. McGUIRT et al. (1995a) reported on the identification of benign versus malignant parotid masses. PET identified all malignant lesions (sensitivity 100%) but made the correct categorization between benign and malignant in only 69% of the 26 cases. Six benign lesions (Warthin's tumours, pleomorphic adenomas and a toxoplasmosis adenopathy) showed false-positive FDG uptake. Therefore, caution should be exercised when confronted with a positive focal lesion in the parotid salivary gland.

In conclusion, PET seems to provide an at least comparable or slightly higher accuracy for lymph node staging of head and neck SCCa compared to the conventional imaging modalities, including CT and MRI. The cost-effectiveness of FDG-PET for primary staging has not yet been proven. Therefore, its use has to be restricted to selected patients in whom the treatment choice strongly depends on the exact nodal status, or in whom conventional work-up yields equivocal results. The major reason why FDG-PET should be included in the routine work-up of these selected patients presenting with head and neck cancer is its high sensitivity and negative predictive value. Therefore acquisition parameters have to be optimized to result in maximal diagnostic sensitivity, i.e. longer acquisition times, longer waiting time post-tracer injection, myorelaxation with diazepam, attenuation correction, as described in the previous section.

The imperfect specificity due to false-positive FDG uptake in inflamed lymph nodes has to be neutralized through the use of ultrasound-guided biopsy or fine needle aspiration. In order to reduce sampling errors, the exact anatomical localization of the PET hot spot is essential. This is often difficult because of the lack of anatomical landmarks provided by the metabolic images. Therefore, we recommend that careful correlation, including software- or hardware-based fusion of the PET and CT images, should be performed as a routine practice (Fig. 10.4).

10.2.5
Detection and Staging of Recurrent Disease

The basic rationale for the use of PET in the postoperative surveillance of patients with previously treated head and neck SCCa is that earlier and more accurate detection of cancer recurrence may improve survival. Several reports indicate that metabolic imaging using FDG-PET, as compared with struc-

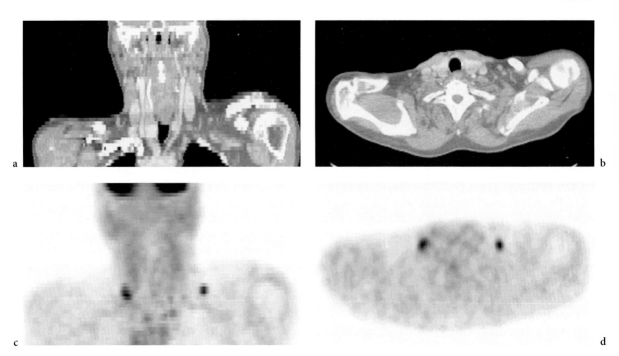

Fig. 10.4a–d. Registration of the PET (**c, d**) and CT images (**a, b**) using software algorithms is essential for accurate anatomic localization of the lesions seen on the FDG-PET images. The slice thickness of both modalities is set to 5 mm. In this patient, PET-CT correlation allowed the lymph node involvement seen on PET to be defined as a right prescalenic and a left retroclavicular lymph node metastasis. The latter was of subcentimetre size and not reported on the diagnostic CT scan

tural imaging methods, has improved diagnostic accuracy for recurrent head and neck SCCa. The structural imaging modalities are severely hampered by their specificity limitations resulting from anatomic distortions, tissue thickening, fibrosis and the presence of postsurgical flaps. Indeed, the findings of CT and MRI are all too often equivocal in the detection of recurrent/residual tumours in the irradiated or postsurgical head and neck region, and therefore further diagnostic evaluation is required.

REGE et al. (1994) demonstrated a sensitivity of 90% and a specificity of 100% for FDG-PET compared to 70% and 59% for MRI, respectively, in 18 patients imaged 2.5 to 192 weeks after radiation therapy. McGuirt et al. (1995b) reported an accuracy of 85% for PET and 42% for CT/MRI in 13 patients with a history of laryngeal cancer. ANZAI et al. (1996) studied 12 patients with previously treated head and neck SCCa and a clinical suspicion of recurrence. FDG-PET was compared with CT and/or MRI. FDG-PET yielded a sensitivity and specificity of 88% and 100%, respectively. This was significantly superior to MRI and/or CT with 25% and 75%, respectively.

Receiver-operating characteristic analysis has shown significantly better diagnostic accuracy with PET than with MRI/CT imaging ($P<0.03$). FARBER et al. studied 28 patients with SCCa of the head and

neck who had undergone radiation therapy with or without surgery. These patients had a clinical suspicion of recurrence, but no obvious mass or lesion to biopsy on physical examination or anatomic imaging. The sensitivity and specificity of FDG-PET was 86% and 93%, respectively. The overall accuracy was 89%. GREVEN et al. (1997) found a sensitivity and specificity of 80% and 81%, respectively, for FDG-PET in detecting laryngeal cancer recurrence in patients after irradiation. In this population, CT was equivocal in 25% of the patients and its sensitivity was only 58%.

The accuracy of FDG-PET for the detection of subclinical recurrence has been studied by LOWE et al. (2000). For this, serial post-therapy FDG-PET imaging was prospectively performed in 44 patients with advanced cancer who had been treated according to a neoadjuvant organ-preservation protocol that included chemotherapy, radiation therapy, and surgical salvage. PET was performed twice during the first post-treatment year (at 2 and 10 months after therapy) and thereafter as needed. PET was studied in comparison to physical examination (including endoscopy) and helical, contrast-enhanced CT. In the postoperative year, 16 patients were found to have recurrent disease. The sensitivities and specificities were calculated to be 44% and 100% for physical examination, 38% and 85% for CT, and 100% and 93% for PET. PET had a statistically significant advantage over the other techniques.

Finally, LAPELA et al. (2000) reported the FDG PET results obtained in 56 patients with 81 lesions which were clinically suspected as recurrent carcinoma. The purpose of the study was to compare qualitative image interpretation with quantitative (using SUV) analysis. The visual image analysis was preferred, because the SUV values showed a significant overlap between benign and malignant lesions.

In conclusion, the studies summarized above indicate that PET may play an important role in the early detection of clinically occult recurrent head and neck SCCa. If the clinical suspicion for recurrence is high, FDG-PET may be the first imaging study performed to identify the patients who need to undergo further examination. The high sensitivity of FDG-PET justifies a wait and see approach in cases of a negative result. In cases of a positive PET, further dedicated structural imaging methods have to be performed in order to provide the anatomical landmarks necessary for defining the optimal diagnostic and therapeutic approach.

10.2.6
Therapy Monitoring

Histologically similar tumours may respond to irradiation at different rates, and in vitro assays indicate remarkable differences in inherent radiosensitivities of SCCa of the head and neck (PEKKOLA-HEINO et al. 1992). Since radiosensitivity assays are technically demanding and too slow to be used in routine clinical practice, a reliable and clinically feasible method to predict the outcome of radiotherapy would be of great value. A method capable of early recognition of patients likely to fail standard radiotherapy would give an opportunity for a more individualized therapy, and save those patients with radiosensitive tumours from mutilating surgery. The use of metabolic imaging techniques in this regard looks very appealing because using these techniques, early metabolic changes induced by the treatment may relate to the final response of a particular tumour to a particular treatment.

10.2.6.1
Radiotherapy

An accurate early assessment of tumour response to radiation therapy is of utmost importance because it enables treatment modification early in the course of therapy. The use of conventional diagnostic modalities for identification of residual or recurrent disease during and after radiation therapy is severely hampered by radiation-induced facial plane distortion, dense scarring, and fibrosis. In brain tumours several investigators have shown that metabolic imaging techniques, particularly PET, can accurately depict residual or recurrent tumours after irradiation.

MINN et al. (1988) were the first to indicate the utility of FDG-PET for the assessment of the effects of radiation on head and neck SCCa. They studied 19 patients before and during radiation therapy (at 30 Gy). Of the 19 patients, 14 had decreased FDG uptake in the treated neoplasm after radiotherapy, and of these 14, 12 had a marked subjective response to radiotherapy. The three patients with increasing FDG activity had stable or progressive disease. It was found that among the responders the administered dose of radiotherapy correlated with the decrease in FDG activity.

REGE (1993) reported on the effects of radiotherapy on the FDG uptake by normal structures within the radiation port. For this, 11 patients were studied with FDG-PET before, during and 6 weeks after a 6-week course of radiation therapy. It was shown that the average FDG uptake in the tonsils, nasal turbinates, soft palate, and gingiva did not change significantly with treatment. These findings were in marked contrast to the FDG uptake by SCCa in the head and neck, which decreased dramatically with treatment. Glucose metabolism, as reflected by FDG uptake, decreased in all patients who responded to the treatment, but increased after 6 weeks of treatment in those resistant to treatment. There was no relationship found between the intensity of pretreatment FDG uptake and the response to radiation therapy.

CHAIKEN et al. (1993) described the post-treatment PET scans of 15 patients. Among seven patients with elevated FDG activity after completion of radiotherapy, 86% showed persistent or recurrent disease. Importantly, in some patients who underwent FDG-PET imaging at 10 days after the initiation of therapy, an increase in tracer uptake was observed, although a complete response was finally achieved. Similar observations were reported by BRUN et al. (1997). This early "flare" phenomenon could be explained as a stress reaction of the tumour cells themselves, which has been observed in vitro during chemotherapy, or as the reactive infiltration of FDG avid inflammatory and scavenging cells.

GREVEN et al. (1994) studied 22 head and neck SCCa patients before and 1 and 4 months after high-dose irradiation. The tumours of all the patients showed decreased levels of FDG uptake. Postradiation PET scans were interpreted as normal in 16 patients, of whom 3 had histologically documented persistent or recurrent disease. Of six patients with decreased but persistent FDG uptake, persistent disease was documented in all. Thus, this study also indicates that negative 1-month PET scans are not accurate indicators of absence of disease, and that persistent FDG uptake is an infant prognostic sign.

10.2.6.2
Chemotherapy

The use of FDG-PET to assess the metabolic response of head and neck SCCa to chemotherapy was first reported by HABERKORN et al. (1993). A group of 11 patients underwent FDG-PET imaging before and 1 week after a first chemotherapeutic cycle (5-FU and cisplatinum). It was found that the chemotherapy-induced change in FDG uptake was correlated with the growth rate as measured by CT. It was observed that multiple lymph nodes in the same patients showed different baseline metabolisms and also different changes following therapy. This can be explained by the concept of cell heterogeneity in human tumours. Different metastatic clones can lead to metastases with a different biological behaviour. Also, primary tumours were more sensitive to therapy than the metastatic lymph nodes. In the same study it was found that lesions with higher FDG uptake prior to therapy had a higher decrease in volume after chemotherapy. It was postulated that the lesions with higher FDG uptake represented lesions with a higher propensity to divide, and these lesions also showed a better short-term response to the chemotherapeutic agent.

LOWE et al. (1997) performed serial FDG-PET imaging in 27 patients with stage III/IV head and neck SCCa before and after (1–2 weeks) chemotherapy. The sensitivity and specificity of PET for detection of residual disease was 90% (19/21) and 83% (5/6), respectively. Two patients showed false-negative PET images for residual disease at the primary tumour site, one of whom had only microscopic disease below the detection limits of the PET camera and the other had a complete normalization of the primary tumour but a persistent hypermetabolic cervical lymph node. The change in FDG uptake between pre- and post-treatment PET scans was 34±29% (mean ± SD) in patients with pathological proof of residual disease, and 82±5% in patients with a pathological complete remission.

10.2.6.3
Chemoradiation Therapy

A study on the effects of combined radiochemotherapy was reported by SAKAMOTO et al. (1998). Patients were scanned before treatment and 1 month after radiotherapy and/or chemotherapy (carboplatin). The mean radiation dose was 57 Gy for the patients undergoing radiation therapy alone and 42 Gy for those undergoing combination therapy. Interestingly, when the FDG uptake after treatment and the clinical response (CT, MRI, and macroscopic findings) were compared, there were no significant differences in SUV among those with a complete response, partial response and stable disease (no response). This indicated that SUV is an indicator independent of clinical response. Histopathological examination revealed that patients with residual viable tumour cells had significantly higher SUVs (range 8.3–2.9) than those without viable tumour cells (range 3.3–1.9).

KITAGAWA et al. (1999) evaluated the use of FDG-PET in the assessment of the effectiveness of combined intra-arterial chemotherapy and radiotherapy of head and neck SCCa. Of 14 patients who completed the treatment regimen and underwent FDG-PET before and 4 weeks after chemoradiotherapy, it was found that the pretreatment FDG uptake was predictive of the response to treatment. On the other hand, post-treatment FDG uptake predicted the presence or absence of residual viable tumour cells. The specificity of FDG-PET, however, was low (64%). This was due to high FDG uptake in four benign inflamed tissues after therapy in patients showing severe mucositis at the time of the post-treatment PET. No false negatives were reported.

10.2.6.4
Conclusion

In conclusion, on first impression, the usefulness of sequential FDG-PET imaging during or immediately after radio- and/or chemotherapy of head and neck cancer seems to be compromised because the initial decrease in FDG uptake seen soon during or soon after therapy does not seem to correlate with the final outcome of the patients. However, these PET signs should not necessarily be considered as "false negatives". They certainly do reflect a positive response to therapy but incomplete elimination of tumour cells, as well as the possibility of differentiation of cells between those that are responsive to the treatment and those that are not. It is becoming increasingly clear that the limited ability of FDG-PET to predict the responsiveness of a tumour to a treatment is severely hampered by the limitations of the treatments themselves which allow rapid tumour regrowth after an initial period of response.

Therefore, the relationship between early response as measured by PET and the ultimate survival of the patients is hard to demonstrated using the presently available treatments. The use of carbon-11 labelled methionine has similar limitations, as was reported by NUUTININ et al. (1999). Therefore, using the presently available therapies, the evaluation of disease with FDG seems more reliable if 2–3 months from irradiation is allowed to elapse in order to detect early recurrent disease foci. The use of PET for treatment monitoring should therefore mainly aim at the early selection of those patients *not* responding to a given treatment, in whom the FDG uptake remains stable or decreases only slightly. This is particularly important in monitoring chemotherapy treatments because in head and neck SCCa, the nonresponse rate to chemotherapy is much higher compared to the one to radiotherapy.

The use of PET for patient selection and monitoring the effects of new experimental therapies, with regard to so-called molecular medicine, will certainly constitute the major part of the future role of metabolic imaging in head and neck SCCa. The use of FDG will probably be complemented by other radiotracers which will provide more specific information about other elements of tumoral metabolism, such as proliferation (^{18}F-deoxyfluorothymidine, ^{11}C-thymidine) or ischaemia (^{18}F-misonidazole, FMISO; see Fig. 10.5).

An example of such a use of PET is a report by RISCHIN et al. (2001). In this phase I trial the toxicity and effects of tirapazamine, a bioreductive compound that demonstrates differential toxicity for hypoxic cells, was under study. It was shown that 14 out of 15 studied patients had detectable hypoxia on baseline FMISO scans, with focal abnormality corresponding to a region of increased FDG uptake in either the primary lesion or a nodal mass. The pattern of FMISO uptake was consistent with the expected pattern of hypoxia in tumour tissue being either adjacent to areas of tumour necrosis or in the centre of nonnecrotic lesions. In all but one of the 14 patients with initially positive FMISO PET, complete resolution of the abnormality was apparent within 4 to 5 weeks of commencing treatment. This rapid normalization of FMISO PET suggests successful treatment of the hypoxic component. The authors concluded that on the basis of these preliminary data, FMISO should be further evaluated as a technique for selecting patients for tirapazamine-containing regimens and for monitoring such therapy.

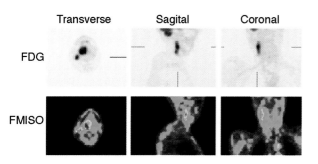

Fig. 10.5. Multitracer PET study in a patient with regionally advanced head and neck squamous cell carcinoma. Registration of the FDG-PET (*upper row*) and the FMISO-PET (*lower row*) allows precise comparative analysis of the two data sets. Both primary tumour and lymph node metastases show increased FDG and FMISO uptake indicating significant ischaemia at these sites

References

Anzai Y, Carroll WR, Quint DJ, et al (1996) Recurrence of head and neck cancer after surgery or irradiation: prospective comparison of 2-deoxy-2-[F-18]fluoro-D-glucose PET and MR imaging diagnoses. Radiology 200:135–141

Benchaou M, Lehmann W, Slosman D, et al (1996) The role of FDG PET in the preoperative assessment of N staging in head and neck cancer. Acta Otolaryngol 116:332–335

Braams JW, Pruim J, Freling N, et al (1995) Detection of lymph node metastases of squamous-cell cancer of the head and neck with FDG-PET and MRI. J Nucl Med 36:211–216

Brun E, Ohlsson T, Erlandsson K, et al (1997) Early prediction of treatment outcome in head and neck cancer with 2-^{18}FDG-PET. Acta Oncol 36:741–747

Chaiken L, Rege S, Hoh C, et al (1993) Positron emission tomography with fluorodeoxyglucose to evaluate tumor response and control after radiation therapy. Int J Radiat Oncol Biol Phys 27:455–464

Conti PS, Lilien DL, Hawley K, et al (1996) PET and (^{18}F)-FDG in oncology: a clinical update. Nucl Med Biol 23:717–735

Dahlbom M, Hoffman E, Hoh C, et al (1992) Whole-body positron emission tomography, part 1. Methods and performance characteristics. J Nucl Med 33:1191–1199

Di Chiro G, De La Paz R, Brooks RA (1982) Glucose utilization of cerebral gliomas measured by (^{18}F) fluordeoxyglucose and positron emission tomography. Neurology 32:1323–1329

Di Martino E, Nowak B, Hassan H, et al (2000) Diagnosis and staging of head and neck cancer. Arch Otolaryngol Head Neck Surg 126:1457–1461

Eichhorn T, Schroeder HG, Glanz H, et al (1987) Histologisch kontrollierter Vergleich von Palpation und Sonographie bei der Diagnose von Halslymphknotenmetastasen. Laryngol Rhinol Otol 66:266–274

Farber LA, Benard F, Machtay M, et al (1999) Detection of recurrent head and neck squamous cell carcinomas after radiation therapy with 2-18F-fluoro-2-deoxy-D-glucose positron emission tomography. Laryngoscope 109:970–975

Flier JS, Mueckler MM, Usher P, et al (1987) Elevated levels of glucose transport and transporter messenger RNA are induced by ras or src oncogenes. Science 235:1492–1495

Greven KE, Williams DW, Keyes JW, et al (1994) Positron emission tomography of patients with head and neck carcinoma before and after high dose irradiation. Cancer 74:1355–1359

Greven KM, Williams DW 3rd, Keyes JW Jr, et al (1997) Can positron emission tomography distinguish tumor recurrence from irradiation sequelae in patients treated for larynx cancer? Cancer J Sci Am 3:353–357

Griffeth LK, Dehdashti F, McGuire AH, et al (1992) PET evaluation of soft tissue masses with fluorine-18 fluoro-2-deoxy-D-glucose. Radiology 182:185–194

Haberkorn U, Strauss LG, Reiser C, et al (1991) Glucose uptake, perfusion, and cell proliferation in head and neck tumors: relation of positron emission tomography to flow cytometry. J Nucl Med 32:1548–1555

Haberkorn U, Strauss LG, Dimitrakopoulou A, et al (1993) Fluorodeoxyglucose imaging of advanced head and neck cancer after chemotherapy. J Nucl Med 34:12–17

Haberkorn U, Bellemann ME, Altmann A, et al (1997) PET 2-fluoro-2-deoxy-D-glucose uptake in rat prostate adenocarcinoma during chemotherapy with gemcitabine. J Nucl Med 38:1215–1221

Higashi K, Clavo AC, Wahl RL (1993) In vitro assessment of 2-fluoro-2-deoxy-D-glucose, L-methionine and thymidine as agents to monitor the early response of a human adenocarcinoma cell line to radiotherapy. J Nucl Med 34:773–779

Jabour BA, Choi Y, Hoh CK, et al (1993) Extracranial head and neck: PET imaging with 2-[F-18]fluoro-2-deoxy-D-glucose and MR imaging correlation. Radiology 186:27–35

Jones T (1996) The imaging science of positron emission tomography. Eur J Nucl Med 23:807–813

Kao J, Hsieh J, Tsai S, et al (2000) Comparison of 18-fluoro-2-deoxyglucose positron emission tomography and computed tomography in detection of cervical lymph node metastases of nasopharyngeal carcinoma. Ann Otol Rhinol Laryngol 109:1130–1134

Kau RJ, Alexiou C, Laubenbacher C, et al (1999) Lymph node detection of head and neck squamous cell carcinomas by positron emission tomography with fluorodeoxyglucose F 18 in a routine clinical setting. Arch Otolaryngol Head Neck Surg 125:1322–1328

Kitagawa Y, Sadato N, Azuma H, et al (1999) FDG PET to evaluate combined intra-arterial chemotherapy and radiotherapy of head and neck neoplasms. J Nucl Med 40:1132–1137

Kubota R, Yamada S, Kubota K, et al (1992) Intratumoural distribution of fluorine-18-fluorodeoxyglucose in vivo: high accumulation in macrophages and granulation tissues studied by microautoradiography. J Nucl Med 33:1972–1980

Lapela M, Eigtved A, Jyrkkio S, et al (2000) Experience in qualitative and quantitative FDG PET in follow-up of patients with suspected recurrence from head and neck cancer. Eur J Cancer 36:858–867

Laubenbacher C, Saumweber D, Wagner-Manslau C, et al (1995) Comparison of fluorine-18 fluorodeoxyglucose PET, MRI and endoscopy for staging head and neck squamous cell carcinomas. J Nucl Med 36:1747–1757

Leskinnen-Kallio S, Ruotsalainen U, Nagren K, et al (1991) Uptake of carbon-11-methionine and FDG in non Hodgkins lymphoma: a PET study. J Nucl Med 32:1211–1218

Lowe V, Stack B (2001) PET's role in head and neck cancer. Nucl Med Ann 2001:1–21

Lowe VJ, Dunphy FR, Varvares M, et al (1997) Evaluation of chemotherapy response in patients with advanced head and neck cancer using [F-18]fluorodeoxyglucose positron emission tomography. Head Neck 19:666–674

Lowe V, Kim H, Boyd JH, et al (1999) Primary and recurrent early stage laryngeal cancer: preliminary results of 2-(fluorine 18)fluoro-2-deoxy-D-glucose PET imaging. Radiology 212:799–802

Lowe VJ, Boyd JH, Dunphy FR, et al (2000) Surveillance for recurrent head and neck cancer using positron emission tomography. J Clin Oncol 18:651–658

McGuirt W, Keyes J, Greven K, et al (1995a) Preoperative identification of benign versus malignant parotid masses: a comparative study including positron emission tomography. Laryngoscope 105:579–584

McGuirt WF, Williams III DW, Keyes J, et al (1995b) A comparative diagnosis study of head and neck nodal metastasis. Laryngoscope 105:373–375

Minn H, Joensuu H, Ahonen A, et al (1988) Fluorodeoxyglucose imaging: a method to assess the proliferative activity of human cancer in vivo – comparison with DNA flow cytometry in head and neck tumors. Cancer 61:1776–1781

Minn H, Lapela M, Klemi PJ, et al (1997) Prediction of survival with fluorine-18-fluorodeoxyglucose and PET in head and neck cancer. J Nucl Med 38:1907–1911

Myers LL, Wax MK, Nabi H, et al (1999) Positron emission tomography in the evaluation of the N0 neck. Laryngoscope 108:232–236

Nuutinen J, Jyrkkiö S, Lehikoinen P, et al (1999) Evaluation of early response to radiotherapy in head and neck cancer measured with ^{11}C-methionine-positron emission tomography. Radiother Oncol 52:225–232

Pauwels E, McCready VR, Stoot JH, et al (1998) The mechanism of accumulation of tumour-localising radiopharmaceuticals. Eur J Nucl Med 25:277–305

Pekkola-Heino K, Kulmala J, Grenman R (1992) Sublethal damage repair in squamous cell carcinoma cell lines. Head Neck 14:196–199

Rege SD, Chaiken L, Hoh CK, et al (1993) Change induced by radiation therapy in FDG uptake in normal and malignant structures of the head and neck: quantitation with PET. Radiology 189:807–812

Rege S, Maas A, Chaiken L, et al (1994) Use of positron emission tomography with fluorodeoxyglucose in patients with extracranial head and neck cancers. Cancer 73:3047–3058

Rigo P, Paulus P, Kaschten B, et al (1996) Oncological applications of positron emission tomography with fluorine-18 fluorodeoxyglucose. Eur J Nucl Med 23:1641–1674

Rischin D, Peters L, Hicks R, et al (2001) Phase I trial of concurrent tirapazmine, cisplatin, and radiotherapy in patients with advanced head and neck cxancer. J Clin Oncol 19:535–542

Sakamoto H, Nakai Y, Ohashi Y, et al (1998) Monitoring of

response to radiotherapy with fluorine-18 deoxyglucose PET of head and neck squamous cell carcinomas. Acta Otolaryngol Suppl 538:254–260

Schiepers C, Hoh CK (1998) Positron emission tomography as a diagnostic tool in oncology. Eur Radiol 8:1481–1494

Schuller DE, McGuirt WF, McCabe BF, et al (1980) The prognostic significance of metastatic cervical lymph nodes. Laryngoscope 90:557–570

Slevin NJ, Collins CD, Hastings D, et al (1999) The diagnostic value of positron emission tomography (PET) with radio-labelled fluorodeoxyglucose (^{18}F-FDG) in head and neck cancer. J Laryngol Otol 113:548–554

Strauss LG (1996) Fluorine-18 deoxyglucose and false-positive results: a major problem in the diagnostics of oncological patients. Eur J Nucl Med 23:1409–1415

Uematsu H, Sadato N, Yonekura Y, et al (1998) Coregistration of FDG PET and MRI of the head and neck using normal distribution of FDG. J Nucl Med 39:2121–2127

Warburg O (1956) On the origin of cancer cells. Science 123:309–314

Weber WA, Avril N, Schwaiger M (1999) Relevance of positron emission tomography (PET) in oncology. Strahlenther Onkol 175:356–373

Wong WL, Chevretton EB, McGurk M, et al (1997) A prospective study of PET-FDG imaging for the assessment of head and neck squamous cell carcinoma. Clin Otolaryngol 22:209–214

Young H, Baum R, Cremerius U, et al (1999) Measurement of clinical and subclinical tumour response using ^{18}F-fluorodeoxyglucose and positron emission tomography: review and 1999 EORTC recommendations. Eur J Cancer 35:1773–1782

11 Recent Advances in Laryngeal Imaging

ILONA M. SCHMALFUSS, EMANUELE NERI, CARLO BARTOLOZZI, MARK RIJPKEMA, AND
JOHANNES KAANDERS

11.1 Dynamic Imaging of the Larynx

ILONA M. SCHMALFUSS

CONTENTS

11.1.1 Introduction

The introduction of CT and MRI a few decades ago revolutionized static imaging of the larynx. Suddenly, normal anatomy could be clearly delineated, pathological processes encountered at significantly less advanced stages and necessary biopsies of lesions could be better guided, particularly of lesions in submucosal locations. However, evaluation of laryngeal motion still remained an almost impossible task.

In recent years, a number of different tools have been used in an attempt to better understand changes in vocal tract configuration during speech production or deglutition, including clinical tools such as frequency analysis of acoustic recordings and endoscopy as well as different radiographic techniques such as single-frame radiography (MOLL 1965; SUNDBERG 1969), cineradiography (HEINZ and STEVEN 1964; KENT 1972), videofluorography (MCCALL et al.

I.M. SCHMALFUSS, MD
Department of Radiology, University of Florida, 1600 SW
Archer Road, Gainesville, FL 32610, USA

1971) or ultrasound. Inherent to almost all of these tools is the inability to directly acquire objective measurements of laryngeal structures predominantly due to calibration issues. Frequency analysis of acoustic recordings only indirectly reflects the level of abnormality and does not give any anatomical information. Endoscopic evaluation in contrast, provides excellent anatomical detail, but is somewhat invasive and has limitations due to imaging of the laryngeal motion in an axial plane as a two-dimensional image only. The vertical motion of the larynx is not appreciated (GILBERT et al. 1996). Additionally, certain areas of the vocal tract remain inaccessible to endoscopic assessment such as the laryngeal ventricle and subglottic region. It is also unknown to what degree the normal laryngeal function is altered by the presence of the endoscope or the local anesthetic administered. The radiographic methods listed above are limited due to the difficulty in clearly identifying the different parts of the larynx because of the reduced inherent contrast between the various soft tissue components and their small size. As with endoscopy, only two-dimensional images are acquired. In addition, these studies involve significant radiation exposure of the patient. Ultrasound remains a subjective method and is limited in quality by user experience and available scanning window.

Until recently, the long acquisition times of CT and, particularly, of MRI prohibited dynamic imaging of the vocal tract. A number of attempts were made to overcome this problem with the majority ending up in imaging of sustained vowel production and/or interruption of data acquisition for respiration (MATHIAK et al. 2000; MOORE 1992; STORY et al. 1996). Recent advances in both technologies, particularly the introduction of multislice helical CT scanners and echoplanar technology, have brought dynamic imaging of the vocal tract a large step forward and significantly widened clinical applications and research opportunities.

11.1.2
Imaging Techniques

11.1.2.1
Computer Tomography

Multislice helical CT scanners have been commercially available for a few years. They currently allow simultaneous acquisition of four CT images within 0.5 to 1 second depending on the manufacturer of the equipment. Multislice helical CT allows coverage of the entire true vocal cords within this time frame at a reasonable slice thickness (2.5–5 mm), particularly when a pitch of greater than 4:1 is chosen. As laryngeal motion is a much faster process, the temporal resolution remains insufficient. Therefore, imaging has to be performed during sustained maintenance of a task such as vowel production, Valsalva's maneuver etc. Since image acquisition happens within seconds it is usually possible for the patient to maintain the task throughout the scanning time, even when the patient is significantly compromised by the underlying disease process.

The main advantages of CT are its wide availability, very good spatial resolution (512×512 matrix), and significantly fewer contraindications as well as costs compared to MRI. One of the main disadvantages of CT is the radiation exposure. As scanning during multiple different tasks is performed in an individual patient, the total radiation dose depends upon the number of tasks and their repetition. In addition, CT does not have the multiplanar capabilities of MRI – a minor drawback since reformations in any plane can be easily performed in a very short time. As mentioned above, the temporal resolution of current CT scanners is still suboptimal. Since some manufactures have already announced the next generation of multislice CT scanners with a capability of 16–32 simultaneous images, it is just a question of time as to when the acquisition times will be short enough to enable true dynamic images of the vocal tract to be obtained with CT.

11.1.2.2
Magnetic Resonance Imaging

Currently, two major types of MRI sequences are used to perform dynamic imaging of the larynx: FLASH (fast low-angle shot) (CRARY et al. 1996; HAGEN et al. 1990; SCHMALFUSS et al. 2000) and EPI (echoplanar imaging) (GILBERT et al. 1996; FLAHERTY et al. 1995). Both techniques are available on all new MRI scanners. EPI, however, cannot be performed on older types of scanners. The FLASH sequence should be available on almost all MRI scanners currently in use but may need to be optimized by a physicist for this purpose. It allows imaging of the larynx at a reasonable image quality with a temporal resolution of up to five images per second corresponding to a minimal acquisition time of 200 ms per image (CRARY et al. 1996; HAGEN et al. 1990; SCHMALFUSS et al. 2000). This is significantly faster than multislice CT scanners but much slower than EPI.

An acquisition time of 67 ms per image with EPI has recently been reported (FLAHERTY et al. 1995; GILBERT et al. 1996). Theoretically, even faster imaging within a few tens of milliseconds could be achieved but at a significant cost to image quality. The main problems encountered with EPI is the susceptibility artifacts caused by the high contrast interfaces of the larynx (air-soft tissues-cartilage/bone), flow effects in vessels and magnetic field inhomogeneities. Therefore, careful shimming and the use of a glove-like encasement filled with chlorinated fluorocarbon placed around the neck are crucial (FLAHERTY et al. 1995; GILBERT et al. 1996).

The main advantages of these MRI sequences are obviously the speed, lack of radiation exposure and direct multiplanar capabilities when compared to CT. To some degree, these sequences also have somewhat better soft tissue delineation. The main disadvantages include lower spatial resolution (maximal matrix of 128×128), thicker image slices (4–8 mm), higher costs, and significantly more contraindications compared to CT. Claustrophobia is typically considered a relative contraindication for MRI since patients can be given some type of sedation prior to scanning. This is not possible for dynamic imaging of the larynx since full cooperation of the patient to perform the different tasks is essential. The use of chlorinated fluorocarbon-filled pads for EPI can exaggerate the feeling of claustrophobia. Additionally, it is also feasible that it might somewhat affect laryngeal motion.

11.1.2.3
Practical Issues of Cross-sectional Dynamic Imaging of the Larynx

Currently, CT and MRI both have similar significant issues to be considered when scanning the larynx in a dynamic fashion in the axial plane. During quiet breathing, no significant problems are encountered. Both modalities record the changes in vocal cord position. However, when imaging is attempted during the performance of various tasks, e.g., vowel production or Valsalva's maneuver, axial imaging becomes a challenge. The larynx significantly moves during these tasks in craniocaudal dimension and therefore moves out of the axial imaging plane (Fig. 11.1.1). Tracing of the laryngeal motion would be feasible, but this requires the use of a trigger mechanism as well as significant planning for each individual patient and task. Nevertheless, the subsequently performed axial images may still be suboptimal because of inconsistency in task performance (see 11.1.3.1 Physiological Changes of the Larynx). An easier way to account for this type of laryngeal motion is to acquire a scout for CT or sagittal images for MRI during the performance of a specific task and than obtain the axial images at the desired level and subsequently adjacent levels if needed. As the first option, this also requires strict consistency in task performance but is significantly less time-consuming even when multiple repetitions are needed to capture the appropriate level.

With the expected advances in CT, this problem will be solved in the near future. The significant increase in simultaneously performed CT images will cover a much larger area allowing the up-and-down motion of the larynx to be captured without any difficulty.

The use of EPI may be the solution for MRI. Four interleaved images spread throughout the larynx can be acquired in the coronal plane with an acquisition

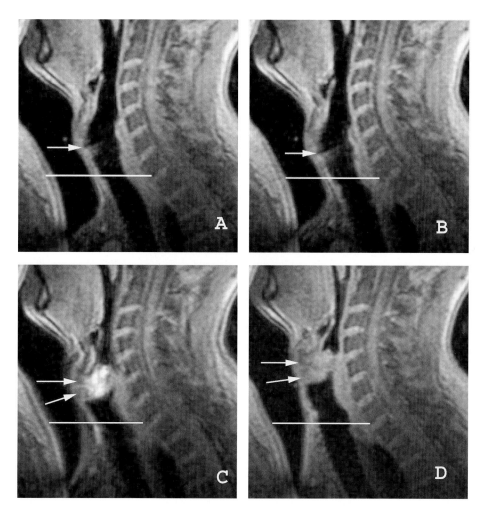

Fig. 11.1.1. Mid-sagittal MRI images through the larynx performed with the Turbo-FLASH sequence (TR 3.3 ms, TE 1.4 ms and a flip angle of 8°) (**B** obtained 400 ms after **A**, **C** obtained 200 ms after **B** and **D** obtained 800 ms after **C**). The images demonstrate significant craniocaudal motion of the larynx during the performance of Valsalva's maneuver in a healthy male volunteer. During deep inspiration, the larynx descends (from **A** to **B**) and the true vocal cords open widely (**B**). During valsalva's maneuver the true and false vocal cords are completely closed (**C, D** *arrows*) and the larynx ascends to above the level of normal breathing (**D**). A horizontal *reference line* is provided to assist in visualization of the craniocaudal motion of the larynx. Notice also the mild changes in anterior to posterior position of the larynx (**A, B** *arrow* laryngeal ventricle)

time of 67 ms per image (FLAHERTY et al. 1995; GIL-BERT et al. 1996). This coronal image set can be repeated multiple times. Since MRI does not allow simultaneous acquisition of these four images using the EPI technique at this time, images obtained at certain coordinates in the coronal plane will actually be 4×67 ms apart. Reformations of these images in the axial plane can subsequently be performed (FLAHERTY et al. 1995; GILBERT et al. 1996). The quality of reformations can be increased by performing more interleaved coronal images spread throughout the larynx, but this will occur at the expense of temporal resolution.

11.1.3
Potential Current and Future Applications

11.1.3.1
Physiological Changes of the Larynx

The introduction of endoscopy revolutionized the understanding of laryngeal motion. It not only pro-

hibits evaluation of the vocal cords as a three-dimensional structure but it also prevents visualization of the larynx during certain maneuvers, e.g., swallowing or Valsalva's maneuver. CT and MRI have the great potential to qualitatively and quantitatively capture these changes in a more physiological setting, since no foreign body is in place.

As is well known, different degrees of adduction and length of the true vocal cords are observed during different tasks: maximal widening and lengthening with deep inspiration (Fig. 11.1.2B and F), almost complete closure of the true vocal cords with vowel production (Fig. 11.1.2C, D, G, H, K and L) and complete closure and maximal foreshortening of the vocal cords during Valsalva's maneuver. The length of the true vocal cords during phonation depends upon the pitch. During phonation at low pitch, the true vocal cords are significantly shorter and thicker than during vowel production at high pitch (Fig. 11.1.2C, D, G and H) (SODERSTEN et al. 1995). Additionally, the so-called posterior laryngeal gap may be seen during high pitch phonation (Fig. 11.1.2D and H). These changes can be easily and qualitatively better assessed with endoscopy. However, CT and MRI are

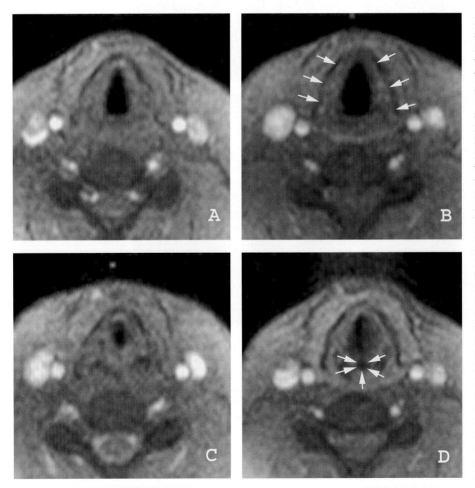

Fig. 11.1.2. Axial (**A–D**) and coronal (**I–L**) MRI images through the true vocal cords performed with the Turbo-FLASH sequence (TR 3.3 ms, TE 1.4 ms, flip angle 8° and an acquisition time of 200 ms per image). Semidynamic axial MRI images (**E–H**) obtained with fast spin echo T2-weighted sequence (TR 3000 ms, TE 120 ms, flip angle 140° and an acquisition time of 9 s) of the same healthy volunteer are provided for comparison. All images were done during different maneuvers including quiet breathing (**A, E, I**), deep inspiration (**B, F, J**), vowel production using low pitch (**C, G, K**) and using high pitch (**D, H, L**). Notice the significant widening of the airway and the lengthening of the true vocal cord (*arrows*) during deep inspiration when compared to quiet breathing (**B, F**) as seen on the axial images. In the coronal plane,

▷

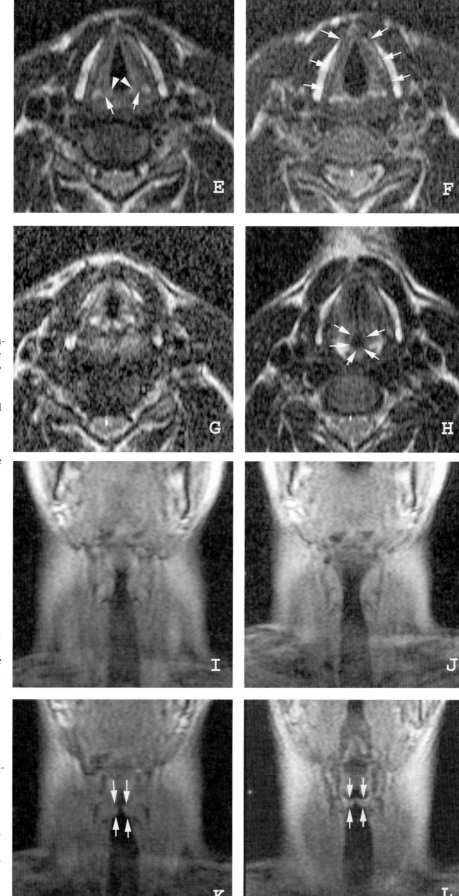

there is complete flattening of the true and false vocal cords during deep inspiration (**J**) when compared to the other tasks (**I, K, L**). The vocal cords are difficult to distinguish from adjacent anatomical structures. As expected, there is variable closure of the true vocal cords during vowel production, but there are also changes in vocal cord length and thickness with different degrees of pitch used during vowel production. With low pitch, the vocal cords are shorter (**C, G**) and thicker (**K** *arrows*) than with high pitch (**D, H, L**, respectively). Notice also the presence of a small posterior gap between the arytenoid cartilages during high pitch vowel production (**G, H** *arrows*). The fast spin echo T2-weighted images (**E–H**) show markedly more anatomical detail when compared to the Turbo-FLASH images (**A–D** and **I–L**), but at a significant expense of temporal resolution with 200 ms versus 9 s acquisition time (**E** *arrowheads* arytenoid cartilage, *arrows* cricoarytenoid joint)

essential in capturing the differences in true vocal cord thickness and laryngeal position in the craniocaudal plane, e.g., during Valsalva's maneuver the larynx is significantly elevated when compared to its position during quiet breathing (Fig. 11.1.1). Mild elevation of the true vocal cords with concurrent adduction is also seen during the first phase of swallowing followed by descent to normal position with concurrent abduction of the true vocal cords during the second phase of swallowing (FLAHERTY et al. 1995). These morphological and physiological changes in laryngeal configuration that are still not very well understood might become essential in development of speech therapy and for planning and development of different and less-extensive laryngeal interventions.

11.1.3.2
Vocal Cord Paralysis

11.1.3.2.1
Presurgical Evaluation

Unilateral vocal cord paralysis results in significant changes in the laryngeal dynamics. The paralyzed vocal cord may be fixed in a variety of positions independently of the underlying etiology: adducted versus abducted as well as at, above or below the normal plane of the larynx (WOODSON 1993). Vocal symptoms are directly related to the position of the paralyzed cord and to the compensatory motion of the nonparalyzed cord. The compensatory position of the normal vocal cord is very variable but often includes shortening, crossing the midline and up or down movement (WOODSON 1993). However, only rarely is this compensatory motion sufficient to result in no or minor symptoms. Therefore, the majority of patients typically undergo one of the different types of medialization procedures, e.g., thyroplasty, prosthesis placement or arytenoid cartilage adduction.

The success of these procedures is dependent upon the correct alignment of the vocal cords in the axial and craniocaudal dimensions. Since the latter is not well seen with endoscopy, presurgical evaluation of the paralyzed and non-paralyzed vocal cords with dynamic CT and/or MRI during performance of different tasks might become essential in surgical planning in the near future. Preliminary results have shown that the complexity of vocal cord motion is not only important for phonation but also for prevention of aspiration during swallowing. GILBERT et al. demonstrated with EPI the reduced elevation and medial motion of the paralyzed vocal cord (GILBERT

et al. 1996). At maximal laryngeal elevation the normal vocal cord assumed a position superior to the paralyzed cord resulting in an interglottic gap in the craniocaudal direction (GILBERT et al. 1996) and increased risk of aspiration. The complex process of swallowing cannot be assessed with endoscopy because of the nature of the procedure emphasizing the importance of dynamic cross-sectional imaging.

11.1.3.2.2
Postsurgical Evaluation

As for presurgical evaluation, cross-sectional studies gain importance in determination of the cause of a failed medialization procedure. Static cross-sectional studies can easily depict the displaced injected material or prosthesis (FORD et al. 1995), but they do not give any information about sufficient adduction during voice production, swallowing etc. Dynamic imaging during performance of different tasks becomes essential to solve this problem (Fig. 11.1.3). It is crucial to include coronal reformations or direct coronal imaging for evaluation of a failed medialization procedure since up-and-down malalignment of the vocal cord will become more apparent and not be mistaken as oblique positioning of the imaging plane or deformity secondary to the prior surgical intervention.

11.1.3.3
Spasmodic Dysphonia

Spasmodic dysphonia is a rare disease process involving postmenopausal women. It can be subdivided into adductor and abductor types. It is characterized by phonatory breaks, aperiodicity and frequency shifts (SAPIENZA et al. 1998). The milder forms are difficult to differentiate clinically or by frequency analysis from muscle tension dysphonia. Since the treatment is very different, with speech therapy for muscle tension dysphonia and botulinum toxin injections for spasmodic dysphonia, there is a constant search for objective measures to make the correct diagnosis.

Preliminary MRI results indicate higher laryngeal position, increased pharyngeal constriction and more vocal tract instability in patients with spasmodic dysphonia when compared to healthy subjects (CANNITO 1989; CRARY et al. 1996). Unpublished data from a few patients studied at the University of Florida with dynamic MRI also suggest smaller cross-sectional subglottic area pretreatment during phonation when

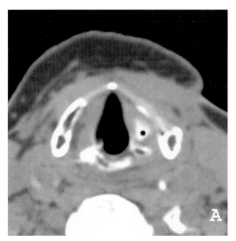
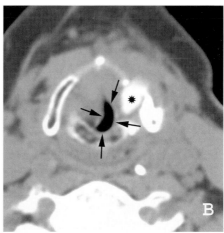

Fig. 11.1.3A, B. Axial CT images performed through the true vocal cords in a patient with persistent dysphonia following thyroplasty on the left side. The images were performed with 1.25 mm slice thickness and a pitch of 3:1 during quiet breathing (**A**) and sustained Valsalva's maneuver (**B**). During quiet breathing (**A**) there is symmetric position of the true vocal cords. The high-density material (*asterisk*) within the left true vocal cord corresponds to the injected Teflon. During Valsalva's maneuver the true vocal cords should be completely closed, which is not the case in this patient. A relatively large airway is seen between the posterior portions of the vocal cords (*arrows*). The thyroplasty did not medialize the left true vocal cord sufficiently to restore normal laryngeal function. In some patients, the normal vocal cord can move across the midline to compensate for the paramedian location of the paralyzed vocal cord, but this was not the case in this patient. The coronal reformations (not demonstrated) showed that both vocal cords were at the same level during both tasks

compared to quiet breathing with some improvement a few weeks following botulinum toxin injection. These preliminary results imply the great potential of MRI and/or CT in this field. The main limiting factor for research in this area is the rarity of the disease process leading to the requirement for multicenter studies for robust results. Additionally, cross-sectional dynamic imaging not only has the potential to confirm the diagnosis but also to determine why some patients with spasmodic dysphonia do not respond at all or poorly to botulinum toxin injections.

11.1.3.4
Chondromalacia/Tracheomalacia

Tracheal or subglottic stenosis and/or chondrotracheomalacia are well-known complications of prolonged intubation or tracheostomy. Numerous other factors, such as type of endotracheal tube, previous trauma to the neck, hypotension, can also increase the incidence of such complications. Most reports emphasize prolonged overdistension of the airway by the endotracheal cuff as well as tracheal infection as the major causes of tracheal or subglottic stenosis and/or chondrotracheomalacia. Stenosis in the subglottic area or of the trachea is easily diagnosed with CT and/or MRI. The cross-sectional dimension of the true lumen in

relation to the expected lumen can be easily calculated since the cricoid cartilage and/or tracheal rings are well seen with both imaging modalities.

In contrast, chondro- or tracheomalacia is very difficult to diagnose with static cross-sectional imaging. Calcifications in the cartilaginous rings can be a sign of underlying chondro- or tracheomalacia on CT studies. Endoscopic evaluation is possible and is currently used to make the diagnosis. However, it is uncertain to what degree the severity of the malacia is influenced by the presence of a foreign body within the upper airway. Additionally, the subglottic area is difficult to assess with this modality because of partial obscuration of the view by the true vocal cords, unless the examination is performed from below through a tracheostomy site.

Currently, dynamic MRI performed in the sagittal and axial planes can give the exact extent and severity of chondro- or tracheomalacia. Repeated imaging of the upper airway in these planes during different tasks is essential. At minimum, the study has to contain dynamic MRI images during quiet breathing and deep expiration, the main trigger of maximal chondro- or tracheomalacia (Fig. 11.1.4). Additionally, individual patient may know other maneuvers causing more pronounced dyspnea and the radiologist should ask for such prior to the study to optimize the imaging protocol.

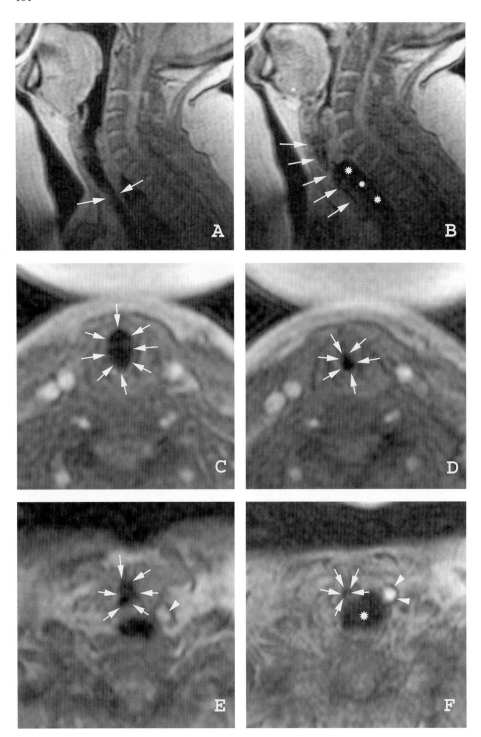

Fig. 11.1.4. Sagittal (**A, B**) and axial (**C–F**) MRI images performed with the same Turbo-FLASH sequence as in Figs. 11.1.1 and 11.1.2 in a patient with suspected tracheomalacia. During quiet breathing there is mild narrowing of the trachea appreciated at the level of the thoracic inlet (**A** *arrow*). During deep expiration there is essentially almost complete collapse of the trachea from the subglottic region to the thoracic inlet (**B** *arrows*). The significant decrease in airway (*arrows*) can be confirmed on the axial images performed during quiet breathing and deep expiration through the subglottic region (**C, D**, respectively) and at the level of the thoracic inlet (**E, F**, respectively). One might mistake the air-filled esophagus (**B, F** *asterisk*) for the trachea, but the relationship to the left carotid artery (**E, F** *arrowhead*) clearly identifies the air-filled structure (**F** *asterisk*) as the esophagus, particularly in comparison with the image performed during quiet breathing (**E**)

References

Cannito MP (1989) Vocal tract steadiness in spasmodic dysphonia. In: Yorkston KM, Beukelman DR (eds) Recent advances in clinical dysarthria. College-Hill Publication, Boston, pp 243–262

Crary MA, Kotzur IM, Gauger J, et al (1996) Dynamic magnetic resonance imaging in the study of vocal tract configuration. J Voice 10:378–388

Flaherty RF, Seltzer S, Campbell T, et al (1995) Dynamic magnetic resonance imaging of vocal cord closure during deglutition. Gastroenterology 109:843–849

Ford CN, Unger JM, Zundel RS, et al (1995) Magnetic resonance imaging (MRI) assessment of vocal fold medialization surgery. Laryngoscope 105:498–504

Gilbert RJ, Daftary S, Woo P, et al (1996) Echo-planar magnetic resonance imaging of deglutitive vocal fold closure: normal and pathological patterns of displacement. Laryngoscope 106:568–572

Hagen R, Haase A, Matthaei D, et al (1990) Oropharyngeale funktionsdiagnostik mit der FLASH-MR-tomographie. HNO 38:421–425

Heinz JM, Steven KN (1964) On the derivations of area functions and acoustic spectra from cineradiographic films of speech. J Acoust Soc Am 36:1037

Kent RD (1972) Some considerations in the cinefluorographic analysis of the tongue movement during speech. Phonetica 26:16–32

Mathiak K, Klose U, Ackermann H, et al (2000) Stroboscopic articulography using fast magnetic resonance imaging. Int J Lang Commun Disord 35:419–425

McCall GM, Skolonick ML, Brewer DW (1971) A preliminary report of some atypical movement pattern in the tongue, palate, hypopharynx, and larynx of patients with spasmodic dysphonia. J Speech Hearing Dis 36:466–470

Moll KL (1965) Photographic and radiographic procedures in speech research. ASHA Rep 1:129–140

Moore CA (1992) The correspondence of vocal tract resonance with volumes obtained from magnetic resonance images. J Speech Hearing Res 35:1009–1023

Sapienza CM, Murry T, Brown WS Jr. (1998) Variations in adductor spasmodic dysphonia: acoustic evidence. J Voice 12:214–222

Schmalfuss IM, Mancuso AA, Melker R, et al (2000) MR imaging of the upper trachea during quiet respiration and valsalva maneuvers. Abstract ASNR 2000, p 170

Sondersten M, Hertegrad S, Hammarberg B (1995) Glottal closure, transglottal airflow, and voice quality in healthy middle-aged women. J Voice 9:182–197

Story BH, Titze IR, Hoffman EA (1996) Vocal tract area functions from magnetic resonance imaging. J Acoust Soc Am 100:537–554

Sundberg J (1969) On the problem of obtaining area functions from lateral X-ray pictures of the vocal tract (STL-QPSR 1). Royal Institute of Technology, Stockholm, pp 43–45

Woodson GE (1993) Configuration of the glottis in laryngeal paralysis. I. Clinical study. Laryngoscope 103:1227–1234

11.2 Virtual Endoscopy of the Larynx

Emanuele Neri and Carlo Bartolozzi

CONTENTS

11.2.1 Virtual Endoscopy: Definition

Virtual endoscopy is a computer-generated simulation of endoscopic perspective obtained by processing digital data sets; it represents one of the applications of virtual reality in the medical field. The simulation can be obtained by dedicated software that reconstructs in three dimensions data obtained from computed tomography (CT) or magnetic resonance imaging (MRI). The reconstruction process produces a virtual volume containing all information relative to the imaged anatomy but, to extract the endoluminal view, an operator-dependent segmentation and visualization action is required.

Two methods of data segmentation are available, based on surface or volume rendering. In surface rendering the endoluminal view is obtained by setting a threshold level which defines the transmission from the luminal air to the wall. In practice, this is represented by a density value in CT and by an intensity value in MRI. In volume rendering the display of

E. Neri, MD
Diagnostic and Interventional Radiology, Department of Oncology, Transplants, and Advanced Technologies in Medicine, University of Pisa, Via Roma 67, 56100, Pisa, Italy
C. Bartolozzi, MD
Professor and Chairman, Diagnostic and Interventional Radiology, Department of Oncology, Transplants, and Advanced Technologies in Medicine, University of Pisa, Via Roma 67, 56100, Pisa, Italy

the lumen is modulated by specific opacity and transparency settings that define the visibility of the imaged anatomical structures according to the corresponding CT density or MRI signal intensity of the individual voxels. A combination of surface and volume rendering may be used for the optimal display of endoluminal views.

Virtual endoscopy can potentially be applied to the study of any anatomical space of the human body. Currently reported applications are in the study of the colon, stomach, trachea and bronchi, nasopharynx, nasal cavity and paranasal sinuses, ear, vessels, biliary tract, urinary tract, brain ventricles and joint spaces (Rogalla et al. 2001; Rubin et al. 1996). The larynx was one of the initial fields of application of virtual endoscopy (Rodenwaldt et al. 1996). To date the study of the larynx with virtual endoscopy is based on CT data sets obtained with a volumetric acquisition. MRI, that could be a potential source of images, has not yet been used for this purpose.

11.2.2 Image Acquisition

To obtain three-dimensional reconstructions of the larynx any given software requires a volumetric dataset (Silverman et al. 1995). Moreover, to reduce motion artefacts in the larynx due to respiration and phonation the image acquisition should be fast. As a consequence the ideal imaging technique for three-dimensional imaging of the larynx is spiral CT.

The image acquisition is performed with the patient in the supine position with moderate extension of the neck. The proper study of the glottic level can be done by asking the patient to phonate the sound of "ee" or "ay"; this brings the true vocal cords more to the midline, making them more easily identifiable on the three-dimensional images.

To demonstrate the true and false vocal cords properly, the acquisition should be made with thin collimation (1–3 mm), pitch 1, and adjacent or overlapping reconstruction spacing (0.5–1 mm). These parameters allow the minimization of blurring and stairstep artefacts that occur in multiplanar reconstruction along the longitudinal axis. The fast acquisition (20–30 s for coverage of the larynx) is necessary for imaging the larynx during phonation.

The parameter settings aim at achieving a maximum volume coverage in a short time-frame. Various authors, having experience in the study of the larynx with single slice CT, report the necessity to accept a compromise in order to avoid artefacts and anatomic distortion on the images. In particular, the visualization of the vocal cords, which are parallel to the axial plane, is mainly influenced by partial volume averaging artefacts, depending on collimation, pitch and reconstruction spacing. Furthermore, the cords continue to vibrate during the acquisition and this intrinsic movement may cause artefacts as well.

RODENWALDT et al. (1997) evaluated the image quality of virtual endoscopy performed in a cadaver phantom, scanned with single slice spiral CT and varying the scanning collimation from 1 to 10 mm, and the pitch from 0.5 to 3. The best correlation between virtual endoscopy and anatomical findings was observed with a collimation of 3 mm and a pitch of 1.5.

Multislice helical CT requires only a fraction of the scanning time required for a single-slice detector system (BRUENING et al. 1999; RODENWALDT et al. 2000). TOYODA et al. (2000) used multislice CT for evaluating the extent of laryngeal tumors in 20 patients, and concluded that with a late-phase contrast-enhanced acquisition and integration of multiplanar reconstructions, multislice CT is superior to endoscopy in diagnosing the extent of laryngeal cancers. MAGLI et al. (2001) reported their experience with multislice CT in the evaluation of 22 patients with suspected laryngeal pathology (10 patients had normal findings, 12 abnormal), incorporating virtual endoscopy. They found a small true vocal cord polyp to be missed. Overall, although a higher sensitivity is expected with multislice CT compared to single-slice spiral CT, similar limitations in the diagnosis of subtle lesions seem to affect both methods.

11.2.3
Anatomy of the Larynx: Laryngoscopy and Virtual Endoscopy

11.2.3.1
Laryngoscopy

The clinical endoscopic evaluation of the larynx implies a combined morphological and functional study.

State of the art laryngoscopes allow easy access to the larynx, causing a minimum of patient discomfort, so that maximum cooperation can be obtained. During the examination patients are asked to alternate quiet breathing with phonation to enable a detailed functional study to be performed.

A more detailed description of the clinical laryngoscopic study can be found in Chap. 1.

11.2.3.2
Virtual Endoscopy of the Larynx

The main advantage of virtual endoscopy is the unrestricted positioning of the virtual endoscope within the air spaces of the larynx. For example, the subglottic area is easily explored by angling the virtual endoscope from the tracheal lumen upwards; such a view is not feasible by direct laryngoscopy.

Clinical laryngoscopy offers a superb view of the mucosal layer of the larynx. The main limitation of virtual endoscopy is that it does not reveal the mucosal aspect, such as colour changes, presence of mucous secretions and so on. Although volume rendering could potentially display the submucosal fat, muscles and cartilages, such use of virtual endoscopy has not been reported.

To describe the three-dimensional endoluminal anatomy of the larynx, as seen by virtual endoscopy, the common subdivision in the supraglottic, glottic and subglottic level can be used.

11.2.3.2.1
Supraglottic Level

At the supraglottic level, positioning the virtual endoscope in the hypopharynx to look toward the glottis allows visualization of most of the laryngeal structures. It displays the epiglottis, with laterally the symmetrical pharyngoepiglottic folds, the median glossoepiglottic fold dividing the right and left valleculae, and the aryepiglottic folds that continue posteroinferiorly. Downwards, the aryepiglottic folds show slight elevations, corresponding with the underlying cuneiform and corniculate cartilages. The aryepiglottic folds are separated by the interarytenoid fold (Fig. 11.2.1a). In some cases the base of the tongue can be an obstacle to the complete visualization of the valleculae. The supraglottic lumen is delineated anteriorly and superiorly by the superior free border of the epiglottis. More inferiorly, the lumen is delineated by the laryngeal face of the epiglottis in the anterior part, laterally by the false vocal cord and posteriorly by the interarytenoid fold (Fig. 11.2.1b).

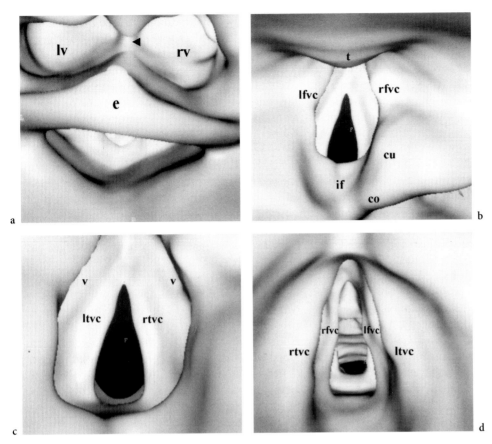

Fig. 11.2.1a–d. Surface-rendered virtual endoscopy of the supraglottic, glottic and subglottic level obtained from a multislice CT data set (slice thickness 1.3 mm, increment 0.6 mm, pitch 0.875, rotation time 0.75 s). The virtual endoscope is progressively moved toward the trachea in four steps (**a, b, c, d**). **a** The endoscope looks toward the epiglottis (*e*) and shows the median glossoepiglottic fold (*arrowhead*) dividing the right (*rv*) and left vallecula (*lv*). **b** The endoscope is positioned in the supraglottic lumen and looks downwards. The lumen is almost completely shown lying between the false vocal cords (*fvc*). From the same perspective the cuneiform (*cu*) and corniculate (*co*) elevations in the posteroinferior part of the aryepiglottic folds, the interarytenoid fold (*if*) and the tuberculum of the epiglottis (*t*) can be appreciated. **c** The ventricular recess (*v*) and then the superior face of both true vocal cords (*tvc*) are visible. **d** Virtual endoscopy without phonation displays the false (*fvc*) and true vocal cords (*tvc*) from the trachea

Posterolateral to the supraglottic compartment, the piriform sinus can be inspected bilaterally. The oesophageal lumen usually cannot be inspected by virtual endoscopy since its lumen only opens during deglutition.

11.2.3.2.2
Glottic Level

The clinical study of the glottic level is the most complex part of the laryngoscopic examination since it implies a combined morphological and functional study. The direct visualization of the larynx with and without phonation allows the adduction and abduction phases to be distinguished. These are visible by observation of the glottic level at laryngoscopy. However, during adduction the true vocal cords vibrate at a specific frequency, and this vibratory movement can only be detected using strobe illumi-

nation (see Chapter 1). Of course, virtual endoscopy cannot be used to perform this kind of evaluation, but can be used to study the morphology of the vocal cords during adduction and abduction.

The preferred phase for morphological study of the glottic level should be the adduction occurring during phonation. In this phase both true vocal cords are symmetrically aligned along the midline of the glottis (Fig. 11.2.1c). In vocal cord paralysis or with the presence of expansive lesions (polyp, tumor, granuloma, laryngocele, etc) the asymmetrical aspect of the glottis is suggestive of pathology.

Moreover, during phonation, the alignment of both true vocal cords allows the laryngeal ventricle to enlarge and become more clearly visible on virtual endoscopy. Incomplete distension of this recess or the presence of a space-occupying lesion in this region can be detected by virtual endoscopy.

11.2.3.2.3
Subglottic Level

Clinically, the subglottic level is quite difficult to study by laryngoscopy. The true vocal cords obstruct the direct visualization of this region, and the endoscope cannot cross the glottic level and turn backward in the caudal-cephalic direction. The assessment of tumor extension or other pathological process below the glottic level is difficult by laryngoscopy alone, and integration with radiological findings is required. The use of virtual endoscopy is helpful in this specific indication. When angling the endoscopy from the tracheal lumen upwards, both inferior faces of the true vocal cords are visible and their symmetry can be easily assessed; even the false vocal cords and vestibule may be seen (Fig. 11.2.1d).

From such a viewpoint, the free borders of the true vocal cords are the main anatomical landmark to evaluate with virtual endoscopy. A symmetrical appearance is expected; an asymmetrical aspect of their free borders or deformation of their inferior face suggest pathological involvement (YUMOTO et al. 1997, 1999).

11.2.4
Imaging Pathology

In comparison to laryngoscopy, virtual endoscopy has the potential advantage of being able to explore any space in the larynx. The main limitation of virtu-

al endoscopy is that it cannot be used to evaluate the mucosal layer; as already mentioned, colour changes due to bleeding, oedema or the presence of mucosal dysplasia, are not detectable. On the other hand, virtual endoscopy enables morphological evaluation of the mucosal surface, such as elevations or depressions, or profile changes of anatomical components (Figs. 11.2.2 and 11.2.3). GALLIVAN et al. (1999) compared virtual endoscopy and laryngoscopy in 21 patients with aerodigestive head and neck tumors, and showed that mucosal irregularities cannot be detected by virtual endoscopy. Another limitation is the possible superposition of normal tissue against tumor; such superposition may be intermittent when caused by movement of, for example, the tongue base or epiglottis. As only the luminal surface is visible, such superposition obstructs direct visualization of the pathological process. Overall, as reported by GALLIVAN et al. (1999), the correlation between the two visualization techniques was very good. FRIED et al. (1999) emphasized that virtual endoscopy if combined with the native images, can be used to assess the transmural extent of tumors and to view the airway distal to areas of luminal compromise. RODENWALT et al. (2000) confirmed the usefulness of virtual endoscopy in exploring the laryngeal lumen distal to a stenosis. GUAZZARONI et al. (2001) also reported virtual endoscopy of the larynx as being valuable particularly in stenotic tumors. In the same study, it was found that small and plane tumors of the vocal cords are not adequately visualized by virtual endoscopy. Similar results have been reported by ASCHOFF et al. (1998), who studied three patients

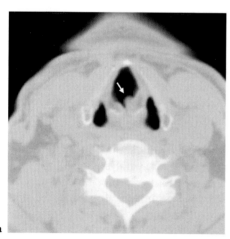
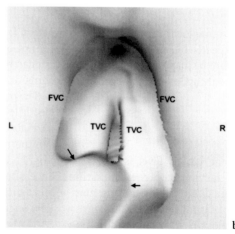

Fig. 11.2.2. a Axial image of single-slice spiral CT obtained at the supraglottic level shows an endoluminal mass arising from the posterior portion of the left false vocal cord (*arrow*). **b** Virtual endoscopy perspective generated by positioning the virtual endoscope in the supraglottic lumen shows the polypoid aspect of the mass, bulging in the lumen (*arrows*) (*FVC* false vocal cord, *TVC* true vocal cord). Granuloma

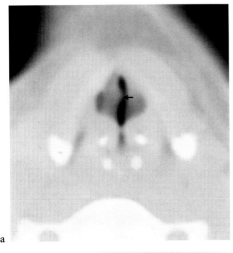
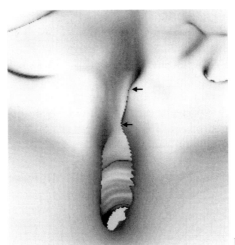

a

b

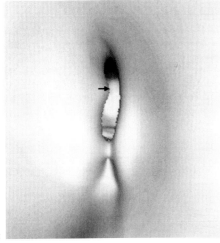

c

Fig. 11.2.3. a At single slice spiral CT, obtained during phonation, the irregular border of the right true vocal cord (*arrow*) can be appreciated. b, c Virtual endoscopy perspectives generated from the supraglottic lumen (b) and trachea (c) show the asymmetry of the true vocal cords with protrusion of the right vocal cord over the midline of the glottic level (*arrows*). The lesion corresponded to a cyst of the true vocal cord

(out of nine with laryngeal pathology) with tumors of the vocal cords. In this work none of the vocal cord cancers was recognized on virtual endoscopy nor on the native cross-sectional CT images, although the acquisition was performed with 1 mm collimation. These authors attribute the missed diagnosis to the motion artefacts resulting from involuntary swallowing by the patient.

Virtual endoscopy is affected by the inherent limitations of CT study: every lesion not depicted on the native CT images is subsequently missed on virtual endoscopy. This is an obvious consideration since this technique is simply a different way to show native images. In a study performed by BURKE et al. (2000), virtual endoscopy was compared to laryngoscopy in the evaluation of airway obstruction. In this study, the cause could not be detected by virtual endoscopy, but it was excellent for the measurement and definition of fixed airway lesions. Precise measurements are quite difficult on axial and reformat-

ted images given the frequent tortuosity of anatomical structures. Also GIOVANNI et al. (1998) demonstrated that virtual endoscopy overcomes this limitation since it directly displays the lumen and allows the measurement of lengths, angles and calibres from the inside. This is useful in the case of laryngeal and tracheal stenosis. Virtual endoscopy is also useful for demonstrating to surgeons the extension of lumen pathology, as the anatomy is displayed in a format familiar to clinicians (GREES et al. 2000).

Most reports on virtual endoscopy of the larynx are of preliminary studies with a small series of patients, but in all cases the value of this technique in laryngotracheal stenosis with unsuccessful laryngoscopy is emphasized. In fact, in the case of stenosis of the laryngeal lumen the laryngoscopic study is often incomplete as the evaluation of the level beyond the stenosis is impossible. In these situations the role of virtual endoscopy is the ability to demonstrate the caudal extension of the pathological process or to identify further surface alterations (Fig. 11.2.4). However, as in case of any other anatomical area, this evaluation must be made in combination of the axial views from which the reformatting has been obtained.

Most available software allows the lumen to be displayed but is also able to correlate each endoluminal perspective with the corresponding axial images. This allows for example a tumor from a benign condition such as a granuloma, laryngocele, etc, to be differentiated.

11.2.5
Conclusion

Virtual endoscopy is a powerful tool for the study of anatomical areas with a complex endoluminal anatomy, and the larynx is certainly one such area. Although in the study of the larynx the exact clinical role of this technique has not yet been defined, it seems that virtual endoscopy may be a valuable tool

in situations where conventional laryngoscopy fails or cannot be performed, such as in severe stenoses.

Acknowledgements. The authors would like to thank Davide Caramella, MD, Paola Sbragia, MD, Tommaso Magli, MD, and Francesco Ursino, MD, for their contribution to this chapter.

References

Aschoff AJ, Seifarth H, Fleiter T, et al (1998) High-resolution virtual laryngoscopy based on spiral CT data. Radiologe 38:810–815
Bruening R, Sturm C, Hong C, et al (1999) The diagnosis of stages T1 and T2 in laryngeal carcinoma with multislice spiral CT. Radiologe 39:939–942
Burke AJ, Vining DJ, McGuirt WF Jr, et al (2000) Evaluation of airway obstruction using virtual endoscopy. Laryngoscope 110:23–29
Fried MP, Moharir VM, Shinmoto H, et al (1999) Virtual laryngoscopy. Ann Otol Rhinol Laryngol 108:221–226
Gallivan RP, Nguyen TH, Armstrong WB, et al (1999) Head and neck computed tomography virtual endoscopy:

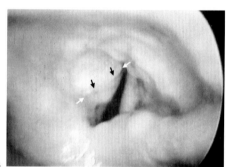

a

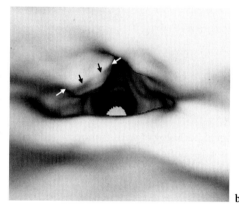

b

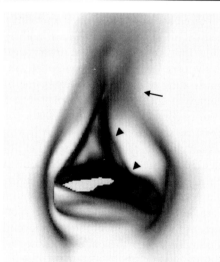

c

Fig. 11.2.4a–c. Laryngeal carcinoma. Direct laryngoscopy (a) demonstrates an irregular endoluminal mass (*between white arrowheads*) altering the profile of the left false vocal cord (*black arrows*) with extension into the ventricle. The virtual endoscopic image obtained from the supraglottic level (b) corresponds nicely with the "true" laryngoscopic image. The retroangled virtual endoscopic image obtained from the trachea (c) shows thickening of the left false (*black arrowheads*) and true vocal cord (*arrow*); the ventricular recess appears effaced. These findings correspond to transglottic tumor spread

evaluation of a new imaging technique. Laryngoscope 109:1570–1579

Giovanni A, Nazarian B, Sudre-Levillain I, et al (1998) Geometric modeling and virtual endoscopy of the laryngo-tracheal lumen from computerized tomography images: initial applications to laryngo-tracheal pathology in the child. Rev Laryngol Otol Rhinol 119:341–346

Greess H, Nomayr A, Tomandl B, et al (2000) 2D and 3D visualisation of head and neck tumours from spiral-CT data. Eur J Radiol 33:170–177

Guazzaroni M, Turchio P, Di Rienzo L, et al (2001) Virtual laryngoscopy of neoplastic pharyngeal and laryngeal pathology. Radiol Med 101:265–269

Magli T, Fella R, Scialpi M, et al (2001) Virtual laryngoscopy with multislice volumetric spiral CT. Preliminary study. Eur Radiol 11 [Suppl 2]:399–400

Rodenwaldt J, Kopka L, Roedel R, et al (1996) Three-dimensional surface imaging of the larynx and trachea by spiral CT: virtual endoscopy. Rofo Fortschr Geb Rontgenstr Neuen Bildgeb Verfahr 165:80–83

Rodenwaldt J, Kopka L, Roedel R, et al (1997) 3D virtual endoscopy of the upper airway: optimization of the scan parameters in a cadaver phantom and clinical assessment. J Comput Assist Tomogr 21:405–411

Rodenwaldt J, Schorn C, Grabbe E, et al (2000) Virtual endoscopy of the upper airway with spiral CT. Radiologe 40:233–239

Rogalla P, Terwisscha van Scheltinga J, Hamm B (eds) (2001) Virtual endoscopy and related 3D techniques. Springer, Berlin Heidelberg New York

Rubin GD, Beaulieu CF, Argiro V, et al (1996) Perspective volume rendering of CT and MR images: applications for endoscopic imaging. Radiology 199:321–330

Silverman PM, Zeiberg AS, Sessions RB, et al (1995) Three-dimensional imaging of the hypopharynx and larynx by means of helical (spiral) computer tomography – comparison of radiological and otolaryngological evaluation. Ann Otol Rhinol Larngol 104:425–431

Toyoda K, Kawakami G, Fukuda Y, et al (2000) Dynamic multidetector CT of laryngeal and hypopharyngeal cancers. Radiology 217:177

Yumoto E, Sanuki T, Hyodo M, et al (1997) Three-dimensional endoscopic mode for observation of laryngeal structures by helical computed tomography. Laryngoscope 107:1530–1537

Yumoto E, Sanuki T, Hyodo M, et al (1999) Three-dimensional endoscopic images of vocal fold paralysis by computed tomography. Arch Otolaryngol Head Neck Surg 125:883–890

11.3 Functional MR Imaging of Laryngeal Cancer

Mark Rijpkema and Johannes Kaanders

CONTENTS

Abbreviations.
AIF: arterial input function
ARCON: accelerated radiotherapy with carbogen and nicotinamide
BOLD: blood oxygen level dependent
DCE-MRI: dynamic contrast enhanced MRI
EES: extravascular extracellular space
Gd: gadolinium-DTPA (meglumine gadopentetate)
k_{ep}: rate constant of contrast medium uptake
K^{trans}: volume transfer constant
T2*: time constant for transverse magnetization decay
v_e: volume of extravascular extracellular space per unit volume of tissue

11.3.1
Introduction

Almost all malignancies of the larynx are squamous cell carcinomas, located at the mucosal surface. The most frequently applied treatment strategies include radiation therapy or total or partial laryngectomy (Curtin 1989). The choice of treatment depends on the initial stage of the tumor. Less-advanced laryngeal tumors can be treated by radiotherapy, whereas more advanced tumors are best treated by surgery. Recently, also accelerated radiotherapy with carbogen and nicotinamide (ARCON) is being used for laryngeal tumors, with promising results (Kaanders et al. 1998).

An important factor in the planning of treatment for laryngeal carcinoma is the accuracy of pretherapeutic staging. Further characterization of the tumor, for example the determination of tumor vascularity, may also assist in the diagnosis and choice of treatment (Endres et al. 1995). To assess the exact tumor extension and characterization, clinical and endoscopic tumor evaluation have clear limitations. Therefore, both computed tomography (CT) and magnetic resonance imaging (MRI) are used in the staging of head and neck tumors. Comparative studies of both imaging techniques show that in general CT and MRI offer comparable accuracy in staging squamous cell carcinoma of the larynx, although MRI yields a slightly better sensitivity (Becker et al. 1995; Castelijns et al. 1996; Zbären et al. 1996). Although estimations of perfusion of head and neck tumors by CT are feasible (Hermans et al. 1999), this is more commonly studied by MRI (see, for example, Baba et al. 1999; Escott et al. 1997; Hoskin et al. 1999).

With conventional MRI, the differences in signal intensity between tumor, muscle, fat and normal cartilage enable the delineation of the tumor. The diagnostic accuracy can be increased with the use of contrast agents, especially in the evaluation of malignant tumors (Hirsch et al. 1998; Vogl et al. 1990; Weber 2001). However, MRI offers techniques to study not only tumor anatomy but also various aspects of tumor physiology in more detail. This may be of importance in treatment selection and may have prognostic significance. In the next section two important techniques are discussed: fast dynamic contrast enhanced imaging to study tumor vascularity and blood oxygen level-dependent imaging to study tumor oxygenation.

M. Rijpkema, MSc
Department of Radiology, University Medical Center Nijmegen, PO Box 9101, 6500 HB Nijmegen, The Netherlands
J. Kaanders, MD, PhD
Professor, Department of Radiotherapy, University Medical Center Nijmegen, PO Box 9101, 6500 HB Nijmegen, The Netherlands

11.3.2
Functional MRI

Functional MRI, defined as MR investigations of dynamic physiological processes, can be applied both to normal and abnormal tissues. A leading application of functional imaging is the study of the normal brain in response to stimuli using imaging techniques that are sensitive to oxygenation. In tumors, several approaches can be used to monitor physiological processes dynamically. Dynamic contrast enhanced MRI (DCE-MRI) and blood oxygen level-dependent (BOLD) MRI are often used nowadays, although other MR techniques, e.g. blood pool contrast-enhanced imaging or diffusion-weighted imaging, can also be used. DCE-MRI can be used to assess changes in vascularity, including vascular permeability, blood flow and blood volume. BOLD MRI can be used to assess changes in blood oxygenation status. In tumors, information about blood supply, vascular architecture and oxygenation status may be important factors determining the choice and outcome of therapy and may be helpful in selecting patients for various treatment strategies.

11.3.2.1
Vascularity

Tumors often feature a more chaotic vascular architecture than normal tissue and a heterogeneous blood supply. Shunting of blood flow within a tumor has been recognized together with variations in vascular permeability (Hoskin et al. 1999; Vaupel 1994). Information on tumor vascularity may aid not only the characterization of tumors, but also treatment planning. Tumor blood perfusion, for example, is of fundamental importance to the efficacy of chemotherapy (drug delivery) and radiotherapy (oxygen supply). Also, assessment of functional changes of tumor vasculature may be used to monitor treatment response.

Various aspects of vascularity, in particular vascular permeability and vascular surface area, can be assessed by DCE-MRI (Delorme and Knopp 1998; Stubbs 1999). Using this technique a contrast agent is administered and its uptake in tumor or normal tissue is monitored by fast imaging (temporal resolution in the order of seconds). Fast MR imaging techniques have not yet been applied frequently to laryngeal tumors. Most dynamic imaging studies so far have employed a temporal resolution of 30 s or more. Using this technique images can be obtained with a high level of anatomical information, but the first-pass effects

of the contrast medium cannot be monitored. A higher temporal resolution can only be achieved at the expense of spatial resolution. DCE-MRI techniques have been widely employed for the assessment of various human tumors in detection, in identification, and in staging (Barentsz et al. 1999; Buckley et al. 1997; Degani et al. 1997; Mayr et al. 1999).

Gadolinium chelates are commonly used as contrast media, in particular meglumine gadopentetate (gadolinium-DTPA, Gd). This exogenous contrast agent remains intravascular in normal brain tissue due to the blood brain barrier, but in all other tissues it diffuses into the extravascular extracellular space (EES). In tumor tissue, the exchange of Gd between blood plasma and the EES and the rate constant of this process can be studied. The rate of Gd uptake provides information about, for example, vascular permeability and vascular surface area. Usually Gd is administered as a bolus to study first-pass effects and fast MRI is applied until the contrast medium in the EES is in equilibrium with the plasma.

In head and neck tumors, investigation of tumor vascularity by DCE-MRI has been used to improve the detection of tumors, to determine the tumor extension, and to aid differential diagnosis (Escott et al. 1997). Time curves obtained from dynamic MRI have been shown to indicate differentiated grades and cell proliferating activity in thyroid tumors (Kusunoki et al. 1998). DCE-MRI has also proven to be useful in the evaluation of therapy of head and neck cancers (Baba et al. 1997). Most malignant lesions of the head and neck show early enhancement and early wash-out of contrast medium on DCE-MRI (Baba et al. 1999). This information may aid in predicting the response of tumors to chemotherapeutic treatment. Also, DCE-MRI studies have been shown to be useful in predicting the response to accelerated radiotherapy for head and neck cancer (Hoskin et al. 1999).

11.3.2.2
Oxygenation

Tumor oxygenation is an important factor in the response of tumors to therapy, especially radiotherapy. Radiosensitivity is directly correlated with the oxygen concentration in the tumor; well-oxygenated cells are more radiosensitive than hypoxic cells (Gray et al. 1953). Increasing tumor oxygen levels may therefore improve the efficacy of radiotherapy. For laryngeal tumors, carbogen breathing and nicotinamide administration result in a significantly improved tumor response to accelerated radiotherapy (ARCON), most likely mediated by improved tumor oxygenation levels (KAANDERS et al. 2001, submitted for publication; KAANDERS et al. 1998, 2000). Thus, information on the tumor oxygenation status is particularly valuable in predicting the outcome of radiotherapy and the effect of oxygenating agents.

Changes in tumor blood oxygenation, e.g. due to an oxygenation protocol, can be assessed by BOLD MRI (OGAWA et al. 1990). This technique makes use of the different magnetic properties of oxyhemoglobin and deoxyhemoglobin. Unlike oxyhemoglobin, deoxyhemoglobin is paramagnetic and shortens the MRI time constant for the transverse magnetization decay (T2*), resulting in an attenuation of MRI signals from tissue adjacent to (venous) blood vessels. Thus, deoxyhemoglobin acts as an endogenous contrast agent which can be monitored by gradient-echo MRI. Although the value of T2* has been shown to be related directly to the concentration of deoxyhemoglobin in normal brain tissue of laboratory animals (PUNWANI et al. 1998), in tumors this value may be mainly governed by the magnetic field distortions caused by tissue inhomogeneity. Especially in laryngeal tumors this may be an important factor, because the border between tissue and air tends to distort the magnetic field to a large extent. However, monitoring changes in the value of T2* due to an oxygenating agent can be used to assess changes in local vascular oxygenation status.

So far, little information is available on BOLD MRI in patients with laryngeal cancer. Using oxygen electrodes, pretreatment oxygenation levels have been shown to be predictive of radiation response in patients with advanced squamous cell carcinomas of the head and neck (NORDSMARK et al. 1996). Oxygenating agents will increase the blood oxygen level, which could result in a decrease in the deoxyhemoglobin concentration and an increase in the value of T2*. Therefore, the oxygenating effects on tumor tissue can be monitored noninvasively by measuring the change in the value of T2*. BOLD MRI of tumors may thus assist in the prediction of radiotherapy outcome and be used to investigate the effect of oxygenating agents on radiosensitivity.

11.3.3
MRI Methods

All data reported in this chapter were recorded on a 1.5 T Siemens Vision whole body system (Siemens Medical Systems, Erlangen, Germany), using a CP-neck-array receive coil. The patients in all studies from which these data were obtained have given their informed consent and approval has been obtained from the local ethics committee.

11.3.3.1
Dynamic Contrast-Enhanced MRI

11.3.3.1.1
MRI Protocol

The procedure for a DCE-MRI measurement is a combination of administration of a contrast agent and recording fast MRI contrast-enhanced images. As a contrast agent, gadolinium-DTPA (Gd) is most commonly used. Intravenous injection of Gd can be applied either by hand or by an automatic injection system. An automatic injection system has the clear advantage that the contrast agent can be administered in a more reproducible way, which may be important in comparing the signal enhancement curves of two measurements of the same patient, for example before and after therapy. Gd is usually administered at a dose of 15 ml of 0.5 M Gd solution. This volume has to be administered as a bolus (e.g. 2.5 ml/s) to be able to study first-pass effects of the contrast medium in the tumor.

Fast dynamic contrast-enhanced MRI techniques can be classified into two methods: T1-weighted and T2*-weighted sequences. For dynamic contrast studies of the head and neck region, T2*-weighted sequences are difficult to implement because of magnetic field inhomogeneity effects. Furthermore, T2*-weighted imaging requires the Gd contrast medium to remain intravascular for reliable assessment of the time-intensity curves (BABA et al. 1999), a prerequisite that is not met by laryngeal carcinomas. Under these conditions, T1-weighted imaging methods such as fast spin-echo and gradient-echo techniques are usually applied (ESCOTT et al. 1997; LARSSON et al. 1994; RIJPKEMA et al. 2001a; TAKASHIMA et al. 1993). To study the dynamics of the contrast medium in the tumor in detail, imaging sequences have to be fast. For the accurate measurement of tracer kinetic parameters the temporal sampling requirement is about 4 s, and if time-intensity curves of large blood vessels also have to be measured, the sampling rate should be even higher (HENDERSON et al. 1998). DCE-MRI data acquired this way are shown in Fig. 11.3.1 for a patient with a laryngeal tumor. The sequence parameters (2D FLASH, TR 50 ms, TE

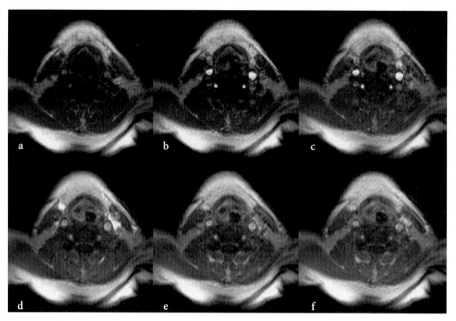

Fig. 11.3.1a–f. Six transversal dynamic contrast enhancement images of a patient with a laryngeal tumor (T3) obtained from a data set of 44 images. The images were acquired as described in Section 13.3.1.1 with a temporal resolution of 2 s. Images **a–f** were recorded at t=4, 14, 16, 24, 60 and 75 s, respectively. Dynamic contrast enhancement in both normal tissue, tumor tissue and large blood vessels can be recognized

4.4 ms, a=60°, slice thickness 7 mm, seven slices, matrix 256^2, FoV 210×280 mm) enabled reconstruction of an image every 2 s. The six images displayed in Fig. 11.3.1 are a subset of a data set of 44 consecutive images. The bolus passage of the contrast medium in the carotid and vertebral arteries can be recognized, as well as the dynamic contrast enhancement in the tumor.

Artifacts may be introduced into the dynamic contrast enhancement images, particularly when a mobile organ like the larynx is being imaged. Patients with laryngeal tumors may have trouble breathing, which may introduce motion artifacts. Also, the laryngeal region is extremely sensitive to artifacts caused by swallowing. These artifacts are very difficult to correct for after the data have been recorded. So, to reduce motion artifacts on the images, the total measurement time of the set of dynamic contrast enhancement images should be kept short. The first-pass effects and the washout of the contrast medium, however, have to be sampled for an accurate measurement of dynamic contrast enhancement parameters. In practice, with a short bolus and a sampling rate of 2 s, a total measurement time of 90 s suffices.

11.3.3.1.2
Data Analysis

For clinical purposes, it may be sufficient to perform a parametric analysis of the DCE-MRI data, resulting in values of parameters such as maximum contrast enhancement and rate of enhancement. This approach may yield reliable data of clinical significance (e.g. HUISMAN et al. 2001). However, to minimize variations among patients and different measurements caused by variable systemic blood supply, it is necessary to apply some kind of normalization. As a reference the concentration-time curves of the contrast agent in the feeding vessels (arterial input function, AIF) can be used. The advantage of imaging laryngeal tumors compared to, for example, brain tumors or breast tumors is that multiple arteries are present in a transversal imaging slice through the tumor (vertebral and carotid arteries). Thus, the signal enhancement versus time curves in the tumor and in the arteries can be acquired simultaneously, without any additional measurements. The necessity to record the AIF for quantitative analysis of DCE-MRI data was recently shown by PORT et al. (2001) and RIJPKEMA et al. (2001a) for various tumors, including laryngeal carcinomas. The Gd uptake curve of a laryngeal tumor and the coregistered AIF are plotted in Fig. 11.3.2, which shows clearly the bolus passage of the contrast medium and the (rate of) Gd uptake in the tumor. To gain insight into the underlying physiology of the tumor, various physiological pharmacokinetic models have been proposed to describe the dynamic MR contrast enhancement. Using these models DCE-MRI data may be described in physiological terms such as vascular permeability and surface area, extracellular volume and tumor blood perfusion.

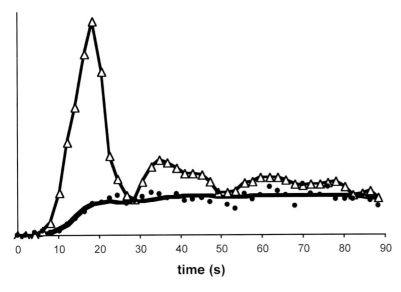

Fig. 11.3.2. Gd uptake curve (*black dots*) of 1 pixel of the tumor region and the fit of this curve (*solid line*) according to the physiological model of LARSSON et al. (1990). The arterial input function (*open triangles*) is also shown. The data were obtained from the same patient as in Fig. 11.3.1

time (s)

11.3.3.1.3
Physiological Pharmacokinetic Models

The most commonly used physiological models in DCE-MRI are those described by LARSSON et al. (1990) and TOFTS and KERMODE (1991). The measured concentration-time curves of the contrast medium in the tumor and the AIF serve as input for these models. The output consists of quantified physiological parameters like the rate constant of contrast medium uptake, which is directly related to, for example, the vascular permeability and surface area.

In its simplest form a physiological pharmacokinetic model describing dynamic contrast medium uptake contains two compartments: blood plasma and EES. A rate constant defines the exchange of contrast medium between these compartments. This rate constant k_{ep} (TOFTS et al. 1999) is one of the three principle parameters in the analysis of T1-weighted contrast enhancement data. The two other parameters are the volume transfer constant between blood plasma and EES (K^{trans}) and the volume of EES per unit volume of tissue (v_e). These three physiological parameters are related according to the expression

$$k_{ep}=K^{trans}/v_e$$

(Tofts et al. 1999). When a physiological model is applied to DCE-MRI data on a pixel-by-pixel basis, maps can be reconstructed in which these parameters are displayed. In Fig. 11.3.3 a contrast enhancement image is displayed, together with maps of k_{ep} and K^{trans}, for the same patient as in Fig. 11.3.1. The tumor can readily be distinguished from the sur-

rounding tissue in all three images. However, spatial inhomogeneity within the tumor is more easily recognized in the parameter maps (Fig. 11.3.3b, c).

The characterization of tumors by quantification of physiological parameters enables the direct comparison of the characteristics of the tumor with those of other tumors. In Table 11.3.1 the rates of the Gd uptake in laryngeal tumors are shown for eight patients. The T classification of the tumor according to the TNM classification system (SOBIN and WITTE-KIND 1997), describing the extent of the tumor, is also shown. Because the amount of quantified physiological DCE-MRI data on laryngeal tumors is still limited, no correlation with tumor TNM classification can yet be found. This correlation is complicated further since histological data obtained by biopsy may not be representative of the whole tumor, especially when a tumor is heterogeneous, whereas the physiological parameters obtained by DCE-MRI so far are an average of the whole tumor.

11.3.3.2
Blood Oxygen Level-Dependent MRI

MRI techniques to study tumor vascular oxygenation usually employ the BOLD effect. Using gradient-echo MRI, changes in the value of the relaxation time T_2^* can be determined, which correlate with changes in the deoxyhemoglobin concentration. Although changes in T2* are sensitive to changes in both blood volume, hematocrit, and oxygenation (NEEMAN et al. 2001), the decrease in T2* during hyperoxygenation has been shown to be strongly correlated with increased tumor pO_2 levels, as mea-

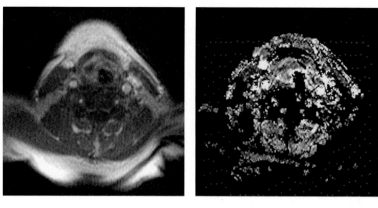 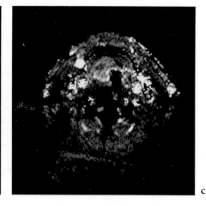

a,b   c

Fig. 11.3.3. a T1-weighted dynamic contrast enhancement image of the same patient as in Fig. 11.3.1 recorded 75 s after Gd contrast medium administration. The DCE-MRI data were analyzed using the physiological model of LARSSON et al. (1990). The results are shown as (**b**) a map of the Gd uptake rate (k_{ep}) and (**c**) a map of the volume transfer constant (K^{trans}) of the same patient

Table 11.3.1. The contrast medium uptake rate k_{ep} (min^{-1}) in laryngeal tumors of eight patients (±SD). The T classification of the tumor according to the TNM classification system is also indicated. The contrast medium uptake rate may provide information on, for example, vascular permeability and surface area

Patient	T category	k_{ep} (min^{-1})
1	T4	2.3±0.7
2	T3	1.3±0.6
3	T2	3.0±1.3
4	T3	2.8±0.9
5	T4	1.9±1.7
6	T3	2.4±2.5
7	T3	2.3±1.0
8	T4	2.9±1.5

sured using oxygen electrodes (AL HALLAQ et al. 1998). Conventional T2*-weighted MRI cannot distinguish accurately changes in blood oxygenation from changes in blood flow, because of inflow effects (ROBINSON et al. 2001). To overcome this disadvantage a multigradient echo MRI technique can be applied, which can quantify T2* independently of effects of blood flow. In Fig. 11.3.4 data obtained with a multiple-gradient echo sequence is presented from a patient with a laryngeal tumor. In this figure, 6 out of 16 images obtained with a 16-echo sequence are shown (sequence parameters: 16 echo FLASH, TR 65 ms, TE 6–51 ms, a=20°, 5 mm slice). Values of T2* (ms) can be calculated from the monoexponential signal decay at increasing echo times. This calculation can be performed on a pixel-by-pixel basis, enabling reconstruction of a map of T2*. In Fig. 11.3.5 a map is shown of the relaxation rate R2* (R2*=1/T2*) obtained from

the data set shown in Fig. 11.3.4. In this way, spatial information about tumor blood oxygenation changes can be visualized. (R2* is used here instead of T2* for display convenience.)

In Table 11.3.2 the values of T2* in laryngeal tumors are listed for eight patients. The tumor values were obtained by averaging all pixels within a selected tumor region on the T2* maps. Although absolute T2* values are difficult to interpret directly in terms of tumor oxygen levels (see Section 11.3.2.2 Oxygenation), they may serve as "baseline values" in the investigation of the effect of oxygenating agents on tumor blood oxygenation. An increase in the value of T2* caused by an improved blood oxygenation may indicate the radiotherapeutic usefulness of the oxygenating agent. For example, changes in T2* caused by breathing hyperoxic hypercapnic gas mixtures (e.g. 95–98% O_2 plus 5–2% CO_2) might predict whether the patient could benefit from radiotherapy treatment using these gas mixtures as a hyperoxygenation medium.

11.3.4
Laryngeal Cancer: Application of Functional MRI Approaches

An important treatment option for laryngeal cancer is radiotherapy. Although radiotherapy produces a high local control rate, in advanced carcinomas the radiation response is less good. Traditional prognostic factors, such as clinical staging, tumor size, and tumor extent, may not sufficiently predict results of radiotherapy (BABA et al. 1999). Blood flow and the

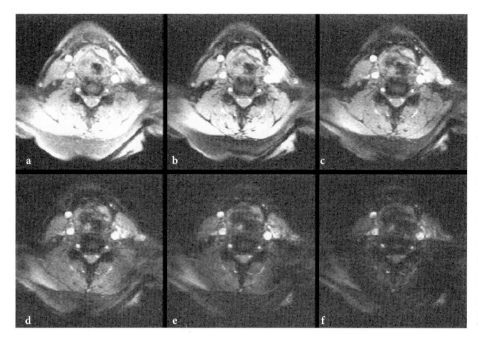

Fig. 11.3.4a–f. Six transversal T2*-weighted images from a data set of 16 images recorded using a multiple-gradient echo sequence. The data were obtained from the same patient as in Fig. 11.3.1. Images **a–f** were recorded with an echo time of 6, 9, 15, 21, 27 and 36 ms, respectively. The signal decay at increasing echo times was used to calculate the value of T2* (ms)

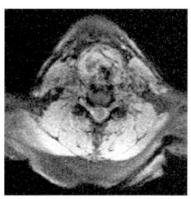

Fig. 11.3.5. Map of the relaxation rate R2* (R2*=1/T2*) obtained from pixelwise analysis of the multiple-gradient echo data shown in Fig. 11.3.4. The R2* map is shown instead of the T2* map for display convenience

Table 11.3.2. The MRI time constant for the transverse magnetization decay (T2*) (ms) in laryngeal tumors of eight patients (±SD). These values are particularly important in the investigation of the effects of oxygenation agents on tumor blood oxygenation

Patient	T2* (ms)
1	29.1±1.8
2	26.9±0.9
3	30.8±2.0
4	32.5±2.8
5	43.9±2.5
6	37.2±1.3
7	34.2±2.7
8	24.5±2.1

presence of hypoxia in the tumor have long been considered important factors influencing the response to radiotherapy. Because functional MRI provides a way of assessing tumor hypoxia by studying both functional changes in tumor vasculature and oxygenation status, the potential radiosensitizing effect of oxygenating agents can be investigated.

For laryngeal tumors, increased tumor oxygenation levels achieved by carbogen breathing and nicotinamide administration result in a significantly improved tumor response to accelerated radiotherapy (ARCON), as has been demonstrated by KAANDERS and coworkers (submitted for publication; 1998, 2000). Breathing a hyperoxic hypercapnic gas mixture such as carbogen was hypothesized to increase the blood oxygen level which may reduce hypoxic regions in the tumor. The first results of their study show an actuarial local control rate at 3 years of 79% for T3 laryngeal carcinomas and 84% for T4 laryngeal carcinomas, higher than any previous report in the literature for this category of patients (KAANDERS et al., submitted for publication). Currently a randomized phase III trial of this treatment is ongoing for laryngeal tumors.

Breathing a hyperoxic hypercapnic gas mixture may have an effect on both blood flow and oxygenation (BUSSINK et al. 1999; HORSMAN et al. 1994). To study these effects in the clinic, a combination of BOLD MRI and DCE-MRI techniques seems suitable. Recently, the effects of breathing a hyperoxic hypercapnic gas mixture (98% O_2 plus 2% CO_2) were assessed by functional MRI techniques in patients with head and neck tumors (RIJPKEMA et al., submitted for publication). The main conclusion of this study was that breathing this gas mixture improved tumor blood oxygenation in these patients. No changes in tumor vascularity were found as assessed by the Gd uptake rate. Furthermore, functional MRI proved to be a promising tool to investigate both tumor oxygenation and vascularity and might be developed into a predictive tool for testing treatments using hyperoxygenation for other types of tumors as well.

As an example to show the use of different functional MRI techniques to monitor the effects of hyperoxygenation in laryngeal tumors, a case is presented of a patient with a T4 laryngeal tumor. In Fig. 11.3.6

the results of the MRI study of this patient is shown. To investigate the effects of breathing a hyperoxic hypercapnic gas mixture on tumor oxygenation and vascularity, this patient was measured twice, once breathing air and once breathing a gas mixture consisting of 98% O_2 and 2% CO_2. Tumor vascularity was assessed by DCE-MRI as described in Section 11.3.3.1. Physiological parameter maps (e.g. K^{trans}, Fig. 11.3.6b) were obtained from both the air-breathing session and the session breathing the hyperoxic hypercapnic gas mixture. The values of the Gd uptake rate, k_{ep}, are displayed in Table 11.3.3. No significant differences could be detected, indicating that no dramatic changes in vascularity occurred due to breathing the hyperoxic

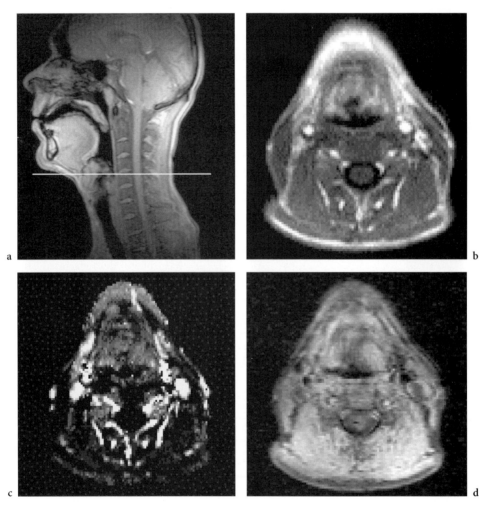

Fig. 11.3.6a–d. Functional MR images of a patient with a laryngeal tumor (T4). The images were recorded while the patient was breathing a hyperoxic hypercapnic gas mixture. **a** Sagittal image of the head and neck region showing the position of the transversal imaging slice used in both BOLD MRI and DCE-MRI. **b** Transversal dynamic contrast-enhancement image of the same patient, recorded 1 min after Gd contrast medium administration. The image was acquired as described in Section 11.3.3.1.1. **c** Volume transfer constant (K^{trans}) map the of the same patient, providing information on tumor vascularity (see Section 11.3.3.1.3 for details). **d** Relaxation rate (R2*) map of the same patient (see Section 11.3.3.2 for details).

hypercapnic gas mixture.

Tumor oxygenation was assessed using BOLD MRI as described in Section 11.3.3.2. The map of the relaxation rate R2* is shown in Fig. 11.3.6d. The values of T2* for the tumor obtained during air breathing and breathing the hyperoxic hypercapnic gas mixture proved to differ significantly (Table 11.3.3); the value of T2* increased during hypercapnic hyperoxygenation. Although the T2* increase may seem small, it may reflect a much larger decrease in deoxyhemoglobin concentration (PUNWANI et al. 1998).

Table 11.3.3. The contrast medium uptake rate k_{ep} (min^{-1}) and the MRI time constant for the transverse magnetization decay (T2*) (ms) of a patient with a laryngeal tumor. Data were obtained during air breathing and during breathing a hyperoxic hypercapnic gas mixture. The increased value of T2* during breathing this gas mixture indicates an improved tumor blood oxygenation. Statistical significance is shown (*NS* not significant) (Student's *t*-test)

	Air	Carbogen	Significance
k_{ep} (min^{-1})	2.3	2.2	NS
T2* (ms)	29.1	31.4	$P=0.02$

A powerful approach would be to combine the maps containing data on vascularity and oxygenation. A spatial relationship of the BOLD effect and the dynamic Gd enhancement could provide a useful physiological insight. However, in practice spatial correlation of the maps of the Gd uptake rate and (the changes in) T2* is problematic. Even small shifts of the patient position between the measurements could dramatically affect a pixel-to-pixel correlation.

In this patient Gd uptake did not reveal any effect on tumor vascularity due to breathing of the hyperoxic hypercapnic gas mixture. However, as the blood oxygenation level increased in the tumor during breathing the gas mixture, this patient could benefit from radiation treatment using this hyperoxygenating agent. In fact, this patient was treated using the ARCON therapy and had not shown tumor recurrence after 3 years. Of course, this case only is no proof of the benefit of breathing a hyperoxic hypercapnic gas mixture or the validity of the MRI methods as a predictive tool. A more robust study to prove this is currently ongoing.

11.3.5
Conclusion

Functional MRI approaches to laryngeal cancer can be applied to study dynamic physiological processes and may aid in characterizing physiological features of the tumor. Using dynamic contrast-enhanced MRI various aspects of tumor vascularity can be assessed. Blood oxygen level-dependent MRI enables investigation of blood oxygen levels in the tumor. Because for laryngeal carcinomas radiation treatment with hyperoxygenating agents has proven to be successful, studying the radiosensitizing effects of these agents may provide valuable information. In this respect, functional MRI may be developed into a predictive tool for testing treatments using hyperoxygenation of laryngeal cancer.

Acknowledgements. The authors would like to thank Frank Joosten, Arend Heerschap, Albert van der Kogel, and the ARCON and MRI technicians of the Departments of Radiology and Radiotherapy for their assistance.

References

Al Hallaq HA, River JN, Zamora M, et al (1998) Correlation of magnetic resonance and oxygen microelectrode measurements of carbogen-induced changes in tumor oxygenation. Int J Radiat Oncol Biol Phys 41:151–159

Baba Y, Furusawa M, Murakami R, et al (1997) Role of dynamic MRI in the evaluation of head and neck cancers treated with radiation therapy. Int J Radiat Oncol Biol Phys 37:783–787

Baba Y, Yamashita Y, Onomichi M, et al (1999) Dynamic magnetic resonance imaging of head and neck lesions. Top Magn Reson Imaging 10:125–129

Barentsz JO, Engelbrecht M, Jager GJ, et al (1999) A fast dynamic gadolinium-enhanced MR imaging of urinary bladder and prostate cancer. J Magn Reson Imaging 10:295–304

Becker M, Zbaren P, Laeng H, et al (1995) Neoplastic invasion of the laryngeal cartilage: comparison of MR imaging and CT with histopathologic correlation. Radiology 194:661–669

Buckley DL, Drew PJ, Mussurakis S, et al (1997) Microvessel density of invasive breast cancer assessed by dynamic Gd-DTPA enhanced MRI. J Magn Reson Imaging 7:461–464

Bussink J, Kaanders JH, van der Kogel AJ (1999) Clinical outcome and tumour microenvironmental effects of accelerated radiotherapy with carbogen and nicotinamide. Acta Oncol 38:875–882

Castelijns JA, Becker M, Hermans R (1996) Impact of cartilage invasion on treatment and prognosis of laryngeal
cancer. Eur Radiol 6:156–169

Curtin HD (1989) Imaging of the larynx: current concepts.
Radiology 173:1–11

Degani H, Gusis V, Weinstein D, et al (1997) Mapping patho-
physiological features of breast tumors by MRI at high
spatial resolution. Nat Med 3:780–782

Delorme S, Knopp MV (1998) Non-invasive vascular imaging: assessing tumour vascularity. Eur Radiol 8:517–527

Endres D, Manaligod J, Simonson T, et al (1995) The role of
magnetic resonance angiography in head and neck surgery. Laryngoscope 105:1069–1076

Escott EJ, Rao VM, Ko WD, et al (1997) Comparison of dynamic contrast-enhanced gradient-echo and spin-echo
sequences in MR of head and neck neoplasms. Am J
Neuroradiol 18:1411–1419

Gray LH, Conger AD, Ebert M, et al (1953) The concentration
of oxygen dissolved in tissues at the time of irradiation as
a factor in radiotherapy. Br J Radiol 26:638–648

Henderson E, Rutt BK, Lee TY (1998) Temporal sampling requirements for the tracer kinetics modeling of breast disease. Magn Reson Imaging 16:1057–1073

Hermans R, Lambin Ph, Van der Goten A, et al (1999)
Tumoural perfusion as measured by dynamic computed
tomography in head and neck carcinoma. Radiother
Oncol 53:105–111

Hirsch JA, Loevner LA, Yousem DM, et al (1998) Gadolinium-
enhanced fat-suppressed T1-weighted imaging of the
head and neck: comparison of gradient and conventional
SE sequences. J Comput Assist Tomogr 22:771–776

Horsman MR, Nordsmark M, Khalil AA, et al (1994) Reducing
acute and chronic hypoxia in tumours by combining nicotinamide with carbogen breathing. Acta Oncol 33:371–376

Hoskin PJ, Saunders MI, Goodchild K, et al (1999) Dynamic
contrast enhanced magnetic resonance scanning as a predictor of response to accelerated radiotherapy for advanced head and neck cancer. Br J Radiol 72:1093–1098

Huisman HJ, Engelbrecht MR, Barentsz JO (2001) Accurate
estimation of pharmacokinetic contrast-enhanced dynamic MRI parameters of the prostate. J Magn Reson Imaging 13:607–614

Kaanders JH, Pop LA, Marres HA, et al (1998) Accelerated
radiotherapy with carbogen and nicotinamide (ARCON)
for laryngeal cancer. Radiother Oncol 48:115–122

Kaanders JHAM, Bussink J, Pop LA, et al (2000) Accelerated
radiotherapy with carbogen and nicotinamide (ARCON):
from mouse to man. Int J Radiat Oncol Biol Phys 46:705

Kusunoki T, Murata K, Hosoi H, et al (1998) Malignancies of
human thyroid tumors and dynamic magnetic resonance
imaging (MRI). Auris Nasus Larynx 25:419–424

Larsson HB, Stubgaard M, Frederiksen JL, et al (1990)
Quantitation of blood-brain barrier defect by magnetic
resonance imaging and gadolinium-DTPA in patients
with multiple sclerosis and brain tumors. Magn Reson
Med 16:117–131

Larsson HB, Stubgaard M, Sondergaard L, et al (1994) In vivo
quantification of the unidirectional influx constant for
Gd-DTPA diffusion across the myocardial capillaries with
MR imaging. J Magn Reson Imaging 4:433–440

Mayr NA, Hawighorst H, Yuh WT, et al (1999) MR microcir-
lation assessment in cervical cancer: correlations with
histomorphological tumor markers and clinical outcome.
J Magn Reson Imaging 10:267–276

Neeman M, Dafni H, Bukhari O, et al (2001) In vivo contrast
MRI mapping of subcutaneous vascular function and
maturation: validation by intravital microscopy. Magn
Reson Med 45:887–898

Nordsmark M, Overgaard M, Overgaard J (1996) Pretreatment oxygenation predicts radiation response in advanced squamous cell carcinoma of the head and neck.
Radiother Oncol 41:31–39

Ogawa S, Lee TM, Nayak AS, et al (1990) Oxygenation-sensi-
tive contrast in magnetic resonance image of rodent brain
at high magnetic fields. Magn Reson Med 14:68–78

Port RE, Knopp MV, Brix G (2001) Dynamic contrast-enhanced MRI using Gd-DTPA: interindividual variability
of the arterial input function and consequences for the
assessment of kinetics in tumors. Magn Reson Med
45:1030–1038

Punwani S, Ordidge RJ, Cooper CE, et al (1998) MRI measure-
ments of cerebral deoxyhaemoglobin concentration
[DHb] – correlation with near infrared spectroscopy
(NIRS). NMR Biomed 11:281–289

Rijpkema M, Kaanders JHAM, Joosten FBM, et al (2001a)
Method for quantitative mapping of dynamic MRI contrast agent uptake in human tumors. J Magn Reson Imaging (in press)

Robinson SP, Rodrigues LM, Howe FA, et al (2001) Effects of
different levels of hypercapnic hyperoxia on tumour R(2)*
and arterial blood gases. Magn Reson Imaging 19:161–166

Sobin LH, Wittekind C (eds) (1997) TNM classification of
malignant tumors, 5th edn. Wiley-Liss, New York, pp 33–
37

Stubbs M (1999) Application of magnetic resonance techniques for imaging tumour physiology. Acta Oncol
38:845–853

Takashima S, Noguchi Y, Okumura T, et al (1993) Dynamic
MR imaging in the head and neck. Radiology 189:813–821

Tofts PS, Kermode AG (1991) Measurement of the blood-
brain barrier permeability and leakage space using dynamic MR imaging. 1 Fundamental concepts. Magn Reson
Med 17:357–367

Tofts PS, Brix G, Buckley DL, et al (1999) Estimating kinetic
parameters from dynamic contrast-enhanced T(1)-
weighted MRI of a diffusable tracer: standardized quanti-
ties and symbols. J Magn Reson Imaging 10:223–232

Vaupel PW (1994) Blood flow, oxygenation, tissue pH distribution, and bioenergetic status of tumors. Ernst Schering
Research Foundation, Berlin

Vogl T, Dresel S, Bilaniuk LT, et al (1990) Tumors of the nasopharynx and adjacent areas: MR imaging with Gd-
DTPA. Am J Roentgenol 154:585–592

Weber AL (2001) History of head and neck radiology: past
present and future. Radiology 218:15–24

Zbären P, Becker M, Lang H (1996) Pretherapeutic staging of
laryngeal carcinoma clinical findings computed tomography and magnetic resonance imaging compared with histopathology. Cancer 77:1263–1273

Subject Index

List of Contributors

Carlo Bartolozzi, MD
Professor and Chairman
Diagnostic and Interventional Radiology
Department of Oncology, Transplants,
and Advanced Technologies in Medicine
University of Pisa
Via Roma 67
56100 Pisa
Italy

Giuseppe Battaglia, MD
Department of Radiology
University of Brescia
Piazza Spedali Civili 1
25 123 Brescia
Italy

Minerva Becker, MD
Privat-docent, Médecin adjoint résponsable
de la radiologie tête et cou
Department of Radiology
Division of Diagnostic and
Interventional Radiology
Geneva University Hospital
24, Rue Micheli-du-Crest
1211 Geneva 14
Switzerland

Jonas A. Castelijns, MD, PhD
Professor, Department of Radiology
Free University Hospital Amsterdam
P.O. Box 7057
1007 MB Amsterdam
The Netherlands

Pierre R. Delaere, MD, PhD
Professor, Department of Otolaryngology
Head and Neck Surgery
University Hospitals Leuven
Kapucijnenvoer 33
3000 Leuven
Belgium

Kathelijne G. Delsupehe, MD
Department of Otolaryngology
Head and Neck Surgery
University Hospitals Leuven
Kapucijnenvoer 33
3000 Leuven
Belgium

Davide Farina, MD
Department of Radiology
University of Brescia
Piazza Spedali Civili 1
25 123 Brescia
Italy

Patrick Flamen, MD, PhD
Department of Nuclear Medicine
University Hospitals Leuven
Herestraat 49
3000 Leuven
Belgium

Pawel P. Gruca, DO
Departments of Radiology and Surgery School of
Medicine. Department of Diagnostic Sciences
School of Dentistry
University of North Carolina at Chapel Hill
Chapel Hill, NC 27599-7510
USA

Robert Hermans, MD, PhD
Professor, Department of Radiology
University Hospitals K.U. Leuven
Herestraat 49
3000 Leuven
Belgium

Varsha Joshi, MD
Departments of Radiology and Surgery School of
Medicine. Department of Diagnostic Sciences
School of Dentistry
University of North Carolina at Chapel Hill
3324 Infirmary CB 7510
Chapel Hill, NC 27599-7510
USA

JOHANNES KAANDERS, MD, PhD
Professor, Department of Radiotherapy
University Medical Center Nijmegen
P.O. Box 9101
6500 HB Nijmegen
The Netherlands

PATRIZIA MACULOTTI, MD
Department of Radiology
University of Brescia
Piazza Spedali Civili 1
25 123 Brescia
Italy

ROBERTO MAROLDI, MD
Professor, Department of Radiology
University of Brescia
Piazza Spedali Civili 1
25 123 Brescia
Italy

SURESH K. MUKHERJI, MD
Section Chief, Neuroradiology
Department of Radiology
University of Michigan Health System
1500 East Medical Center Drive
Ann Arbor, MI 48109-0030
USA

EMANUELE NERI, MD
Division of Diagnostic and Interventional Radiology
Department of Oncology, Transplant
and Advanced Technologies in Medicine
University of Pisa
Via Roma 67
56100 Pisa
Italy

LAURA PALVARINI, MD
Department of Radiology
University of Brescia
Piazza Spedali Civili 1
25 123 Brescia
Italy

FRANK A. PAMEIJER, MD, PhD
Department of Radiology
The Netherlands Cancer Institute
Antoni van Leeuwenhoek Hospital
Plesmanlaan 121
1066 CX Amsterdam
The Netherlands

MARK RIJPKEMA, MSc
Department of Radiology
University Medical Center Nijmegen
P.O. Box 9101
6500 HB Nijmegen
The Netherlands

ILONA M. SCHMALFUSS, MD
Department of Radiology
University of Florida
1600 SW Archer Road
Gainesville, FL 32610
USA

ROBERT SIGAL, MD, PhD
Professor, Department of Radiology
Institut Gustave Roussy
39, rue Camille-Desmoulins
94800 Villejuif Cédex
France

MEDICAL RADIOLOGY
Diagnostic Imaging and Radiation Oncology

Titles in the series already published

 Springer

MEDICAL RADIOLOGY
Diagnostic Imaging and Radiation Oncology

Titles in the series already published

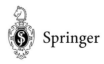

Springer

Printing and Binding: Stürtz AG, Würzburg